HEALTHCARE SYSTEM ACCESS

STEVENS INSTITUTE SERIES ON COMPLEX SYSTEMS AND ENTERPRISES

Title: *Modeling and Visualization of Complex Systems and Enterprises: Explorations of Physical, Human, Economic, and Social Phenomena*
Author: William B. Rouse
ISBN: 9781118954133

Title: *Perspectives on Complex Global Challenges: Education, Energy, Healthcare, Security, and Resilience*
Editors: Elisabeth Pate-Cornell and William B. Rouse with Charles M. Vest
ISBN: 9781118984093

Title: *Universities as Complex Enterprises: How Academia Works, Why It Works These Ways, and Where the University Enterprise Is Headed*
Editors: William B. Rouse
ISBN: 9781119245889

Title: *Emergent Behavior in Complex Systems Engineering: A Modeling and Simulation Approach*
Editors: Saurabh Mittal, Saikou Diallo, and Andreas Tolk
ISBN: 9781119378853

Title: *Healthcare System Access: Measurement, Inference, and Intervention*
Author: Nicoleta Serban
ISBN: 9781119601319

HEALTHCARE SYSTEM ACCESS

Measurement, Inference, and Intervention

NICOLETA SERBAN
Georgia Institute of Technology
Atlanta
GA, USA

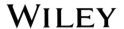

Registered Office
John Wiley & Sons, Inc., 111 River Street, Hoboken, NJ 07030, USA

Editorial Office
John Wiley & Sons, Inc., 111 River Street, Hoboken, NJ 07030, USA

For details of our global editorial offices, customer services, and more information about Wiley products visit us at www.wiley.com.

Wiley also publishes its books in a variety of electronic formats and by print-on-demand. Some content that appears in standard print versions of this book may not be available in other formats.

Library of Congress Cataloging-in-Publication Data

Names: Serban, Nicoleta, 1975- author.
Title: Healthcare system access : measurement, inference, and intervention
 / Dr. Nicoleta Serban.
Other titles: Stevens Institute series on complex systems and enterprises.
Description: First edition. | Hoboken, NJ : Wiley, 2020. | Series: Stevens
 Institute series on complex systems and enterprises | Includes
 bibliographical references and index.
Identifiers: LCCN 2019035345 (print) | LCCN 2019035346 (ebook) | ISBN
 9781119601319 (hardback) | ISBN 9781119601357 (adobe PDF) | ISBN
 9781119601364 (epub)
Subjects: MESH: Health Services Accessibility | Socioeconomic Factors |
 Healthcare Disparities | Outcome and Process Assessment (Health Care) |
 United States
Classification: LCC RA418 (print) | LCC RA418 (ebook) | NLM W 76 AA1 |
 DDC 362.1–dc23
LC record available at https://lccn.loc.gov/2019035345
LC ebook record available at https://lccn.loc.gov/2019035346

Cover Design: Wiley
Cover Image: © Josh Rios/Getty Images

Set in size of 10/12pt and TimesLTStd by SPi Global Ltd, India, Chennai

Printed in the United States of America

V10015257_103119

CONTENTS

PREFACE

My interest in healthcare access arose in the context of exploring service distribution and access within a research program funded by a NSF CAREER award. It did not take long to realize that access to fundamental services is a broad topic, which requires a more focused approach, depending on the service network to be accessed, for example, financial, healthcare, education, among others. Because my research interests also are in the field of healthcare system and engineering, I bridge two areas of research, access modeling and healthcare systems, to come to what this book is about.

My approach to healthcare access is inspired by both mathematical modeling (my training) and engineering (my current research home) along with an understanding of the healthcare system in terms of constraints, trade-offs and public health policy. The mathematical modeling approach highlights fundamental approaches on measurement of and inference on healthcare access. Modeling methodologies facilitate translating data into knowledge accounting for structures and dependencies in a system, to make data-driven estimates and projections about parameters, patterns and trends in the system. Complementally, the engineering approach informs efforts to design systems that will yield better outcomes using estimates and projections about the system.

One overarching challenge is that the healthcare system is a socio-technical system poised by behaviors of people, organizations and other stakeholders, and by intricacies of the health policies at the national and state levels. Healthcare access in the healthcare system will thus not be rigorously understood and effectively managed without the integration of knowledge across the fields of statistics, operations research, engineering, health economics, and health services research. This book is intended to illustrate how crosspollination of research fields and integration of data and knowledge provide a framework for decision making in transforming access to healthcare.

I am pleased to acknowledge many colleagues who have worked with me on one or more of the research projects discussed in this book. Many of the research studies included in this book are collaborative with former students and postdoctoral fellows in the H. Milton School of Industrial and Systems Engineering at Georgia Tech including Shanshan Cao, Stewart Curry, Erin Garcia, Monica Gentili, Pravara Harati, Ross Hilton, Ben Johnson, Ilbin Lee, Mallory Nobles, Zihao Li, Jessica Heir Stamm, and Yuchen Zheng. I was also fortunate to collaborate with health economists, public health decision makers and health services researchers including Susan Griffin, Jean O'Connor, Anne Fitzpatrick, Carol Smith, Michael Schechter, and Scott Tomar. I am very grateful for the advice and guidance of Paul Griffin and Julie Swann; both have been very supportive of my research program on healthcare access and have encouraged me to pursue new research opportunities in areas outside of my former training. My friend and collaborator Julie Swann has given me the foundation for deriving knowledge about healthcare, in general. Last, I want to thank my mentor, William B. Rouse, who has encouraged me during the writing of this book and has inspired me to aspire to high achievements in life.

NICOLETA SERBAN
ATLANTA, GA, USA
MARCH 2019

1

INTRODUCTION

Will I be able to get the care I need if I become seriously ill?

(Institute of Medicine 1993)

This fundamental question is at the basis of healthcare access. It implies the opportunity of gaining appropriate healthcare when needed, where needed, and at the level needed. It involves utilization of healthcare services and provision of appropriate services. Toward this end, health systems must achieve health(care) of all individuals and populations by delivering healthcare services to those who need them and benefit from them.

Local and national resources as well as personal resources must be available for the materialization of healthcare access. First, health policies set the stage for various approaches to healthcare delivery. Secondly, health personnel, facilities, and/or technology must be available where people live, work, or pursue their education. Thirdly, people must have the means and know-how to obtain the services. Thus, healthcare access in all its dimensions impacts all levels of the healthcare system, including people, processes, providers, organizations, and policy makers (Rouse and Serban 2015). This book is intended to present a synthesis of concepts, principles, models, and methods for addressing healthcare access within a system rife with complexity coming from all its levels.

This chapter proceeds as follows: I will first discuss the complexity of the concept of healthcare access, a multidimensional construct, going beyond its (mis)interpretation as a financial barrier in the existing political discourse on healthcare in the United States and beyond. I will address the relevance of understanding access in the context of public health, expanding on the system levelers for change and potential approaches to drive change. Then, I will proceed by pointing out that access is not an end in itself; it moderates healthcare utilization, with both intended consequences, such as improving health outcomes through appropriate utilization, and unintended consequences, such as over-utilization and potentially higher costs. I will subsequently consider methodological approaches to addressing healthcare

Healthcare System Access: Measurement, Inference, and Intervention, Nicoleta Serban.
© 2020 John Wiley & Sons, Inc. Published 2020 by John Wiley & Sons, Inc.

access problems, focusing on the use of quantitative approaches to explore a wide range of solutions. Finally, this chapter provides an overview of the remaining chapters in this book and how they address the framework presented in this chapter.

ACCESS AS A MULTIDIMENSIONAL CONSTRUCT

The current political discourse around healthcare access primarily focuses on financial barriers; it has been taken as synonymous with the availability of financial and health system resources. Limiting the access discussion to affordability or provider availability is understandable. It is however a simplistic approach for regulatory agencies charged with advancing access (Khan and Bhardwaj 1994). Simply measuring affordability or provider availability is neither adequate nor appropriate to understand healthcare access. Construing the conceptual framework for access requires a richer perspective.

There is a very large literature on the conceptual construct of healthcare access. Many organizations have been promoting and publishing on this topic (Healthy People 2020 2010; RAND Corporation 2010; www.kff.org). To distil this entire literature would not serve the reader of this book well, but several references to the existing proposed conceptual approaches will be provided.

One of the earliest access frameworks is the behavioral model by Ronald Andersen (Andersen 1968), initially developed in the late 1960s. In the early literature, access has also been differentiated between realized and potential, where *realized access* refers to the direct utilization of the services and *potential access* refers to the opportunity to utilize services (Khan 1992; Guagliardo 2004; McGrail and Humphreys 2009). Guagliardo (2004) stages first the potential for care delivery, followed by realized delivery of care. Potential access exists when a population in need for specific healthcare services lives in a community with access to "a willing and able healthcare delivery system." Realized care follows when all barriers to provision of healthcare are overcome. Guagliardo (2004) fundamentally describes "access" as both a noun referring to potential for healthcare use, and a verb referring to the act of using or receiving healthcare.

When Andersen revisited the behavioral access model, he introduced the concepts of *effective access*, established when utilization improves health status, and *efficient access*, established when the level of health status increases relative to the amount of healthcare services consumed (Andersen 1995). More generally, access can be placed under the framework of the 3 E's: Efficiency, Effectiveness, and Equity (Aday et al. 2004), discussed further in Chapters 2 and 3.

Penchansky and Thomas (1981) have usefully grouped access barriers into five dimensions: availability, accessibility, affordability, acceptability, and accommodation. Healthy People 2020 redefines the five dimensions of access, including insurance coverage, health services, and timeliness of care. Access as a multidimensional construct has been defined within multiple other frameworks as reviewed by Ansari (2007) and the Rural Policy Research Institute (MacKinney et al. 2014), among others. Further references to other multidimensional constructs will be

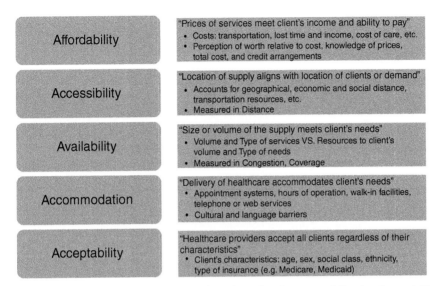

FIGURE 1.1 The access framework as a five-dimensional construct following the model by Penchansky and Thomas (1981).

provided in Chapter 2, however this book will primarily employ the simple but relevant framework provided by Penchansky and Thomas (1981). The diagram in Figure 1.1 shows the five dimensions of access within a service science framework for a broader understanding of service access. This access framework can apply to other fundamental services, for example, education, financial services, and healthy food stores, among others.

ACCESS FOR PUBLIC HEALTH

Urban and rural communities face many challenges to improving public health. Economic initiatives, changing demographics, and growth at the community level have resulted in changes that offer new opportunities for improving health while requiring that health systems be adapted to residents' health needs. One important integration of the community health needs into the directions of the healthcare system transformation is redesigning public healthcare delivery to achieve equitable, efficient, and effective access to healthcare.

Materialization of healthcare access in public health can take many forms, including prevention of emergency department visits and hospitalizations; quality of life of those with unmet health needs and with delays in receiving appropriate care; a cumulative decline in mortality and disability; and an overall improvement in mental health status, life expectancy, and general sense of wellbeing, among others.

While it is well understood that healthcare access is an actionable approach to improving public health, its conceptualization suggests the type of actions that need to be taken. For example, the current understanding of access as a financial barrier (affordability dimension) has brought forward national and state policies with a focus on coverage of healthcare benefits and insurance. As highlighted in the conceptualization of access as a multidimensional construct in this chapter, there are multiple dimensions of access that are interrelated; affordability is one of them but other dimensions are equally relevant to public health.

Importantly, access dimensions also have different relevance depending on the sub-population in need for care. For example, children in the United States are generally insured through commercial or public insurance, with only about 3.2% of children being uninsured (National Center for Health Statistics 2016). Thus, for the child population, affordability is not the primary dimension of relevance. Since children access the healthcare system with the effort and time commitment of their parents, accessibility and availability of the services may have a higher priority over other dimensions. Parents need to take time away from work and the children may miss school days. Timeliness through reducing travel and wait time may be essential to the decision as to whether to seek care.

There is also a wide variation in the relevance of access dimensions by healthcare services sought and/or needed. Mental and behavioral health services present challenges in access across all five dimensions for the majority of the population in the United States. In contrast, dental care is viewed as an axillary service for most health benefits programs hence insurance coverage is low. In many cases, dental care is an out-of-pocket expense; however, for children from low-income families, it is covered by Medicaid. But Medicaid participation by dentists is low (Serban and Tomar 2018). In one of my recent studies for Georgia, USA, my collaborators and I showed that there is a very large gap in accessibility and availability of dental care services between children with public insurance and those whose parents have other forms of affordability (Cao et al. 2017).

Compared with specialized care, primary care has become more available due to comprehensive coverage across all healthcare insurance programs, with a denser network of providers, including physicians. Scope of practice and/or independence practice acts have added supply to the network in many states due to the availability of licensed healthcare providers. Participation in public insurance programs by primary care providers is also higher than specialized care. In one of my recent studies on access to primary care for seven states in the United States, my collaborators and I have found that there is not a significance gap in access to pediatric primary care when comparing public and private insurance access (Gentili et al. 2018).

Thus, each access dimension cannot be considered in isolation from other dimensions in the public health setting. For example, accessibility and availability will be highly dependent on whether providers participate in public insurance programs, one form of acceptability. Affordability precedes other types of access dimensions; however, there are community-focused and federally funded programs opening the door to gaining healthcare for the uninsured, thus such programs must be where most needed; moreover, the population in need for such programs must be knowledgeable about the extent of care provided in these programs.

This discussion points to the fact that access is actionable through targeted policies and interventions taking various forms, depending on the population in need, the healthcare service needed, the access priorities established by policy makers, and the status quo of the healthcare system. Policies and interventions include scope of practice and independence practice acts, integration of services, mobile health, tele-health, home healthcare, community-based care, location and relocation of service providers, school programs, among many others. Such access interventions will be discussed in more detail in Chapter 5.

Most importantly, healthcare access goes beyond enabling healthcare for pub-lic health. When policymakers debate the merits of increasing access to healthcare, they must also consider improvements in the education of the population, economic opportunities, and a general sense of wellbeing. Healthcare access for public health is healthcare access for public wellbeing. Public health policies and interventions must reach the population in need for care holistically. Local initiatives such as the Two Georgias Initiative (Healthcare Georgia Foundation 2010) and California's Center for Collaborative Planning (Public Health Institute 2010) are test beds for learning how the integration of life priorities and opportunities can empower a population and individual health.

ACCESS FOR IMPROVING HEALTH OUTCOMES

Much has been said about the importance of healthcare access; but access is not an end in itself. Access to healthcare does not guarantee good health and appropriate health outcomes. Nevertheless, access to healthcare is necessary to ensuring that society enjoys optimal health, economic opportunities, productivity, and well-being.

The link between improving healthcare access and health outcomes depends greatly on the healthcare services needed, the geographical location, national and state policies in place, the population in need for healthcare services, among many others. In one study, my collaborators and I assessed the impact of access to pediatric asthma specialists on the rate of emergency department visits and hospitalization (Garcia et al. 2015). The study found that geographic access is explained by the rate of severe pediatric asthma outcomes, but the association varies with other geographic factors. Thus, interventions to improve access can be targeted to the areas with the greatest potential for improvement and tailored to each community's health needs. In another study, my collaborators and I analyzed the impact of geographic distance to cystic fibrosis care centers on lung function in children, young adults, and adults with cystic fibrosis (Johnson et al. 2018). We found that geographic access measured by travel distance was not associated with health outcomes among patients who do not change their geographic access over the study period. In fact, we found that overall socioeconomic and genetic factors appeared to be associated with health outcomes to a greater extent. The findings were also different for children, young adults, and adults.

It is not surprising that there are not consistent findings on the relationship between different dimensions of access and health outcomes. In fact, it may also be possible that improving access could lead to over-utilization of services, increasing costs of care while bringing little improvement in the outcomes.

The Rural Policy Research Institute (MacKinney et al. 2014) has provided a synthesis of the existing literature on access measurement and outcomes. The report differentiates access measures into process measures or outcome measures where *process measures* quantify how the system works and *outcome measures* quantify results or final products. However, the outcome measures are not necessarily directly influenced by healthcare access as I pointed out in the examples above. The access measurement alone will not provide an understanding of the impact of interventions for improving access on outcomes; such a relationship can be established by assessing the relationship between access and outcomes in the presence of many other factors potentially influencing outcomes. I will expand more on this topic in Chapter 4 of this book.

ANALYTICAL APPROACHES

Measures do not define access, but rather evaluate access. As described earlier in this chapter, the existing literature on access differentiates between realized and potential access.

On one hand, realized access can be directly measured based on the observed utilization, for example, the travel distance one has incurred to utilize a service or the time one has waited for an appointment. However, it does not reflect access since it does not account for latent barriers that can hamper demand based on true need for care. Realized access or utilization of services will be hindered if access does not fully materialize (Khan 1992; McGrail and Humphreys 2009).

On the other hand, potential access indirectly measures access to services. It requires knowledge about the network of healthcare providers called *supply* for most of this book in the spirit of economic engineering and service science. It also requires understanding and knowledge about the network of the population needing or demanding a service, called *need* for most of this book. Potential access can be measured by overlaying the two networks given one or more access objectives, for example, improving affordability, expanding *spatial access* referring to accessibility and availability together (Guagliardo 2004; McGrail and Humphreys 2009), or increasing acceptability of public insurance.

Conceptualizing access as a multidimensional construct within the decision-making framework is particularly important when deciding which objective is to be achieved (Ansari 2007). Should access be thought of as a multidimensional construct while the access dimensions are viewed as separate pillars of the construct? Or, is access a single concept, with the access dimensions playing the role of influencing barriers or enablers? Depending on the perspective on access, one could influence one access dimension where all other dimensions can be viewed as constraints of the system, or one could influence multiple objectives defined by the access dimensions differently weighted. For example, if spatial access is to be optimized, in other words, reducing travel distance while ensuring some pre-specified maximum wait time, the objective is then a weighted aggregate of accessibility and availability where the weights can be fixed for the entire population or can be different across sub-populations, for example, different for rural and urban communities. Such considerations are significant in the understanding of the access frameworks, and the actionable policies and interventions to be implemented.

In conceptualizing and measuring access, the challenges are on specifying the *assumptions* on the two networks, the *constraints* of the system under which the two networks interact, and the *preferences* of those participating in the two networks. Assumptions are often specified by policies or standards, for example, travel access standards established by states for the Medicaid programs (Department of Health and Human Services 2014). Constraints reflect access barriers for the population in need, for example, whether a provider participates in public insurance or not, or system supply restrictions, for example, restricted scope of practice for nurse practitioners.

Preferences are most difficult to integrate into estimation and evaluation of access since they can be subjective to biases or beliefs. Nonetheless, they are real and can influence one's access to care to a great extent. Examples are one's preference to seek care from a physician instead of a nurse practitioner, if one is available within access constraints (Dill et al. 2013); one's preference to have all care performed by one system or clinic due to integration and coordination of services (Corrigan and Adams 2003); one's choice of recommended physician even if out-of-network, hence incurring higher out-of-pocket expenses; or one's choice not to seek care at all due to religious beliefs.

Another important challenge is availability of data on the supply and need networks, financial resources, and of data and knowledge on system constraints and preferences as expanded in Chapter 6. Figure 1.2 illustrates a sample of potential data sources that can be used to specify the supply and need/demand networks and the associated constraints. The specification of supply includes the location of the

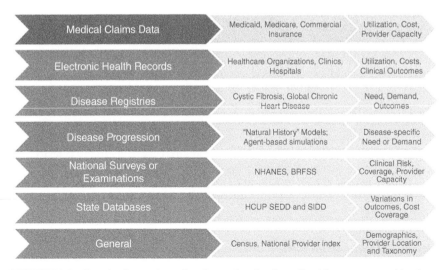

FIGURE 1.2 Data landscape for estimation and evaluation of healthcare access, with a focus on data for specifying the supply and need networks. BRFSS, Behavioral Risk Factor Surveillance System; HCUP, Healthcare Cost and Utilization Project; NHANES, National Health and Nutrition Examination Survey.

healthcare providers and their potential caseload to provide the services needed to be accessed. The specification of demand requires estimation of the population in need, the quantity of services needed, and the health risk influencing the level of service utilization.

Knowledge about system and access constraints can be specified by state policies, providing information on enacted laws, differences across similar legislation acts if enacted in multiple states (e.g. supervision of licensed providers), and standards imposed by states, among others. Such constraints can also be informed by surveys, data repositories or medical records that can provide information on provider-level or patient-level constraints, for example, Medicaid participation of a provider.

Considerations of the access objectives to be achieved with specifications of the assumptions, constraints, and preferences are at the core of measuring potential access. But specifications of the constraints and preferences often come with some level of uncertainty, which will further propagate into the estimation and evaluation of the access measures. In most existing studies on access measurement, uncertainty of the input parameters, thus uncertainty in the access measures, is not accounted for, assuming access is deterministic, meaning no variation due to small changes in the model parameters or assumptions.

While more challenging, decision making can be more statistically reliable and accurate when considering access within an uncertain environment. Insights on the uncertainty of a decision can come in various forms, for example, an estimate of the risk of making the decision or a measure of the plausibility of the decision made to address the issue at hand. Such inferences are essential in decision making because in some cases they may suggest that more data need to be acquired to provide stronger evidence for a decision; in others, they may prompt not making a decision at all because of the high uncertainty of the decision environment.

While access measures alone can make for nice maps, in order to make statistical statements on whether there are disparities in access across communities and sub-populations, or to identify communities and sub-populations for targeted interventions, statistical inference plays a key role. In most studies, access measures are estimated, but most commonly, statistical inferences are not provided. This last step is essential for actionable policies and interventions.

To conclude, while there is an extensive literature on access frameworks and access measurement approaches, there is a need for bridging the conceptualization of healthcare access to the access measurement and inference using rigorous analytical approaches. At the core of this endeavor is a cross-disciplinary approach, integrating many areas of research including health services research, health policy, operations research, and statistical learning, among others.

PEDIATRIC HEALTHCARE

Most of my research on healthcare access has been centered on pediatric healthcare as illustrated by most of the case studies presented in this book. It is particularly important to eliminate health disparities among children because investing in pediatric healthcare will have the highest long-term return as it will reduce the burden of future healthcare costs and foster a healthy and productive population. Child development affects subsequent life, education and occupational opportunities, and the risks of unhealthy behaviors, chronic diseases, malnutrition, mental-health problems, and criminality in later life. Along with good nutrition and wellness, healthcare is a paramount ingredient for healthy child development.

ACCESS IN THE TWENTY-FIRST CENTURY

The diseases of the twenty-first century will be chronic conditions, "those that steal vitality and productivity" (Jackson and Kochtitzky 2012). Managing chronic and high-risk conditions is a complex enterprise, requiring the right balance between best outcomes and limited resources. Improving access particularly is important in the management of chronic conditions; regular and appropriate care can reduce severe outcomes, can slow down the progression of a condition, and/or maintain the well-being of those burdened with chronic conditions.

For best outcomes, improving access has to be aligned with the goal of maximizing value. Thus, additional value and cost constraints have to be integrated into the overall access interventions to make the most out of the return on investment. Many case studies in this book focus on chronic conditions, emphasizing the added value of integrating improvement in access to care into the overall healthcare system.

OVERVIEW OF THE BOOK

The foregoing has provided a broad outline of the comprehensive framework for studying healthcare access from measurement to inference to decision making. The remainder of this chapter provides an overview of each of the other chapters in this book.

A Multidimensional Framework for Measuring Access (Chapter 2)

This chapter begins with an overview of frameworks, models, and definitions, with the focus on their applicability to measurement of and inference on healthcare access. This overview will provide the basis for the general model for access measurement, emphasizing the importance of considering all model components: objective, assumptions, constraints, and preferences. The general model will be contrasted to existing measurement approaches and will be demonstrated with approaches for spatial access. Last, the general model will be applied to one specific case study, measuring access to asthma care.

Disparities in Healthcare Access (Chapter 3)

This chapter first summarizes the concept of systematic disparities, with an overview of various measures, differentiated into social-group disparity measures and disproportionality measures, introduced in the existing literature. It then follows with a statistical framework for making inference on disparities with application to geographic disparities in healthcare access. I will illustrate the statistical inference approach to identify systematic disparities using two case studies, one on access to pediatric primary care with an emphasis on geographic disparities between sub-populations differentiated by the health insurance status, and another case study related to the 2009 H1N1 campaign with a focus on an analysis of disparities with respect to demographic and economic factors.

Linking Access to Health Outcomes (Chapter 4)

This chapter begins with a taxonomy of health outcomes, specifically those targeted through improvements in healthcare access. Access is then introduced as a moderator of healthcare utilization, with potentially both intended and unintended consequences for improving utilization. Discussions on the link between access and outcomes will include methodological considerations and statistical models, depending on the type of outcome, and with an overview of factors influencing outcomes. Two case studies will be provided, one in which I consider the link between healthcare outcomes and access to specialized pediatric asthma care, and another study in which I consider the link between clinical outcomes and access to care centers for patients with cystic fibrosis.

Healthcare Interventions for Improving Access (Chapter 5)

This chapter first introduces a taxonomy of interventions, distinguished into health policy, in-home and in-school healthcare, telemedicine and mobile healthcare, and network interventions, with multiple illustrations of interventions discussed with reference to the access dimensions. Particularly, the challenge of addressing access to improve outcomes holistically will be highlighted. The chapter will continue with a presentation of statistical modeling to address a series of important questions in decision making: Are interventions needed? Where are the interventions needed and for what population groups? What interventions are needed? How to evaluate interventions? Case studies on access to dental care will be used to illustrate approaches to study policy and network interventions toward improving access, addressing substantive questions: *Why*, *Where*, and *How* to intervene? *Which* intervention?

Data Analytics (Chapter 6)

This chapter begins with a discussion of the complexity of the data analytics for studies on healthcare access, highlighting the importance of integrating all data processes from data acquisition and processing to data translation, to data modeling and finally decision making. Multiple data sources are described in detail, covering protected health information (PHI) data, survey data collected by public and private organizations and secondary health and healthcare data. The chapter will continue with data analytics for the primary components of access measurements, supply, need and constraints of healthcare. Then it will focus on data analytics for the analysis of health outcomes commonly employed in the analysis of targeted interventions for improving access. Challenges on data science, data modeling and dissemination are discussed in the more general context of healthcare data analytics. The chapter will illustrate data analytics with a case study on the derivation of the provider-level caseload of mental and behavioral health for the Medicaid-insured population nationwide. Two data portals are also briefly presented within the context of advancing community health.

REFERENCES

Aday, L.A., Begley, C.E., Lairson, D.R. et al. (2004). *Evaluating the Healthcare System: Effectiveness, Efficiency and Equity.* Chicago, IL: Health Administration Press.

Andersen, R.M. (1968). *Behavioral Model of Families' Use of Health Services.* Chicago, IL: Center for Health Administration Studeis, University of Chicago.

Andersen, R.M. (1995). Revisiting the behavioral model and access to medical care: does it matter? *Journal of Health and Social Behavior* **36**: 1–10.

Ansari, Z. (2007). A review of literature on access to primary health care. *Australian Journal of Primary Health* **13**(2): 80–95.

Cao, S., Gentili, M., Griffin, P.M. et al. (2017). Disparities in preventive dental care among children in Georgia. *Preventing Chronic Disease* **14**: 170176.

Corrigan, J.M. and Adams, K. (2003). *Priority Areas for National Action: Transforming Health Care Quality.* National Academies Press.

Department of Health and Human Services (2014). State Standards for Access to Care in Medicaid Managed Care.

Dill, M.J., Pankow, S., Erikson, C., and Shipman, S. (2013). Survey shows consumers open to a greater role for physician assistants and nurse practitioners. *Health Affairs* **32**(6): 1135–1142.

Garcia, E., Serban, N., Swann, J. et al. (2015). The effect of geographic access on severe health outcomes for pediatric asthma. *Journal of Allergy and Clinical Immunology* **136** (3): 610–618.

Gentili, M., Serban, N., Harati, P. et al. (2018). Quantifying disparities in accessibility and availability of pediatric primary care with implications for policy. *Health Services Research* **53**(3): 1458–1477.

Guagliardo, M.F. (2004). Spatial accessibility of primary care: concepts, methods and challenges. *International Journal of Health Geographics* **3**(3): 1–13.

Healthcare Georgia Foundation (2010). The Two Georgias Initiative. http://www.georgiaerc .org/the-two-georgias.asp (accessed June 2019).

Healthy People 2020 (2010). About healthy people. http://www.healthypeople.gov/2020/ about/default.aspx (accessed July 2018).

Institute of Medicine (1993). *Access to Health Care in America.* Washington, DC: National Academy Press.

Jackson, R.J. and Kochtitzky, C. (2012). *Creating A Healthy Environment: The Impact of the Built Environment on Public Health.* Centers for Disease Control and Prevention.

Johnson, B., Ngueyep, R., Schechter, M. et al. (2018). A study of the impact of geographic access on health outcomes for cystic fibrosis. *Pediatric Pulmonology* **53**(3): 284–292.

Khan, A.A. (1992). An integrated approach to measuring potential spatial access to health care services. *Socio-Economic Planning Sciences* **26**(4): 275–287.

Khan, A.A. and Bhardwaj, S.M. (1994). Access to health care. A conceptual framework and its relevance to health care planning. *Evaluation & the Health Professions* **17**(1): 60–76.

MacKinney, A. C. , Coburn, A., Lundblad, J. et al. (2014). Access to Rural Health Care – A Literature Review and New Synthesis. Rural Policy Research Institute.

McGrail, M. and Humphreys, J. (2009). Measuring spatial accessibility to primary care in rural areas: Improving the effectiveness of the two-step floating catchment area method. *Applied Geography* **29**(4): 533–541.

National Center for Health Statistics (2016). *Health Insurance Coverage*. Centers for Disease Control and Prevention.

Penchansky, R. and Thomas, J.W. (1981). The concept of access: definition and relationship to consumer satisfaction. *Medical Care* **19**(2): 127–140.

Public Health (2010). Center for Collaborative Planning. http://www.connectccp.org/ (accessed January 2019).

RAND Corporation (2010). Explore health care access. https://www.rand.org/topics/health-care-access.html (accessed February 2019).

Rouse, W.B. and Serban, N. (2015). *Understanding and Managing the Complexity of Healthcare*. Cambridge, MA: MIT Press.

Serban, N. and Tomar, S. (2018). ADA Health Policy Institute's methodology overestimates spatial access to dental care for publicly insured children. *Journal of Public Health Dentistry* **78**(4): 291–295.

2

A MULTIDIMENSIONAL FRAMEWORK FOR MEASURING ACCESS

Service access is the ability of an individual or community to overcome the barriers of utilizing services in a network consisting of multiple sites spatially distributed over a geographic area. Research on measurement and inference on service access has emerged as economic and social equity advocates recognized that where people live influences their opportunities for economic development, access to quality health-care, and political participation (Jackson and Kochtitzky 2002; Frumkin et al. 2004; Flournoy and Treuhaft 2005; Lee and Rubin 2007; Blackwell and Treuhaft 2008).

Access to fundamental services is a well-studied and debated area, with the first policies dating to as early as 1935 when President Franklin D. Roosevelt signed Title V of the Social Security Act, which is the U.S. national program accountable for the health and well-being of all mothers and children. Title V for higher education was signed in 1998. Other similar laws and acts have targeted improving access to fundamental needs of society such as education, healthcare, financial services, and other public services.

Access has been studied and evaluated for many types of fundamental services, both public and private. Examples are access to healthy foods (Apparicio et al. 2007), to grocery stores (Dunkley et al. 2004), to elementary schools (Talen 2001), to public playgrounds (Talen and Anselin 1998), to emergency services (Ball and Lin 1993; Felder and Brinkmann 2002), for the Medicare populations (Barton et al. 2001), to pediatric primary care (Chang and Halfon 1997; Guagliardo et al. 2004), and to pediatric sub-specialties (Mayer et al. 2004, 2009; Mayer 2006) among many others.

Access to a service network is dependent on barriers and facilitators that reflect multiple dimensions, where each dimension is critical for service delivery, albeit with different relevance across service systems. For example, for education, young children and adolescents are required to attend school, thus they have to travel to school

Healthcare System Access: Measurement, Inference, and Intervention, Nicoleta Serban.
© 2020 John Wiley & Sons, Inc. Published 2020 by John Wiley & Sons, Inc.

no matter what the effect of distance might be. Thus an important access dimension for education is the ability to travel to schools within a reasonable amount of time. Busing children long distances has less of a bearing on utilization of the education services but it may lead to disparities in access to education, since it can negatively impact children as a function of lost opportunity time. Another important dimension is the ability to be accepted in a school that meets one's needs. Public schools primarily accept students on the basis of their school district residence; charter schools have more complex acceptance schedules, while private schools require ability to pay and often have opaque acceptance rules.

For healthcare on the other hand, access comes with different system constraints. For example, while there is not an explicit constraint on which provider to access for a specific healthcare need, affordability of healthcare insurance or out-of-pocket expenses can deem the service inaccessible. Moreover, the healthcare needs are also complex, from wellness to specialized care to acute and complex care. How one accesses the healthcare system is highly dependent on such needs.

Because of the complexity of service systems, defining, measuring, and making inferences about service access requires system-specific considerations, for example, different access constraints. Moreover, improving access can be addressed by system-targeted facilitators, interventions, and policies. While the focus of this book is healthcare access, the access frameworks and the modeling approaches introduced in this chapter will also apply to other service systems.

OVERVIEW OF ACCESS FRAMEWORKS AND MODELS

Fundamentals of Access Modeling

In the introduction, I provided multiple frameworks and definitions of healthcare access. In this section, I will expand on this topic since it is the basis of the measurement models discussed later in this chapter as well as the basis of the intervention approaches discussed in Chapter 5.

One of the very first access models was introduced by Andersen (1968), initially developed in the late 1960s. Aday and Andersen (1974) conceptualized access as being identified by interrelationships among five domains: (i) health policy; (ii) characteristics of the healthcare delivery system; (iii) characteristics of populations at risk; (iv) utilization of health services; and (v) consumer satisfaction. The initial model (Andersen 1968), a behavioral access approach, focused on people's use of healthcare services as a function of their *predisposition* to use services, *enablers* or *barriers* to healthcare utilization as well as their *need* for care. Those are further expanded upon in later research of Andersen and Davidson (2007), differentiated into contextual and individual factors. For example, predisposition to utilize healthcare can be determined by the existing conditions, for example, demographics, social characteristics and beliefs. Enablers and barriers may include health policies and financial characteristics, for example. Need characteristics include environmental need (e.g. housing), and population health (e.g. the prevalence of a health condition).

While additional considerations to the behavioral access approach have been proposed by other frameworks by Andersen (1995) and Andersen and Davidson (2007), the underlying premise of this approach is at the core of defining and understanding healthcare access. In this book, I will bring forth the idea of constraints and preferences along with individual and system objectives to build on this premise.

In relation to this initial behavioral model on healthcare access, it is challenging to account for health behaviors (e.g. smoking, nutrition, self-care, alcohol use) when modeling access. Such behaviors are often "aggregated" as part of the population's prevalence and predisposition to a given condition, also reflected in the population's constraints and preferences for a specific service.

This model also points out that the three components, *predisposition, enablers* or *barriers*, and *need,* influence differently one's behavior to utilize healthcare services depending on the services sought. This suggests that access measurement models must incorporate specific characteristics of an individual's behaviors in relation to the healthcare service to be accessed. This is a very important aspect of measurement of and inference on access to specific services as it suggests tailoring the access frameworks and models to the healthcare service of interest. In this section, I will describe general modeling approaches, but I will point out differences in the approaches depending on the services of interest.

In a more recent exposition, Andersen and Davidson (2007) describe healthcare access as a multidimensional construct, where the defined dimensions are potential access (enabling factors), realized access (use of services), equitable access, inequitable access, effective access, and efficient access. However, these are not dimensions of access but represent the various attributes access can take as discussed next.

A thorough account of definitions, measures, barriers, and frameworks is a report by the Rural Policy Research Institute (RUPRI) (MacKinney et al. 2014), and in reviews by Ansari (2007) and by Guagliardo (2004). Specifically, Guagliardo (2004) highlights that "it [access] is both a noun referring to potential for healthcare use, and a verb referring to the act of using or receiving healthcare." Thus, a first challenge in distilling the concept of access is the differentiation between potential and realized access, where *realized access* refers to the direct utilization of the services where *potential access* refers to the opportunity to utilize services (Khan 1992; Guagliardo 2004; McGrail and Humphreys 2009).

Realized access is the utilization of services once barriers to provision of care are overcome (Guagliardo 2004). Appropriate utilization of healthcare services is a positive tenet in preempting severe health outcomes, particularly important in chronic disease management and with significant implications on healthcare expenditure. Healthcare utilization can reflect behaviors in attaining wellness, treatment, and disease management. Studies on healthcare utilization can also point out behaviors in seeking care in an environment of reduced access to care. For example, the Medicaid-insured population had historically utilized the care system disparately (Pylypchuk and Sarpong 2012), without following recommended care practices (Piecoro et al. 2001; McGrady and Hommel 2013; Chang et al. 2014), because of various access barriers.

Potential access is the focus of this book since access measurement and evaluation should account for healthcare services that are utilized or realized as well as those that are non-utilized, that is, healthcare services desired but not received (MacKinney et al. 2014). Potential exists when a population in need for specific healthcare services overlaps in space with "a willing and able healthcare delivery system" (Guagliardo 2004), thus it is a measure of the *fit between a population's need for healthcare services and the supply of services by healthcare providers* as defined by Penchansky and Thomas (1981). This definition of access is at the core of the measurement models presented in this book.

The most important delineating aspect between realized and potential access is that realized access reflects demand for care and potential access reflects need for care. *Demand* measures the quantity of health services the population is willing to consume and to purchase given cost and access constraints, preferences or other related behaviors. A sub-population's demand for healthcare services depends on cultural, religious, educational, and social status as well as on perceived physical or mental distress (Jeffers et al. 1971). In contrast, *need* consists of services that a healthcare professional finds necessary to delivery following specific health indicators or recommended care guidelines. Need for a particular service is determined by healthcare professionals based on demographics, clinical risk factors, health status, and genetic background among others. Need for healthcare can also be "felt need," when an individual assesses his/her health status and finds a lower or higher need for healthcare than recommended by a medical professional. This is different from demand in that felt need may not be pursued or consumed due to access or cost constraints, for example. Generally, "demand" is most frequently used by medical economists, while "need" is most frequently used by health professionals, commissions, and agencies (Jeffers et al. 1971).

Other definitions of access refer to specific dimensions, such as the timely use of services, opportunity to gain access when healthcare is needed, effectiveness of access and equity of the distribution of services (MacKinney et al. 2014). The approach in this book takes a more general perspective in defining access, assuming that it is an actionable facet of the healthcare system, influencing delivery of care across multiple dimensions jointly. When influencing the healthcare system, specific attributes of the access measures are to be considered, such as effectiveness, efficiency, and equity, the so called 3 E's framework in this book. Thus, such characteristics of access are not defined as dimensions of access as suggested by Andersen and Davidson (2007). The dimensions of the access construct target different access objectives, depending on the outcomes sought to attain.

The 3 E's framework, or the trade-off between effectiveness, efficiency, and equity of access is at the core of decision making on improving access. Generally, *efficiency* measures how well the system is utilizing its resources ("Are we doing things the right way?"). *Effectiveness* is a measure of how well the system meets a need or achieves an objective ("Are we doing the right things?"). *Equity* refers to the fairness of delivery, allocation of resources, and achievement of outcomes ("Are we affecting all people or places in need of care?"). An optimal trade-off between the 3 E's may be desirable but may not always be possible. The decision on which facet of the 3 E's to emphasize depends on the policy agenda, the availability of resources, the existing health policy environment, the type of services, and the population in need, among other factors. It is therefore important to establish a measurement approach that allows for integrating such factors in the trade-off between the 3 E's. The measurement approach discussed in this section will be further explored from the angle of the 3 E's framework in this book.

I will conclude this sub-section with Figure 2.1, which is a synthesis of access perspectives as provided in the existing qualitative research on healthcare access. The endpoint of this synthesis is to inspire actionable and effective policy and practice, with later reference to access measures and inferences on policy and outcomes. While there are many potential confounding factors to good health and many mediators that could result in improving health outcomes, appropriate utilization to healthcare is a major component. Similarly, while there are many potential mediators that could hamper or facilitate healthcare utilization, healthcare access has been the most cited causal factor of utilization of healthcare access; in fact, it is one of the few ways policy makers have addressed improving appropriate use of healthcare services. Nonetheless, access is actionable only if decision makers clearly define what actions need to be targeted. Toward this end, many multidimensional frameworks of access have been introduced in the existing literature, five of them are highlighted in Figure 2.1. Further descriptions and considerations on these different perspectives will be detailed in the next sub-section.

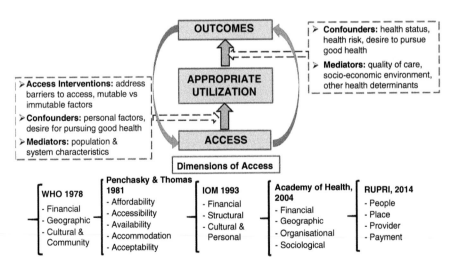

FIGURE 2.1 A synthesis of access frameworks, with causal relationships between access and outcomes. The synthesis is intended to introduce access as a multidimensional construct for measurement and inference. Five different perspectives into access as a multidimensional construct are given by: World Health Organization (1978), Penchansky and Thomas (1981), Institute of Medicine (1993), Academy for Health Services Research and Health Policy (2004), and RUPRI (MacKinney et al. 2014).

Overview of Spatial Access Models

The discussion so far has emphasized definitions and attributes of healthcare access but has not yet fully provided the framework for describing access as a multidimensional construct. I will continue here with a more detailed account of the five frameworks of access as a multidimensional construct presented in Figure 2.1. An early account is by the World Health Organization (1978), later revisited in World Health Organization (2008). The three dimensions refer to financial access, geographic access, and culturally and functionally within reach of all members of a community. In Penchansky and Thomas (1981), financial access is referred to as affordability, geographic access as accessibility with an additional dimension called availability, and the cultural and community dimensions reduced to two concrete dimensions, acceptability and accommodation. The Institute of Medicine (1993) accounted for more general dimensions of access than financial access, called structural, including the affordability and availability dimensions in the framework by Penchansky and Thomas (1981), but more broadly referring to system barriers. The Academy for Health Services Research and Health Policy (2004) summarizes access with a similar set of dimensions, distinguishing organizational and sociological access dimensions, referring to the cultural, community, and structural dimensions as described in the previous accounts of access dimensions. All four frameworks refer to the same set of dimensions although differently grouped or defined.

A new synthesis of access dimensions, referring to people, place, provider, and payment dimensions, is defined by the framework introduced by the RUPRI (MacKinney et al. 2014). The "people" dimension refers to access barriers or facilitators represented by characteristics of a population at risk for inadequate or inappropriate healthcare, including demographics, socioeconomic factors but also personal and cultural characteristics. The "place" dimension refers to spatial barriers to care, geographic as well as place-related characteristics, for example, the rurality of a community. The "provider" dimension refers to not only the location and distribution of the providers but also the "diversity" of care available to a community, e.g. specialized vs primary care; the organizational infrastructure, e.g. hours of operation, patient-centeredness; and policy, e.g. scope of practice. Last, the "payment" dimension is in a nutshell the affordability dimension but taking into account insurance coverage, benefits available for a given insurance coverage, co-pay, deductible, out-of-pocket care among many other aspects of affordability.

This new synthesis of the access dimensions hints to the multilevel system perspective of the healthcare access by Rouse and Cortese (2010) presented in Figure 2.2. My collaborator and I have provided a detailed account of this multilevel framework of the healthcare system in a book expanding on the complexity of the healthcare system (Rouse and Serban 2015).

Since access is pervasive throughout the entire healthcare system, characterizing the access dimensions in relation to the system levels, people, processes, organizations, and society is a timely approach to understanding healthcare access. However, I will focus on a more traditional framework for describing access as a multidimensional construct, specifically that of Penchansky and Thomas (1981).

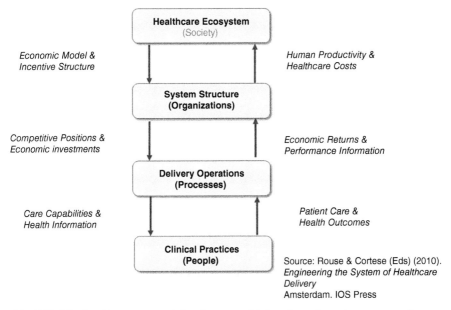

FIGURE 2.2   Healthcare as a multilevel system with interdependence between people, processes, organizations, and society. *Source*: Rouse and Cortese (2010).

The *5 A's framework* as I will refer to throughout the book (see Figure 1.1 for a detailed description) does not have a one-to-one mapping with the four levels of the healthcare system described in Figure 2.2 but they encompass all the measureable aspects of healthcare access. To this end, my objective is to focus on measurement and inference of healthcare access from a quantitative perspective. The 5 A's framework is actionable in the sense that the access dimensions defined by this framework are clearly delineated and measurable, providing a clear mapping between the concept of access and decision making in health policy and healthcare delivery.

Specifically, I will illustrate the measurement and inference approach with a focus on *spatial access*, consisting of two of the dimensions, accessibility and availability (Guagliardo 2004; McGrail and Humphreys 2009). *Availability* refers to scarcity or congestion of healthcare providers. *Accessibility* or proximity is travel impedance (distance or time) between patient location and service points.

Spatial access is important for managing chronic diseases where regular visits can reduce severe outcomes, particularly, for children whose health outcomes accrue over many years and for low income populations covered by public insurance, which is not accepted by all providers. Spatial access has high relevance to systems and/or sub-populations with universal healthcare coverage where spatial access becomes one of the primary barriers to care. For example, in the United States, the majority of children have access to healthcare insurance benefits, private or public, with only 3.2% of children being uninsured, 53.8% having a private insurance, and 43% having a public insurance in 2016 (National Center for Health Statistics 2016). Most of the research case studies provided in this book are addressing important challenges in pediatric healthcare delivery, hence the focus on spatial access.

To conclude, the study of healthcare access has many complexities, however for the purpose of quantifying access into actionable policies and interventions, I will focus on potential access within the 5 A's multidimensional framework. While considering this simpler framework may not capture the rich relationships between the access determinants fully, it is measurable and thus actionable, which is the overarching objective of this book.

ACCESS MEASUREMENT APPROACH

I will begin with the introduction of a general modeling approach for measuring potential access under the 5 A's framework. The model is described by four components:

i. Objective
ii. Assumptions
iii. Constraints
iv. Preferences

In what follows, I will expand on all these components, from a more general modeling perspective but also in a case study for illustration.

General Model

The goal is to measure access for communities within a geographic region. I will begin with some basic notation that will be used throughout the book:

- *Index of the communities*: $s = 1, \ldots, S$ where S is the number of communities within the region of interest.
- *Index of the sub-populations*: $p = 1, \ldots, P$ where P is the number of sub-populations within the region of interest.
- *Index of the providers available*: $j = 1, \ldots, J$ where J is the number of providers available within the region of interest.
- $\theta_{s,p,j}$ is the *access opportunity*, or lack of it, experienced by the sub-population p to provider j defined for all providers $j = 1, \ldots, J$.
- $A_{s,p}$ is the *access opportunity cost or measure* for the community s and for the sub-population p, being a function of the access opportunity to providers in the region, depending on the access objective to be achieved.

The division of the geographic region into communities can be a division of contiguous areas, e.g. census tracts within a state in the US or districts in the UK. It is preferable to use a geographic division that is a proxy of how neighborhoods/communities are delineated to better capture populations with similar characteristics. However, we cannot assume homogeneity in the population of a neighborhood regardless of how well we divide the region into communities. Generally, we should expect people to be of different ages, gender, race, ethnicity, and/or backgrounds. Because of this, we divide the population of a community into sub-populations, for example, by age groups.

The set of providers available in a region depends on the type of services to be accessed. If, for example, the focus is on insurance coverage, the set of providers consists of those accepting specific health insurance plans. If the healthcare services sought are more specific, for example, specialized asthma care, the set of providers consists of all specialized care such as asthma specialists.

The potential access opportunity of a community s and a sub-population p to a provider j is defined by $\theta_{s,p,j}$. It can be expressed as the percentage of the sub-population p in community s selecting provider j. However, other specifications can be considered, for example, a binary (0 or 1) value, e.g. whether provider j provides care at all to the sub-population p in community s since it may not serve the area of a given health insurance plan.

The access opportunity cost or measure can take multiple forms depending on the objective to be achieved or the access dimension to be targeted. Examples of measures are *quantitative* measures such as length of time to appointment, geographic proximity to provider, and percent of adults with health insurance; or *qualitative* measures such as ease of getting an appointment or of contacting the provider, having a regular source of care. Quantitative measures can be derived given multiple sources of data while qualitative measures require surveying the population of interest then obtaining some average or overall population summaries over the surveyed population. In this book, I will primarily focus on quantitative measures since they can be estimated using modeling techniques based on available data.

The access measure can also target one or more access dimensions. For example, one objective is to balance affordability and acceptability of health insurance. Given that an individual incurs higher expenses if accessing out-of-network providers than if accessing in-network providers while possibly experiencing lower travel cost, the access objective will include information about travel cost and expenditure of care together. For spatial access, the objective can be a weighted aggregate between travel distance/time to a provider of choice and the availability or congestion experienced when accessing a provider.

However, such access objectives are materialized under many constraints in the system along with preferences of those interacting in the system. Thus when deriving the access objectives, constraints and preferences need to be considered. Odoki et al. (2001) provided a series of realistic constraints that can be incorporated in many access models, as discussed below.

Transportation constraints: circumscribing access by limiting the distances an individual can travel within a particular time window using the available transportation system.

Temporal constraints: determining when and how long an individual needs or is willing to spend to access services.

Spatial constraints: determining the availability of services within geographic areas and the locations of specific services.

Social and cultural constraints: determining who has or has not access to specific services at specific times as a result of system laws, income levels, gender, and social relationships.

Economic constraints: income is the most important economic constraint, which limits behavioral autonomies due to time and/or place constrains.

Other constraints are system-specific, for example, the scope of practice of a provider as specified by state policies, independence practice for licensed providers, ability of a provider to treat specific conditions or to serve sub-populations with specific needs, participation of healthcare providers in public insurance programs, reduced benefits of healthcare plans, and access to specific insurance plans within a region. Access preferences can be healthcare provision-specific, for example, the preference to seek care from a physician over a nurse practitioner or physician assistant, the preference to see the same provider for both primary and specialized care, or the choice of a provider because of recommendations or cultural accommodation.

Some of the constraints and preferences are not specific enough at the population level, and thus assumptions about access behaviors and system constraints need to be made. Assumptions are often driven by system standards and policies. For example, many states established access standards specifying the maximum travel distance/time to reach a primary or specialized care provider (Murrin 2014); these standards are often used in contracts with organizations to provide managed care. Other assumptions specify the need of basic primary care policies that have been put in place to create a set of comprehensive primary care and wellness services mandated to be part of all health insurance plans.

Given this framework, the analytical question is: *How to derive the access measure or opportunity cost $A_{s,p}$ for the community s and the sub-population p?* Generally, we need a model that incorporates constraints, preferences, and assumptions, along with the data needed to specify them. The model can be used to estimate the value of each opportunity available to an individual or to a sub-population. The overall access opportunity cost that a sub-population derived from the entire set of opportunities available can be obtained by imposing specific constraints that the sub-population experiences when accessing the system and possible preferences on the selection of the service provider.

The modeling approach needs to mimic one's opportunity to access healthcare in order to estimate his/her potential access. In principle, the decision made assuming a rational behavior will be *optimal* given constraints and preferences. This suggests using an operations research approach, where one would optimize an access objective, subject to a set of constraints that also include preferences and assumptions about the model (Li et al. 2015).

To be more specific, given an access objective, the approach is to optimize an opportunity cost function that a sub-population p from the community s would experience when/if accessing care from a provider j for all $j = 1, \ldots, J$, defined here by $f(\theta_{s,p,j})$. This is equivalent to an individual making a decision based on the opportunity cost. Thus, it is important to pay particular attention to how the opportunity cost is defined since it reflects one's decision making for a given access objective. However, simply optimizing (minimizing) one's cost without consideration of other people accessing the system is not realistic. People compete for a limited supply of care. Therefore, instead of considering individual decisions for all providers in the system, we can seek to achieve an overall opportunity cost across the system while accounting for individual constraints and preferences. More generally, if a centralized planner determines all the actions within the system, then the planner seeks to attain a minimal overall opportunity cost across all communities to achieve a system-wide objective,

$$\sum_{s=1}^{S} \sum_{p=1}^{P} \sum_{j=1}^{J} f(\theta_{s,p,j}).$$

Alternatively, individuals can make decisions to optimize local objectives, but the choices of users of the healthcare system impact the entire system. Obtaining individual choices in a decentralized way is computationally challenging, especially if allowing for the flexibility that not everyone in a sub-population within a community visits the same providers (Heier Stamm 2010). The centralized modeling approach, while not "optimizing" at the individual/local level, can account for constraints and preferences of the individuals thus getting a personalized or individually tailored decision, not necessarily being the most optimal one if there would be no consideration of the overall system cost. Thus, in this book, I will primarily focus on approaches to measure access assuming that an individual will only make his/her "best" decision in the context of the overall system costs and constraints as well as his/her preferences. Note that the overarching goal is to estimate potential access and thus these considerations are appropriate in public health decision making under limited resources.

The constraints and preferences given an access objective can be specified based on knowledge about the healthcare system, such as the maximum number of patients or visits (called *caseload* herein) a provider can have within a time period (e.g. a month); whether a provider accepts a specific health insurance plan (e.g. public insurance); availability of transportation means to the population seeking care; a maximum willingness to travel to reach a provider for healthcare (e.g. as assumed by access standards); and whether licensed mid-level providers can provide services without supervision among many others.

Model Specifications: Overview of Existing Approaches

The framework in the previous section can be used to obtain estimates of the *access opportunity parameters*, $\theta_{s,p,j}$, defined for all communities $s = 1, \ldots, S$, sub-populations $p = 1, \ldots, P$ across the set of providers $j = 1, \ldots, J$. The estimated access opportunity parameters are denoted herein by $\hat{\theta}_{s,p,j}$, to distinguish between true and estimated parameters. I will highlight that we *do not know the true access opportunity parameters*; specifically, we do not know the proportion of a sub-population within a community with potential access to a given provider since this depends on many factors, some of them known and some unknown, some of them deterministic and some uncertain/variable.

In the spirit of statistical modeling, I will note that I called $\theta_{s,p,j}$'s parameters. Statistically speaking, parameters are unknown numerical or categorical summaries, characterizing a given population, and are assumed unknown but they can be estimated using a (mathematical or statistical) model mimicking how a sub-population accesses the healthcare system, where the model is informed by data. The output of such a model consists of the so called *estimated parameters*, or, simply, *estimators*. This characterization is at the core of statistical estimation and modeling.

Figure 2.3 presents the general approach to measuring access. As illustrated in this figure, we first begin with input data on supply, demand, and system constraints; the mathematical model used to estimate the opportunity access parameters is a function of the input data and thus the estimated parameters are functions of the input data as well. Furthermore, the access measures are informed by both the estimated parameters and the additional input data. While most models are not introduced within this estimation framework, all access measurement models fall under this framework.

Given a community s and sub-population p, the parameters are only defined (non-zero if they represent percentages of accessing a provider) for a small subset of providers; realistically, a sub-population of a community does not have access to all providers in the system because of various constraints. Thus, while we have a total of $S \times P \times J$ total parameters, because an individual or sub-population can access only a small number of providers, the number of non-zero parameters is much smaller – only the non-zero parameters need to be estimated.

Furthermore, the access measures expressed as access opportunity costs depend on the access opportunity parameters; because these parameters are unknown we need to replace them with their estimates. Thus, the access measures are functions of the estimated parameters, $\widehat{\theta}_{s,p,j}$; the access opportunity parameters need to be estimated to derive the access measures. Thus, the next questions are: *How to estimate these parameters?* and *What kind of data can we use for the estimation?*

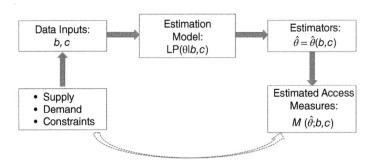

FIGURE 2.3   General approach to measuring access.

I will not distill the entire literature on estimation of such parameters, rather I will focus on: Choice Models, Survey-based Estimates, Gravity Models, and Optimization Models.

Choice Models A first approach is modeling an individual's choices of providers to estimate the opportunity access parameters using discrete choice models (Ben-akiva and Lerman 1985; Train 2009). These models capture an individual's selection from a discrete set of alternatives; in the context of healthcare access, alternatives are the available providers, if any. In healthcare, choice models have been widely used in eliciting preferences about treatments (Ryan and Farrar 2000; Lancsar and Louviere 2008; de Bekker-Grob et al. 2012), but also in specifying patient's choice in receiving healthcare services (Gerard et al. 2004; Porteous et al. 2006; Ahmed and Fincham 2010; Philips et al. 2012). The model statistically relates choices to the attributes of a person (e.g. income) and the attributes of the locations (e.g. distance or quality). It can also be used to forecast choices when there are changes in the system. The general model is a multinomial logit model, where each choice or provider is selected with a probability given individual or sub-population characteristics or other predictors. The higher the probability is, the higher the likelihood to select a provider is. For such models, the parameter $\theta_{s,p,j}$ can be a binary decision, whether to select a provider or not, or the probability of selecting a provider. The choice models provide estimates for the parameter $\theta_{s,p,j}$'s.

However, there is one outstanding challenge in employing the choice models. In order to train a choice model to produce the probabilities of a provider selection given predicting factors, we need extensive data on selecting among tens of thousands of potential providers. Such data are infeasible to acquire unless the model is used to simply characterize general selection criteria for preferred provider type, e.g. primary vs specialized care, physician vs mid-level licensed provider; for willingness to travel (e.g. maximum distance or time to a provider to deem accessible); among others. In this case, the selection criteria can specify constraints and preferences as defined in the general model but it does not directly provide estimates for the opportunity access parameters. Further modeling is needed to obtain these estimates.

Survey-Based Estimates Another widely used approach to estimating opportunity access parameters is based on population surveys, for example, Health Information National Trends Survey (HINTS), National Ambulatory Medical Care Survey (NAMCS), National Health Interview Survey (NHIS), Medical Expenditure Panel Survey (MEPS), or more generally, surveys or data acquisitions by US Census Bureau data, the Centers for Disease Control and Prevention (CDC) or other organizations. Data on healthcare delivery and access have been acquired by many organizations, for example, Centers for Medicare and Medicaid Services (CMS), Agency for Healthcare Research and Quality (AHRQ), Health Resources and Services Administration (HRSA), National Institutes of Health (NIH), Commonwealth Fund, and Kaiser Family Foundation. Such datasets are rich in information, and some provide direct access estimates for some of the access dimensions. However, many such estimates are not provided at a granular level, for example, at the community level or varying by sub-populations. They also capture limited information about access, for example, the percentage of uninsured population or the percentage of those insured by Medicaid. These estimates can inform the models for the supply of healthcare services and the need or demand for the services, however further modeling is needed to capture access as a multidimensional construct. I will illustrate the applicability of such extensive data in many case studies in this book.

Gravity Models Many modeling approaches have been developed for measures of potential spatial access. The two approaches that have dominated the existing research on spatial access are *simple measures* such as distance to nearest service and population-to-provider ratios (Talen and Anselin 1998) and *gravity modeling measures* with the floating catchment area method being the most recent adaptation (Luo and Qi 2009; Wan et al. 2012; Delamater 2013). The two-step floating catchment area (2SFCA) method captures the interaction between two dimensions of access: availability and accessibility (Guagliardo 2004). The catchment methods, which are gravity models of attractions between populations and providers, esti- mate the size of populations served at each provider by using distance zones and estimating accessibility of a community based on the availability of providers in the community's zones. My collaborators and I have recently demonstrated analytically that 2SFCA methods generally overestimate spatial access (Li et al. 2015). Moreover, because selecting a provider depends not only on the travel distance but also whether the provider is too congested (e.g. long wait times or not taking new patients), the 2SFCA methods do not capture cascading effects in the system (Li et al. 2015). In the next section, I will expand more on the 2SFCA methods, with comparison to math- ematical models that provide a mechanism to estimate patient–provider matching, mimicking patient's decision making and considering the system as a whole.

Optimization Models My collaborators and I have developed more advanced methodology for measuring access to healthcare to address some of the limitations of the existing access models (Nobles et al. 2014; Garcia et al. 2015; Gentili et al. 2015, 2018; Harati et al. 2016; Cao et al. 2017; Heir et al. 2017). The model- ing approach is a mathematical optimization model for matching need/demand and supply for particular healthcare services (e.g. preventive dental care). The optimization-based access models capture system effects due to changes based on the wait time or congestion at the provider level. Overall, the optimization models can incorporate many more aspects of access than traditional catchment methods (Li et al. 2015).

Spatial Access Modeling: Overview of Existing Approaches

In this section, I will illustrate the general model described in the previous section for a particular example, measuring spatial access(ibility). As defined before, *spa- tial access* refers to accessibility and availability together (Guagliardo 2004; Wang and Luo 2005; Ansari 2007; McGrail and Humphreys 2009). *Availability* is defined as the opportunity patients have to choose among different providers of healthcare services, varying in the service quality and patient accommodation. *Accessibility* is defined as the time and/or distance barriers that patients experience in reaching their providers. Spatial access is particularly relevant when addressing healthcare disparities for underserved populations such as those with public insurance in the United States because of the reduced network of providers participating in public insurance programs due to low reimbursement rates and the burden of the required paperwork (Berman et al. 1991; Perloff et al. 1995; Berman et al. 2002).

To estimate spatial access, I will consider the definition of access as the *fit between the population's need for healthcare services and the supply of services by healthcare providers* defined by Penchansky and Thomas (1981). Thus potential access is derived from overlaying the networks of need and supply of healthcare services, measuring the opportunity of entry into the healthcare system. The proposed model estimates potential access while accounting for access facilitators and barriers through model constraints, incorporating the trade-offs in the system, supply constraints and potential users' preferences. The proposed access model matches supply of and need for services by incorporating information about the supply of services, need and the overall system.

Since the focus is on modeling spatial access, I will introduce other useful notation:

- Travel distance or time d_{sj} between sth community and jth provider, computed using Geographic Information Systems (GISs) to reflect more realistic traveling routes. It can be expressed in miles for travel distance or in minutes for travel time.

- Caseload $C_{j,p}$ for the jth provider and pth subpopulation, which can be defined by the number of providers at the same location, or the maximum number of patients or visits for the pth subpopulation served by the jth provider within a set amount of time, e.g. year.

- $f_{s,p}$ the potential need or demand for care for the pth sub-population in the sth community, which can be defined by the number of patients/individuals in need of healthcare, or the number of healthcare visits the sub-population needs over a predetermined length of time, e.g. year.

I will begin with some simple spatial access approaches for estimating spatial access, divided into accessibility and availability measures.

Accessibility Measures

Nearest service: $D_s^M = min\{d_{sj}, j = 1, \ldots, J\}$, being the same for all sub-populations. In this case the estimated opportunity parameters $\widehat{\theta}_{s,p,j} = \widehat{\theta}_{s,j}$ are equal to 1 for the closest provider and 0 otherwise. Thus, we can write the measure in terms of these parameters, $D_s^M = \sum_{j=1}^{J} \widehat{\theta}_{s,j} d_{sj}$.

Average nearest distance: $D_s^A = \frac{1}{\#[j \in D_s]} \sum_{j \in D_s} d_{sj}$ where D_s is the travel zone of the sth community. In this case the estimated opportunity parameters $\widehat{\theta}_{s,p,j} = \widehat{\theta}_{s,j}$ are equal to 1 for all providers within the travel zone and 0 otherwise. Thus, we can write the measure in terms of these parameters, $D_s^M = \frac{1}{\#[\theta_{sj} \neq 0]} \sum_{j=1}^{J} \hat{\theta}_{s,j}\, d_{sj}$.

In the accessibility measures above, the opportunity access parameters take binary values only, specifying that the *entire* population in need for service in a community is *matched* or *assigned* to one provider (in the first measure), or one of those providers within a specific distance (the second measure) regardless of whether the provider has sufficient caseload, whether the provider accepts all types of health insurance programs and/or serves all sub-populations. The opportunity access parameters are selected to minimize or optimize travel distance/time only, without accounting for constraints or preferences.

Availability Measures

Container index: $A_{s,p}^M = \sum_{j=1}^{J} C_{j,p} I(d_{sj} \leq T)$ where T is some distance threshold; it defines the total caseload for the pth subpopulation within a given distance (e.g. T) from the community. The estimated opportunity parameter $\hat{\theta}_{s,p,j}$ is then equal to $C_{j,p}$ for all jth providers within distance T or 0 otherwise. It can be further expressed as $A_{s,p}^M = \sum_{j=1}^{J} \hat{\theta}_{s,p,j}$.

Provider-to-patient ratio: $A_{s,p}^R = \sum_{j=1}^{J} \frac{C_{j,p} I(d_{sj} \leq T)}{f_{s,p}}$ defining the ratio between the caseload, or supply of and need for care for the pth subpopulation in the sth community. The estimated opportunity parameter $\hat{\theta}_{s,p,j}$ is then equal to $C_{j,p}$ for all jth providers within distance T or 0 otherwise. It can be further expressed as $A_{s,p}^R = \sum_{j=1}^{J} \hat{\theta}_{s,p,j}/f_{s,p}$.

In the availability measures above, the opportunity access parameters specify that the population in need for service in a community is *matched* or *assigned* to providers within a given catchment area in proportion to the caseload of the providers. Thus, it is assumed that the population seeks care only at these providers, and that their willingness to travel to the providers within the catchment area is the same as long as it is smaller than a given threshold T. The opportunity access parameters are selected to minimize or optimize congestion at the provider level (e.g. wait time) only, without accounting for constraints or preferences on travel time/distance and on various other aspects.

These simpler methods tend to over-estimate or under-estimate spatial access depending on the service for which access is estimated, depending on the density of the service network and the density of the population. Not accounting for demand will simply misrepresent locations with high demand and low density, or low demand and high density of the services sought. For example, in areas with high density of senior population (e.g. large communities in Florida), pediatric practitioners will not be in high demand. A model that accounts for distance only may estimate that these areas will have low access to pediatricians although the need for such services would be sporadic. On the other hand, in many states, large pediatric populations rely on Medicaid insurance system; not accounting for lack of practitioners' participation in Medicaid will definitely over-estimate access in these areas, when in fact they generally have low access.

To address some of these limitations, another stream of spatial access measures has been based on the gravity model, which is perhaps the most widely used model of spatial interaction, similarly to the interaction between objects in Newtonian physics. The "force of attraction" between an individual's location and a service provider is proportional to the attractiveness of the provider and its service, and inversely proportional to the square of the distance between them (Talen and Anselin 1998).

Recent gravity-based models account both for individuals' decreasing willingness to travel as distances increase, and for the interaction between distance traveled and number of people at a facility (also called *congestion* in this book). Most criticism of the gravity model has concentrated on the difficulty in specifying the distance-decay function, a measure of the willingness to travel, most often resulting in an overemphasis of the decay function leading to heavily spatially smoothed access estimate (Joseph and Phillips 1984; Guagliardo 2004). Willingness to travel is not uniform across healthcare services.

One common gravity-based accessibility measure defined for the sth community is

$$A_s = \sum_{j=1}^{J} \frac{C_j d_{sj}^{-\beta}}{\sum_{l=1}^{S} f_l d_{lj}^{-\beta}} \tag{2.1}$$

where β is a disutility coefficient, which defines the decay of willingness to travel and it can be estimated using physician–patient interaction data, although in most research, it is assumed that $\beta = 2$. In this formulation, I suppressed the index corresponding to the subpopulations in $C_{j,p}$ and $f_{s,p}$ to be consistent with the initial formulation of the gravity-based accessibility measure.

The 2SFCA is a descendant of the gravity-based accessibility measure above and it consists of two steps. In the first step, the inverse congestion or service availability (e.g. physician-to-population ratio) at each provider is estimated. In the second step, the accessibility measure is computed as the sum of service availability or congestion-weighted travel cost over all providers within a few miles away from a community. One of the most recent 2SFCA methods is by Luo and Qi (2009), so called Enhanced 2SFCA (E2SFCA), which suggests estimating accessibility by applying weights to differentiate travel time zones, in both the first step and the second step, thereby accounting for distance decay.

In the E2SFCA method, the first step estimates the availability of the service or the physician-to-population ratio at each provider. With the modification that the need/demand may take other forms than the number of patients as defined in the 2SFCA methods, the provider adjusted caseload divided by the need in the region is defined by

$$R_j = \frac{C_j}{\sum_{s \in \{d_{sj} \in D_{1j}\}} f_s w_1 + \sum_{s \in \{d_{sj} \in D_{2j}\}} f_s w_2 + \sum_{s \in \{d_{sj} \in D_{3j}\}} f_s w_3} \tag{2.2}$$

where D_{1j}, D_{2j}, and D_{3j} are catchment areas for the jth provider defining the travel zones within, for example, 5, 10, and 15 miles from the provider's location; and

w_1, w_2, and w_3 are weights calculated from a symmetric statistical distribution (e.g. Normal distribution), capturing the willingness (or lack of it) to travel for accessing the service of interest, for example, $w_r = e^{-d_r}$ where d_r is the rth travel zone radius.

The interpretation of the adjusted caseload R_j of the jth provider is as follows: Only the population or the need for a service within the three catchment areas will be matched to the jth provider. Moreover, not all that need will be assigned to the jth provider; $w_1 \times 100\%$ of the need within the 1st catchment area, $w_2 \times 100\%$ of the need within 2nd catchment area and $w_3 \times 100\%$ of the need within 3rd catchment area will be assigned to the jth provider. Thus, the opportunity cost parameters can be defined as follows:

$$\begin{cases} \hat{\theta}_{s,p,j} = w_1 f_s, if\, d_{sj} \in D_{1j} \\ \hat{\theta}_{s,p,j} = w_2 f_s, if\, d_{sj} \in, D_{2j} \\ \hat{\theta}_{s,p,j} = w_3 f_s, if\, d_{sj} \in D_{3j} \\ 0\ \text{otherwise.} \end{cases}$$

Based on this availability ratio estimates, the spatial access measure is computed as follows:

$$A_s = \sum_{j \in \{d_{sj} \in D_{1s}\}} R_j w_1 + \sum_{j \in \{d_{sj} \in D_{2s}\}} R_j w_2 + \sum_{j \in \{d_{sj} \in D_{3s}\}} R_j w_3 \qquad (2.3)$$

where D_{1i}, D_{2i}, and D_{3i} are catchment areas for the ith community; and R_j is computed as in Eq. (2.2). The formulations in (2.2) and (2.3) can be extended to more than three catchment areas. Note that the access measure is a function of the estimated opportunity access parameters through the weights w_1, w_2, and w_3; and through R_j's, which depend on the weights.

The gravity models as well as the 2SFCA approaches are more challenging to understand within the general modeling framework provided in the previous section. For that, I will illustrate with one particular simple example. I will consider the simplest supply network consisting of n communities in a circular population area with a facility at the center. Let d_s be the distance from community s to a facility and C the number of physicians in the facility. For this system, the matching of the need of services to providers is equivalent to matching need and supply *by shortest distance*. Thus for the simplest system, the 2SFCA method reduces to a simple accessibility measure. For other systems, the method doesn't have a simple mapping to other existing methodologies.

There are a number of variations of the more "traditional" catchment methods. A notable one is the 3SFCA (Wan et al. 2012), which incorporates competitions between multiple providers within the same catchment of a patient and makes assignments of patients by distance. The method by Delamater (2013) modifies the patient level accessibility in (2.3) by multiplying the distance weight twice, while another approach by Mao and Nekorchuk (2013) allows for zones to differ by transportation modes.

My collaborators and I have expanded on some of the limitations of 2SFCA models analytically (Li et al. 2015). I will re-state three of the results here.

Result 1: The total number of visits implied by the 2SFCA catchment methods is overestimated based on the population size, particularly when there are facilities with overlapping catchment zones, commonly in densely populated areas.

Result 2: The 2SFCA methods fail to capture the cascading effects due to lack of availability experienced by those in need at the provider level, where a change in availability for one population leads to different decisions and thus impacts individuals in another location.

Result 3: The composite measures of the 2SFCA are insufficient to distinguish among multiple dimensions of access, such as travel distance/time by patients, congestion at facilities (e.g., visits per physician), congestion or lack of availability experienced by patients, and coverage over an area (how much demand can be met relative to the need).

The analytical proofs along with more specific simple examples of these results are provided in Li et al. 2015.

Spatial Access Modeling: Optimization Approach

Optimization is a mathematical science that is widely accepted in engineering and science, providing a way to account for complex interactions across a system, and it has been applied to many areas including healthcare, transportation, and manufacturing (Barnhart and Laporte 2007; Dempe 2013). In this section, I will demonstrate how optimization models can measure spatial access, on what types of networks they offer the most improvement, and ultimately why they should be used for measuring and improving access.

The three main components of optimization models are (i) the decisions being considered, (ii) the constraints that limit the decisions, and (iii) the criteria that make some decisions better than others (Rardin 1997). Solving an optimization problem returns the decision variables that maximize or minimize the objective function (or performance criteria) under a series of constraints, and the value of the objective function associated with the decision variables. In healthcare, optimization models have been used to determine the best location for a new clinic (Schweikhart and Smithdaniels 1993; Daskin and Dean 2004; Griffin et al. 2008), to ensure that ambulance locations are sufficient to cover the need across a network (Brotcorne et al. 2003), to route nurses for home health services (Begur et al. 1997), and to evaluate policies for pandemic influenza over a network (Ekici et al. 2013), among other examples. Wang (2012) reviewed several examples in which optimization models could be used to improve access or service over a network.

In the formulation of the general access model presented in the previous section, the decisions being considered are the opportunity access parameters and the criteria to make such decisions specify the opportunity cost across the system. The constraints that limit the decisions are not only access constraints or barriers but also preferences in selecting a provider over another.

The decisions or the opportunity access parameters, defined by $\theta_{s,p,j}$ for all locations $s = 1, \ldots, S$, all sub-populations $p = 1, \ldots, P$, and all providers $j = 1, \ldots, J$, reflect an individual's or a sub-population's decision to potentially use a provider or not. These decisions can be in turn used to define multiple access measures. However, the decisions are unknown since we measure potential access, which is not observed. Thus, the decisions or the opportunity access parameters need to be estimated. The estimation approach in this section is using an optimization model, which provides a fit of the need/demand (sub-populations seeking healthcare) and supply (healthcare providers) through an optimal matching. The *matching*, also called *assignment* in the optimization nomenclature, consists of the optimal decisions or the estimated opportunity access parameters. Figure 2.4 illustrates the access measurement modeling using a simple example. Access is measured based on "matching" need/demand locations (e.g. demand centroids in census tracts) with supply locations (e.g. individual healthcare providers). In this example, the parameters $\theta_{s,p,j}$ are $\theta_{sj,1}$ and $\theta_{sj,2}$ with $s = 1, \ldots, 5$ communities and $j = 1, \ldots, 3$ providers. Not all sub-populations and communities have access to the network of the three providers thus some parameters are zero and not included in the network matching because of system constraints.

Constraints in the model reflect individuals' and providers' trade-offs and behaviors. From the perspective of the sub-population potentially accessing healthcare, constraints ensure that the sub-population is assigned to healthcare providers by taking into account the obstacles that it encounters when choosing a provider (e.g. travel time, transportation, co-payment). Individuals or sub-populations may also have preferences, for example, the preference of a particular provider type if available and accessible. From the perspective of the provider, constraints are primarily related to their caseload devoted to a particular sub-population (e.g. child population); their level of accommodation of the patient population (e.g. after hour care), and their participation in various health insurance programs (e.g. public insurance).

The output of the model consists of the optimal matching of demand/need and supply in the healthcare network, or the estimated opportunity access parameters, $\widehat{\theta}_{s,p,j}$, for all locations $s = 1, \ldots, S$; all sub-populations $p = 1, \ldots, P$ and all providers

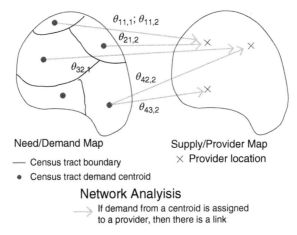

FIGURE 2.4   Access model illustration: a matching between demand and supply locations.

$j = 1, \ldots, J$. To be noted, the demand for care within a community may be assigned to different providers and/or a proportion of the demand may not be served. Hence the model provides estimates of the *served demand*. The difference between the needed and served demand in turn provides *the supply shortage* or *unmet need*, describing patients' (in)ability to find providers who will serve them. Furthermore, multiple availability and accessibility measures can be derived directly from the estimated opportunity access parameters as described below. *Accessibility* can be quantified as the average distance an individual in a community must travel for each visit to his/her matched healthcare provider, thus smaller values of the measure indicate better accessibility. *Availability* is quantified by the congestion a child experiences for each visit at his/her matched provider, where patient congestion is measured as the ratio between all assigned visits to a provider and his/her maximum caseload; thus smaller values indicate better availability. Specific formulae for deriving accessibility and availability as defined above are provided in my collaborative research papers (Harati et al. 2016; Cao et al. 2017; Gentili et al. 2018).

The model is general and can be applied widely to different types of care, different states, and different countries. The methodology is particularly relevant for deriving local estimates because it employs a system approach. The approach characterizes spatial access assuming that not all patients are covered or served by the system of care because of their lack of access in all its forms, and it can separately provide estimates of spatial access for those served by private and public insurance, and/or by age group while accounting for their competition on available resources. It can incorporate timely information specified in the on-going state and national health policy, it can consider all options of care for specific services, with potential preferences, for example, depending on the provider type and patient age, and it can account for a patient's trade-off between accessibility (measured by distance traveled) and availability (measured by congestion at the provider or wait time). Overall, it can integrate contextual information on access, for example, including health organization and provider-related factors as well as community characteristics as suggested by Andersen et al.'s behavioral model (Andersen 1995; Andersen and Davidson 2007).

The modeling approach is data "rich," mathematically rigorous, and computationally scalable, integrating large data and health policy in a systematic manner. As more data become available, the approach has the potential to provide even more specific information to target community-based or state-specific interventions.

Spatial Access Modeling: Data Analytics

A major challenge in access modeling is the extent of data needed to inform the models. The data are divided into: (i) supply; (ii) need/demand; (iii) geographic information; and (iv) constraints and preferences.

One very useful source of data for detailed information on the supply of healthcare services is the National Plan and Provider Enumeration System (NPPES), which includes provider-level information on their unique National Provider Index (NPI) used for reimbursement, their business practice addresses, the taxonomy of their type of services provided, and whether a sole or group provider, specified by the entity field, among other data elements. The NPI coding system was created because the Health Insurance Portability and Accountability Act (HIPAA) of 1996 required a unique healthcare provider identifier to facilitate electronic transmission of claims and other healthcare information. Hence, the NPI of a provider delivering healthcare should be used in every billing claim. Thus, these data provide a snapshot of the entire landscape of healthcare providers reimbursed for their services; however, they do not include information about the mid-level licensed providers working under the supervision of physicians or dentists, thus not directly reimbursed. Another limitation of this dataset is that some providers may practice from different offices, while only the business address is provided with the provider's NPI. Other sources of data on provider census are available (Health Resources and Services Administration April 2013b); however, they particularly target specific types of care and/or are aggregated within specific geographic units, for example, county; they also are not all publicly available. The state boards of physicians and of dentists generally keep a census of the healthcare providers; however, such data are not readily available and/or are not easy to link to medical administrative data, which include information on the NPI providers delivering the healthcare services.

In my research, I used the NPPES data because they are granular (at the provider level), with very detailed information about the providers, and comprehensive across all types of care. Generally, as a provider changes its location and/or other fields in the data, if the provider submits this information to the NPPES, then it is updated immediately. However, providers do not make revisions to their NPI data as soon as they come up and thus there are inconsistencies in the reporting. Moreover, if data are linked to census data, survey data, administrative medical claims and/or electronic health records, then the year of the NPPES data needs to match the year of the additional data to be linked with; NPPES is only available in its more recent form.

Information on the location and taxonomy of the providers is necessary but not sufficient to fully specify supply of healthcare. Providers have different caseloads allocated for specific services (e.g. preventive vs specialized) and/or sub-populations (e.g. children vs adults). Other sources of data can be used to specify the provider-level caseload including the NAMCS (National Center for Health Statistics 2015), administrative claims, or other data sources (Altschuler et al. 2012).

The second data element informing access models is the specification of need or demand for healthcare services. To begin, I will highlight the importance of distinguishing between need and demand for healthcare services. In health economics, *need* is referred as necessity and *demand* as the willingness to operationalize on the need. In my research, I refer to need of healthcare as established by recommended care practices; for example, asthma care guidelines state that children with well-controlled asthma should have a minimum of two visits per year for maintenance of their asthma management plan, and children with more severe or uncontrolled asthma should go to a physician up to twice a month until their asthma is considered to be well-controlled (National Asthma Education and Prevention Program 2007). Demand is actual utilization of healthcare services given the need of care, which can be lower or higher than the need established by the recommended care practices. Demand is often specified by the level of utilization of services observed in the overall population. For example, the average number of asthma visits across all children with asthma in state Medicaid programs over 10 states is about two visits per year, which can be viewed as the demand for asthma care in the pediatric Medicaid population (Garcia 2017). Thus when estimating access, it is important to first establish whether need or demand are considered in the estimation approach. This can have implications in policy making, particularly in the context of the trade-off among the 3 E's (equity, effectiveness, and efficiency).

For both need and demand, demographics data on sub-populations at high geographic granularity are first used to identify the number of potential individuals in need of care within a specific sub-population. The primary data source for demographics is the Bureau Census or the American Community Survey in the United States. For most studies, the need and demand is simply based on the population size or number of patients without consideration of how much healthcare they may need and whether there are differences between sub-populations. For example, care guidelines commonly recommend different levels of care depending on the health risk and/or the severity of a condition. Moreover, there would also be different recommendations by age groups. Such differences may have implications in the specification of need or demand, particularly in areas with higher Medicare and/or Medicaid populations. Data sources used to specify the level of healthcare by need or demand of sub-populations are recommended care guidelines by national associations, surveys on the utilization of healthcare services, or administrative claims data, among others.

The GIS specifies the location of each provider and of each need centroid along with travel distance or travel time between each supply provider and need centroid. As mentioned earlier, the NPPES database includes the practice address which can be geocoded to obtain exact latitude and longitude of the provider's location. Need centroids are commonly specified depending on the division of the geographic space, for example, census tract or block in the census data for the United States. The assumption is that most of the population within one small area of the division is located in the proximity of the centroid; this assumption would be greatly violated if the division of the geographic space is coarse. Further, need centroids are also geocoded so that travel distance or time between the geolocated locations of the supply and need are computed using GIS. In my research, I commonly use the Texas A&M Geocoding Services and the census.gov geocoding services to geocode or derive the latitude and longitude of an address, and the ArcGIS Network Analyst to compute the street-network distances.

Data on supply and need networks along with geographic information for the two networks are commonly integrated in spatial access models; however, many existing models do not incorporate data on the constraints and preferences. I will highlight below two sources of constraints and one source of preferences that can have a significant impact on the accuracy of the access estimates.

Exact location of the providers is useful but it only specifies where providers are located, not whether they provide care for specific sub-populations or health insurance plans, or whether they have a full time or part time caseload, among other specifications of their caseload for healthcare for various sub-populations. Such specifications or caseload constraints require using additional data sources, including

HRSA Bureau of Health Professions, National Center for Health Workforce Analysis (Health Resources and Services Administration 2013a) and Organization for Economic Co-operation and Development (OECD)'s Health Care Resources, for example. Medical claims data such as those available from the CMS can also provide provider-level information on the realized caseload for different sub-populations and services. But realized caseload is not potential caseload; excess caseload may be added and/or some level of uncertainty into the caseload may be considered. Some access denominations assume a pre-specified caseload, for example, the HRSA assumes a provider per-1000-population ratio as one criterion to define medically underserved areas (MUAs). Generally, obtaining provider-level caseload estimates is one of the challenging aspects in estimating access; because of this, few studies incorporate such information in the access estimates although it can impact the accuracy of the access estimates greatly, with implication in deriving policies and interventions (Serban and Tomar 2018; Serban et al. 2019).

One illustration of differencing provider caseload by sub-populations is for private and public insurance health plans. In the United States, Medicaid and the Children's Health Insurance Program (CHIP) are social healthcare programs for families and individuals with low income and limited resources. They constitute the primary sources of coverage for low-income children in the United States. Several requirements need to be met to be eligible in the programs, including total family income which cannot be greater than a fixed threshold. Despite these benefits, children and adults enrolled in these programs have had lower access to healthcare services because not all providers are willing to participate in these programs (Berman et al. 1991, 2002; Perloff et al. 1995; Sebelius 2011). But information on which providers participate in these programs are not readily available. Even when available, such as for dentists accepting public insurance through the InsureKidsNow .gov database, the data may have many inconsistencies and inaccuracies in reporting (Health Policy Institute 2015; Cao et al. 2017). One other potential source of data are administrative claims records; the National Provider indexing was particularly developed for reimbursement and administrative purposes, and thus every provider reimbursed for services for enrollees in specific health insurance programs should have his/her NPI recorded in administrative claims. There may be some limitations however; some providers are reimbursed through a provider group rather as sole providers and thus there will be some potential mis-reporting.

Existing studies show a general preference for physicians with respect to nurse practitioners, but nurse practitioners could be preferred to physicians when the latter are too congested/busy (Freed et al. 2010; Dill et al. 2013). Such information on preferences is not readily available at a granular level, but surveys can provide preferences of provider type as a function of multiple factors, including demographics and socioeconomics. Given the characteristics of a population within a specific small area, one could estimate propensity of preferences for that area using regression models.

The references to the data required for access models in this section are not comprehensive. Data are also specific to the type of services accessed and to the dimensions of access considered. I will expand further on the data analytics for access models in Chapter 6.

CASE STUDY: MEASURING ACCESS TO ASTHMA CARE

Pediatric asthma is one of the most prevalent and costly childhood chronic conditions; Medicaid programs spent more than 272 million dollars on pediatric asthma in 2010 and some southeastern states, such as Georgia, have among the highest expenditures of all states (Pearson et al. 2014; Centers for Disease Control and Prevention 2015). More than 10 million children have had asthma in their lifetime, with 42.9% classified as uncontrolled (Bacharier et al. 2004; Centers for Disease Control and Prevention 2010a). In 2008, children 5–17 years old who had asthma attacks missed 10 million days of school (Akinbami et al. 2011).

The US CDC has identified pediatric asthma as a priority condition for intervention (Centers for Disease Prevention and Control 2015). While asthma is not preventable, the evidence suggests multi-component, multi-trigger (MCMT) approaches can reduce exacerbations and costs associated with pediatric asthma (Community Preventive Services Task Force 2008; Crocker et al. 2011). According to the Community Guide for Preventive Services, one component of the MCMT interventions includes appropriate access to clinical care according to recommended guidelines.

In the case study in this chapter, I will overview the implementation of the general optimization model introduced in the previous section with results on access estimates for pediatric asthma in multiple states. This research is based on a collaborative project with one of the former PhD students, Erin Garcia, in the School of Industrial and Systems Engineering at Georgia Tech (Garcia 2017).

General Model: Notation

For illustration purposes, I will begin with the notation of the general model:

- Geographic division of the need ($s = 1, \ldots, S$): the census tracts for each of the states considered in this study. Census tracts are delineated to be proxies of communities or neighborhoods. The number of communities S varies with each state.

- Grouping the population in need of asthma healthcare ($p = 1, \ldots, P$): the population of children is divided by health insurance access since the sub-populations face different barriers to healthcare; to reflect the sub-populations in further notation, I will use M (Medicaid/CHIP or public insurance) versus O for other health insurance.

- Healthcare providers ($j = 1, \ldots, J$): divided into primary care and asthma specialized care; the primary care providers include Family Medicine physicians, Internal Medicine physicians, General Pediatricians and Nurse Practitioners specializing in pediatrics; the specialized care providers include Allergists and Pulmonologists. I define J^P and J^S the subsets of primary care and specialized care providers, respectively.

- To distinguish between provider types (specialists and primary care) and between those participating in the Medicaid/CHIP versus those who don't, the following types of providers are defined: MD – primary care non-Medicaid, MDM – primary care Medicaid, S – specialist non-Medicaid, SM – specialist Medicaid. Herein J_{type} consists of the four types of providers thus indexing $t \in J_{type}$ to refer to any of the four types.

- Decision or opportunity access parameters: $\theta^M_{s,j}$ and $\theta^O_{s,j}$ the number of patient visits in each census tract s, separated by whether or not they are in the Medicaid system (M for Medicaid/CHIP versus O for other health insurance), that are assigned to each primary or asthma specialist provider j.

The opportunity access parameters were represented by the number of visits rather than the number of patients. This is because when matching supply and demand or need, we took into account that patients do not need the same level of asthma health-care since it depends on the level of severity of the child's asthma condition. Thus, we translated demand/need into number of visits to be matched with the caseload of the healthcare providers, which is often also more accurately measured in number of visits than number of patients.

The decision or opportunity access parameters were further used to derive access measures. However, these parameters are unknown and need to be estimated, as highlighted in the previous sections. In the next section, I will provide the estimation model for the opportunity access parameters and hence the estimation of the access measures.

Access Model: Estimation Approach

I will begin with providing the main model elements: the underlying assumptions, objective function, and model constraints. I will begin with the assumptions at the core of the modeling approach.

A first assumption is that patients prefer to visit nearby and less congested/busy physicians; however, when a provider office has a high patient volume, families prefer physicians farther away and/or mid-level providers. A second assumption is that those with severe asthma need to access a specialist for more targeted healthcare. A third assumption is that the decisions made on which providers to access by those in need for asthma care in one community will affect the decisions made in the communities nearby, thus access for a given sub-population will be similar for nearby communities. These assumptions can be further incorporated into the opportunity cost and/or the access constraints of each community in accessing the network of asthma care providers.

The objective function in the optimization model is specified by the opportunity cost across the communities. When considering the system opportunity cost computed as the aggregate community-level opportunity cost over all communities, another consideration is to "force" similarities in access in neighboring census tracts or communities (Zheng et al. 2018). The objective function shown below in Eq. (2.4) is the sum of the total distance for the matching/fit between supply and need while accounting for the spatial smoothing of access:

$$\sum_{s=1}^{S}\sum_{j=1}^{J}(\theta_{s,j}^{M}+\theta_{s,j}^{O})d_{sj} + \sum_{t\in J_{type}}\sum_{k=1}^{S}\sum_{l=1}^{S}\frac{n_{kl}(d_{k}^{t}-d_{l}^{t})^{2}}{a_{k}^{t}+a_{l}^{t}} \tag{2.4}$$

- The *first term* in the objective function is a weighted sum of travel distances over all communities; thus the overall opportunity cost is in terms of travel distance to care or accessibility. The travel distance in miles from the centroid of census tract s to provider j is defined by d_{sj}.
- The *second term* is a smoothing term, a practical restriction on the system to prevent children in neighboring census tracts to have dramatically different distances to care. Two census tracts are considered to be neighbors ($n_{kl} = 1$ if neighbors and 0 otherwise) if the distance between their centroids is less than 10 miles, for example. The smoothing terms is a weighted sum of the difference in accessibility between neighboring communities (d_{k}^{t} for the tth provider type in the kth census tract), where the weights are provided by the sum of the needed visits for asthma care (a_{k}^{t} for the tth provider type in the kth census tract). We penalize differences in the average distance per visit to a particular provider type between neighboring census tracts. Without this smoothing term, it is possible for the model to assign all of the children in one census tract to one provider and none of the children in a neighboring tract to that same provider, where the more realistic outcome would be that a similar proportion of the children in each tract would visit the provider.

Importantly, the access measure in the smoothing term is a function of the decision or access opportunity parameters since they are obtained as the average travel distance within each community given the fit or match between supply and need. Thus while the first part of the objective function is a linear combination of the decision parameters, the smoothing term makes it (quadratic) nonlinear in the parameters. This has implications in the algorithms used to solve the resulting optimization problem.

While the travel cost is considered here the major determinant of a parent's decision to choose a provider for asthma healthcare of his/her child, there are multiple constraints in the system that restrict one's ability to optimize the travel cost. They are constraints on how the system restricts access to healthcare for pediatric asthma. Below I describe a series of access constraints to be considered for illustration.

- A *first set of constraints* refers to logical constraints, specifically, we cannot serve more demand or need than there is in the system, separately considering the constraints for the Medicaid and non-Medicaid sub-populations and by provider type. These constraints require estimation of the demand for asthma care within each census tract. I will discuss estimation of the demand in the next section.

- A *second set of constraints* refers to caseload of the providers for asthma care. The supply for asthma care may not be sufficient to meet the demand resulting in shortage of supply. These constraints are differentiated by type of provider, whether a provider participated in Medicaid/CHIP and the maximum caseload for the Medicaid-insured children. This later consideration is important since providers limit their caseload devoted to Medicaid programs as I pointed out earlier in this chapter. These constraints require estimation of the caseload for asthma care for each provider location. I will discuss estimation of the supply in the next section.

- The *third constraint* penalizes the opportunity cost if the patients with severe asthma are not seen by specialists. The constraint is: $\sum_{s=1}^{S}(v_s + w_s) < L$. The variables to track the percent of appointments that should ideally be assigned to a specialist but are instead assigned to a primary care provider are defined for non-Medicaid visits (v_s) and for Medicaid visits (w_s) for each census tract s. It is desirable that more severe cases are treated by specialists instead of solely relying on a primary care provider. For this subset of asthmatic children that should receive specialist care, it is possible that they receive some, or all, of their treatment from primary care providers thus we allow for the assignment of these visits to primary care providers with a penalty to account for the preference that the visits be made to a specialist. The penalization depends on the penalty constant L.

- The *fourth constraint* is necessary because there are places where there is insufficient provider caseload to meet the demand and that the overall opportunity cost in the system needs to account for lack of supply in some of the locations. The constraint is: $\sum_{s=1}^{S} \sum_{t \in J_{type}} g_s^t < L_a$, where the variables to track percent of appointments not assigned at all are g_s^t for each census tract s and provider type t. The penalization depends on the penalty constant L_a.

- A *fifth constraint* is that for each census tract, the average distance for visits to a particular provider type for children on Medicaid cannot be lower than the average distance for non-Medicaid children in the same tract. This ensures that we do not assign only the Medicaid patients to one provider when there is insufficient caseload for this sub-population.

I will not provide the formula for all the constraints described above since they are very involved and do not add much to the presentation of the model beyond the description of their meaning. Further descriptions are provided in Dr. Erin Garcia's doctoral thesis (Garcia 2017).

Other constraints can be considered to enforce practical considerations and account for some of the factors that would influence the patient's choice for their provider. An example of constraints I have considered in other access models is related to one's access to means of transportation, for example, personal car. Another example is one's preference of seeking care from a physician rather than a licensed mid-level provider, especially for specialized care such as for pediatric asthma.

Importantly, the constraints described above require input for estimates on demand and supply along with provider participation in Medicaid and a series of pre-specified parameters. Such inputs are challenging to derive, while adding some level of uncertainty in the access measures. Thus careful consideration of what constraints are most important in providing realistic insights about the system is warranted while not undermining the complexity of the healthcare systems. In the next section, I will present the data analytics informing the optimization modeling approach.

Data Sources and Analytics

The states piloted in this study include seven southeastern states: Alabama, Arkansas, Georgia, Louisiana, Mississippi, North Carolina, and Tennessee. The selected states share geographic proximity but vary significantly in implementation of Medicaid/CHIP programs and in population distribution and demographics.

Access models rely on multiple data sources and extensive data analytics to inform estimates of demand and supply and to specify the inputs in the access constraints and preferences. I will briefly illustrate the data analytics involved in the access models for the case study in this section.

Supply Estimation   Access models must provide accurate information about the supply of the healthcare services to be accessed. As mentioned in a previous section of this chapter, supply estimation requires both data for the location and the patient caseload of the healthcare providers and data for their availability to participate in different health insurance plans, incorporated in the model constraints.

The data sources used in this study for estimating supply for pediatric asthma care include the 2012 Medicaid Analytic eXtract (MAX) data files acquired from the CMS, the 2013 NPPES, and publications or reports specifying general information on physician caseloads.

Primary care providers include Pediatricians, Pediatric Nurse Practitioners, and Family Practice or Internal Medicine. Specialist providers include (Pediatric) Allergists and (Pediatric) Pulmonologists. A first step is to identify the corresponding taxonomy codes for these providers; the description for these codes was selected from the website http://www.wpc-edi.com/reference that reports, among other things, the list of Health Care Provider Taxonomy Code Set. A second step is to extract the NPI records from the NPPES database corresponding to the taxonomy codes. Last, the set of NPIs are further matched with the service and billing providers in the MAX claims data identified to have submitted claims with an asthma ICD-9 code (493.X) for reimbursement to the Medicaid programs.

The output of this data analytics step is the set of all potential providers for pediatric asthma healthcare and with the specification whether they participate in Medicaid. Since the NPPES data provide information on the practice business addresses, we also have the exact location of the providers along with their taxonomy. For simplicity, we assumed that if a provider accepts public insurance then he/she will accept any Medicaid patients unless his/her patient caseload is full. This assumption may overestimate access for this sub-population.

Most spatial access models primarily use information about the location of the providers, and only some models use data on full time employment (FTE) as a measure of patient caseload. Importantly, we cannot assume that a provider will dedicate all his/her FTE to only deliver specific healthcare services, such as those services for providing care for pediatric asthma. More specifically, a primary care provider generally dedicates a small portion of his/her caseload to asthma care; moreover, those providers who do not specialize in pediatric healthcare have to divide their effort for caring for both children and adults. Thus, assuming a full caseload dedicated to pediatric asthma care for all providers in the supply network is not realistic.

There are no standard values for what a physician's maximum caseload is because it depends on many factors. Based on the Kaiser Permanente average caseload for primary care and expert opinion, we used a caseload for primary care physicians of 1700 patients per year and for specialists of 1200 patients per year (Weiner 2004; Altschuler et al. 2012; Raffoul et al. 2016). Again for simplicity, we assumed that the percent of the number of visits for pediatric asthma per provider is the same for all children, regardless of whether they are Medicaid or non-Medicaid insured.

To estimate maximum caseload for pediatric asthma, we used the 2012 MAX claims data to derive the percent of the pediatric asthma visits out of the total caseload of each provider, then aggregated by provider type. To account for variations between providers, we added a buffer of 10% caseload to each individual provider's caseload. Last, because pediatric asthma is quite seasonal, we also estimated the supply for each season, by multiplying the available annual visits by the percent of visits for pediatric asthma and the percent of the calendar year in each season.

There are several challenges in the supply estimation, particularly in identifying the potential caseload for pediatric asthma for the two sub-populations. The most noteworthy challenge is that there were providers identified in the MAX data but without an associated NPI. To account for these potentially missing providers, we randomly sampled half of the number of these additional providers from the list of primary care providers and asthma specialists and deemed them as accepting Medicaid. Specialists had varying rates of participation in Medicaid across the states in this study. Thus, for the set of providers without an NPI in the MAX data, the sampling proportion for deeming a provider as participating in Medicaid varied by state.

Demand Estimation   The *demand* is the number of appointments for asthma care demanded for children in each census tract and each season. The study population consisted of children aged 5–17. Children 0–4 are excluded because of the difficulties in obtaining an accurate asthma diagnosis. The number of children in each census tract was obtained from the U.S. Census Bureau (2010).

We divided the population by age group (5–9, 10–14, 15–17) when estimating the demand for pediatric asthma since the asthma prevalence varies by age. We obtained estimates of the number of children with asthma in each census tract by multiplying the number of children in each age group by the asthma prevalence estimates from the Behavioral Risk Factor Surveillance System (BRFSS) (Centers for Disease Control and Prevention 2010). While this provides the population of children with asthma, it does not provide the demand for care, which is specified in number of visits. From the MAX claims data, we identified the Medicaid population with asthma by selecting patients with at least two events with an asthma diagnosis. The resulting Medicaid average of 2.16 asthma visits per year was multiplied by the number of children with asthma in each census tract to obtain the number of asthma visits per tract per year. This is near the lower bound from the asthma care guidelines (National Asthma Education and Prevention Program 2007). We assumed that the average number of asthma visits per year per child is the same for Medicaid and non-Medicaid children. We further computed the percent of Medicaid pediatric asthma visits occurring in the three seasons (fall, spring, summer). These percentages were multiplied by the annual visits per tract to obtain the number of pediatric asthma visits per tract per season. The demand for pediatric asthma visits was further split into demand for primary care and for asthma specialist visits.

Last, we distinguished the demand for Medicaid versus non-Medicaid children. Because we assumed that each child demand was on average the same number of asthma visits, the percent of children with asthma on Medicaid can be assumed to be the percent of visits for asthma care that are demanded by Medicaid patients. For the model input, we then multiplied the number of visits in each tract by the percent of the children with asthma that are on Medicaid in the census tract. This number was subtracted from the total visits needed to give the number of non-Medicaid visits per tract.

Input Data for Model Constraints   There were multiple inputs in the constraints that needed to be specified. The inputs for the model described above were:

- *The percent of children who have a severe asthma and need care from a specialist*: We assumed that 25% of children should be referred to an asthma specialist for care based on the prevalence of severe or uncontrolled asthma (Bacharier et al. 2004; Centers for Disease Control and Prevention 2014) and expert opinion.

- *The penalty constant L specified in the constraint that penalizes the opportunity cost if a child who needs specialist care can only be assigned to a primary care provider*: This constant is meant to "force" children with severe asthma to be assigned to a specialist since they would need more specialized care. To set this value, we assumed that for every non-Medicaid visit that is assigned to a primary care provider instead of a preferred specialist, there is a penalty of 15 miles added to the assignment distance, and for Medicaid patients the penalty is 20 miles. We imposed a higher penalty for Medicaid patients because this population is already underserved and faces greater transportation restrictions, and thus are less likely to be able to travel farther to receive specialist care than non-Medicaid patients. With these penalties, a patient would have no preference between a specialist that is 50 miles and a primary care provider that is 35 miles away.

- *The penalty constant L_a in the constraints that penalizes the opportunity cost for lack of access*: This constant was set to be the largest value at which the optimization is feasible, thus it varies by state. Thus this constant defines the maximum level of access in the system. Note that not all children will have access to primary care and/or specialist.

- *The maximum distance between any two census tracts to deem them "neighbors" in the smoothing penalty*: We set this to be 10 miles. If set too small, then the access measure will not be very smooth. If we set it too high, the access measure will be too smooth.

- *The Medicaid participation of the providers needed in specifying the providers' caseload for the two sub-populations*: The Medicaid participation is binary and it was inferred from the Medicaid claims data. The process of acquiring Medicaid participation was very involved and thus not described here but it was described in detail in the doctoral thesis of Erin Garcia (2017).

- *The maximum willingness to travel to access a provider for asthma healthcare*: Some states have established access standards, specifying the maximum distance Medicaid managed care organizations must secure for their enrollees to access providers. The access standards have been published by the United States Department of Health and Human Services (Murrin 2014). Table 2.1 provides the access standards for three of the states.

Access Measures

In the following, I will use the superscript M to refer to variables related to the Medicaid sub-population and the superscript O to refer to the non-Medicaid sub-population. Three access measures reflecting accessibility and availability dimensions of access are as follows:

1. The *travel distance* measured as the average distance to receive care differentiated by sub-populations:

$$T_s^M = \sum_{j=1}^{J} \hat{\theta}_{sj}^M d_{sj}; T_s^O = \sum_{j=1}^{J} \hat{\theta}_{sj}^O d_{sj}$$

TABLE 2.1   Access Standards for Three States Georgia (GA), Mississippi (MS) and Tennessee (TN) for Urban and Rural Primary and Specialist Healthcare

State	Primary care	Specialist care
GA	Urban: Two providers within 8 miles Rural: Two providers within 15 miles	Urban: One provider within 30 miles Rural: One provider within 45 miles
MS	Urban: Two providers within 30 miles Rural: Two providers within 60 miles	No standard
TN	Urban: One provider within 20 miles Rural: One provider within 30 miles	One provider within 60 miles for 75% of enrollees and one provider within 90 miles for all enrollees

2. The *unmet need for asthma specialists* measured as the percent of visits that are assigned to primary instead of specialist care for treating severe asthma provided by v_s for non-Medicaid visits and w_s for Medicaid visits in the model implementation.

3. The *unmet need* for the overall asthma care measured as the percent of visits that cannot be assigned to a provider within the access standards if provided by the state or using universal access standards, e.g. 30 miles in urban and 45 miles in rural communities, for those states without state-specific access standards. For this we defined the distance thresholds D_u and D_r for urban and rural communities. We also needed additional information on which communities are rural and urban, for example, using the classification based on the rural-urban continuum codes (RUCCs). Differentiating the census tracts by urban and rural, S_u and S_r, then the access measures can be defined as follows:

For urban communities: $s \in S_u : U_s^M = \sum_{j=1}^{J} \widehat{\theta}_{sj}^M I(d_{sj} > D_u)$, $U_s^O = \sum_{j=1}^{J} \widehat{\theta}_{sj}^O I(d_{sj} > D_u)$

For rural communities: $s \in S_r : U_s^M = \sum_{j=1}^{J} \widehat{\theta}_{sj}^M I(d_{sj} > D_r)$, $U_s^O = \sum_{j=1}^{J} \widehat{\theta}_{sj}^O I(d_{sj} > D_r)$

Other access measures can be defined in a similar fashion. The ability to measure multiple dimensions of access is one of the advantages to model potential access using the mathematical assignment models based on optimization as presented in this chapter. Moreover, the model allows for quantifying the impact of interventions by changing various model inputs and estimating the decision or opportunity access parameters given such changes, as I will illustrate in Chapter 5 where I will demonstrate how to design and evaluate interventions using the optimization modeling approach.

Most importantly, all such access measures are functions of the estimated decision parameters $\widehat{\theta}_{sj}^M$ and $\widehat{\theta}_{sj}^O$. The estimated parameters are not true parameters, thus they are derived with some level of error, distinguished between *estimation error* and *modeling error* in statistical terms. The estimation error is due to the uncertainty of the input data. For example, need and supply are estimated based on various data sources. Some of the inputs entering in the constraints also come with some level of uncertainty. The uncertainty level may vary geographically (e.g. urban vs rural communities) and for different sub-populations (e.g. Medicaid vs non-Medicaid). The modeling error comes from the fact that we are using a model to obtain the estimated inputs, which can be reduced if the model captures the potential access appropriately and realistically. Reducing the modeling error is another motivation for developing sophisticated mathematical models to make inferences on access. Decision making on policies and interventions to improve access, and ultimately, outcomes, needs to account for such errors in the estimation of the opportunity parameters as well as of the access measures.

Model Implementation

In this section, I will focus on important considerations in the implementation of the access modeling approach as presented in the previous sections. I will also describe important results derived for this model implementation.

Supply Estimation: Considerations in Estimating Provider Caseload   The percent of visits for pediatric asthma for major classes of providers derived from the MAX data is summarized by provider type in Table 2.2. The percent of the Medicaid caseload for primary care providers for children with asthma is consistently small across all seven states. In Alabama, pediatric pulmonologists have the highest percentage (63.2%) of pediatric asthma patients, followed by non-pediatric allergists and pulmonologists (20% and 25.7%). In Arkansas, the only provider category with more than 7% is for allergists.

These data provide the realized caseload for the Medicaid-insured children with an asthma diagnosis for the corresponding providers. However, this reflects realized not potential caseload. It also captures the caseload for one sub-population only. First, to obtain the caseload together for both the Medicaid and non-Medicaid sub-populations, we assumed the same percent of patients and visits for pediatric asthma for the non-Medicaid patients as for the Medicaid patients. To better reflect potential caseload, a random, non-negative "buffer" caseload was added to the realized caseload and visits. The buffer caseload is based on the empirical distributions of the percent of patients and visits that are used for pediatric asthma among the Medicaid providers. The data for all seven states is combined for this analysis. Among primary care providers, the percent of the caseload and visits for pediatric asthma are very similar across the states, thus combining state-level data

TABLE 2.2   Percent of Visits per Provider in the MAX Claims Files that are Allocated for Pediatric Asthma by State and Provider Type

State/Provider Category	Unknown (%)	PEDIATRICIAN (%)	NP_ PEDIATRIC (%)	FAMILY (%)	INTERNAL (%)	Combined Family and Internal (%)	PULMONOLOGIST (%)	PEDIATRIC_ PULMONOLOGIST (%)	ALLERGIST (%)	PEDIATRIC_ ALLERGIST (%)	Specialist Unknown (%)
AL	1.5	2.4	4.6	1.4	1.9	1.6	25.7	63.2	19.9	—	25.8
AR	0.7	1.3	—	0.5	0.7	0.5	0.2	—	55.1	8.3	7.6
GA	1.0	1.6	2.6	1.2	1.4	1.3	2.6	34.8	14.2	42.6	18.2
LA	0.8	0.75	0.8	0.6	0.6	0.6	0.7	26.5	19.2	1.1	1.3
MS	0.8	1.7	1.9	1.2	1.1	1.2	—	—	—	—	—
NC	0.8	1.1	4.1	0.5	0.7	0.6	0.5	1.2	21.0	10.7	3.5
TN	0.9	1.2	4.5	0.9	0.8	0.9	0.7	17.1	7.5	22.7	5.3

does not have a significant impact on the distributions. While this not the case for specialist providers, all of the states and providers were considered in one sample in order to have a sufficiently large group of providers for the sampling distribution.

Because the sampling distribution for the buffer caseload is bimodal, we considered two distributions for high and low caseload for both the primary and specialized care. Figure 2.5 presents the distribution of the realized caseload for both low and high Medicaid caseload providers.

Supply Estimation: Geographic Variations There is significant geographic variation in the supply of primary and specialist care visits both within each state and between the states as shown in Figure 2.6. The highest concentration of available visits occurs in urban areas, with fewer available in rural areas. As expected, every state has more communities with available primary care visits than communities with available specialist care visits. Arkansas has the lowest percent of communities with available primary care visits (33%) and specialist care visits (5%). Georgia and North Carolina have the highest percent of communities with available primary care visits (59% and 60%), and Georgia, Mississippi and North Carolina have the highest percent of communities with available specialist care visits (14%, 15%, and 15%).

Access Measures: Travel Distance Figure 2.7 presents the maps of the average distance to receive each type of care aggregated at the county level for ease of visualization. Figure 2.8 shows the boxplots of the tract-level travel distance for all seven states and provider types, for the Medicaid and non-Medicaid population. The maps and boxplots are for the fall season; the maps for other seasons are similar since we found that the difference in travel distance among seasons is not statistically significant (p-value <0.05) for most states and provider types.

For all states except Tennessee, the median tract-level distance to primary care for the non-Medicaid population is the lowest, followed by the distance to primary care visits for the Medicaid population, followed by distance to specialist visits for the non-Medicaid population, with the largest distances being to specialist visits for the Medicaid population. The distribution of the tract-level distances to primary care visits are similar across all states, with the differences in distance between the states being higher for primary care visits for the Medicaid population. There is more variation in the distance to asthma specialists than to primary care providers, and the greatest differences between the states occur when considering the driving distance to specialist visits for the Medicaid population.

In all states, the median distance to specialist care is at least twice as high for the Medicaid population as for the non-Medicaid population and the inter-quartile range of the tract-level distance to care is larger for specialist visits for the Medicaid population than for any other type of care.

Access Measures: Unmet Need Table 2.3 provides the number of tracts where all the need for specialist care is met by primary care providers only while lacking access to asthma specialists. In Arkansas, over 20% of the census tracts have all specialist visits served by primary care providers for the Medicaid population, with only 1.3% of the

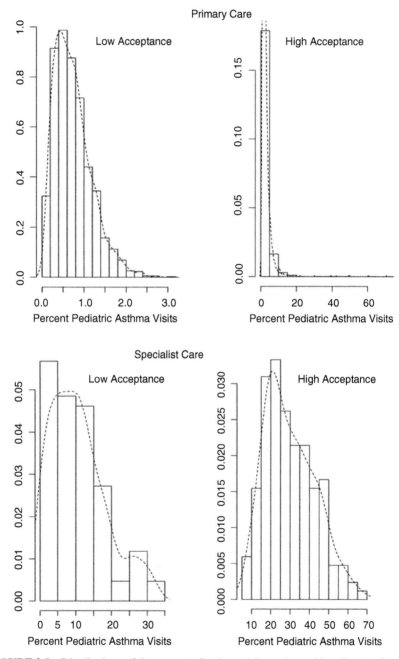

FIGURE 2.5 Distributions of the percent of asthma visits each provider allocates for pediatric asthma by provider type in the Medicaid program.

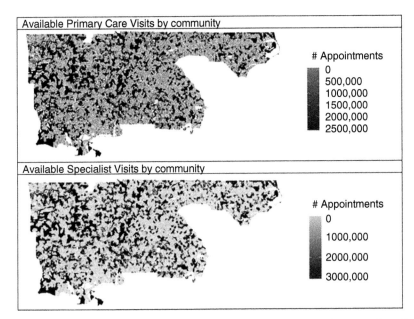

FIGURE 2.6 Number of specialist visits available for primary and specialist care in each zip code. Zip codes that are shown in black have no providers. (a) Available primary care visits by community. (b) Available specialist visits by community. (Note: a community is represented by zip code rather than a census tract due to data availability.)

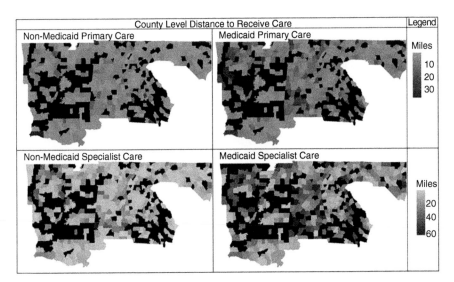

FIGURE 2.7 County level distance for primary and specialist appointments for Medicaid and non-Medicaid patients. Counties shown in black have no met need (the optimization model is unable to assign any visits to providers in these counties).

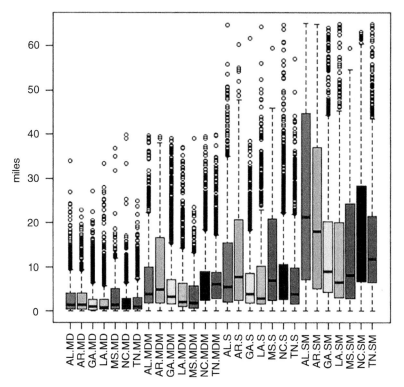

FIGURE 2.8   Distribution of the assigned census tract level distance to primary and asthma specialist care for Medicaid and non-Medicaid patients in each state for the fall season with clearly increasing trend by provider type. Provider type abbreviations: non-Medicaid and Medicaid primary care (MD and MDM); and non-Medicaid and Medicaid specialist care (S and SM).

TABLE 2.3   Number of Census Tracts in Which all Specialist Appointments are Met Instead by Primary Care Providers for Both the Medicaid and Non-Medicaid Population and the Mean Difference and p-values for the Paired t-test Comparing the Tract Level percent of Visits Assigned to Primary (MDM and MD for Medicaid and Non-Medicaid) Instead of Specialist (SM and S for Medicaid and non-Medicaid) Care

State	No. of census tracts	No. of tracts all S visits assigned to MD providers	No. of tracts all SM visits assigned to MDM providers	Mean difference in percent assigned MD/MDM instead of S/SM	p-value
AL	1181	1	138	−0.03873	2.2e-16
AR	686	9	149	−0.04702	2.2e-16
GA	1969	0	10	−0.00743	4.6e-12
LA	1148	7	20	−0.00472	4.9e-07
MS	664	0	0	0.00219	0.00246
NC	2195	4	60	−0.01600	2.2e-16
TN	1497	1	16	−0.00562	8.7e-13

tracts for the non-Medicaid population. In contrast, in Mississippi, there are no such census tracts. The same table also provides the average difference and the p-values for the paired t-tests comparing the percent of specialist visits that have been assigned to primary care visits due to lack of access to specialized care between the Medicaid and non-Medicaid populations. In every state except for Mississippi, the percent of asthma care visits provided by primary care providers that should have been provided by specialist providers due to severity of asthma is significantly higher among the Medicaid than the non-Medicaid population.

Table 2.4 summarizes the unmet need in number of visits by provider type for the seven states. The most substantive result from this table is the difference in the estimated number of unmet number of visits for the Medicaid-insured children versus those with private insurance. Table 2.5 shows a conservative estimate for the unmet need for each state in the fall season for the urban and rural populations. The results for the spring and summer are similar. The unmet need for non-Medicaid visits in rural areas (>5.4%) is the highest in Alabama, Louisiana, and Mississippi. For rural Medicaid children, Tennessee has the highest unmet need of 10.3%. In urban areas, the greatest unmet need, estimated at 2.1%, occurs in Arkansas and Mississippi. Unmet

TABLE 2.4 Unmet Need in Number of Visits by Provider Type in Each State and the Ratio of Unmet Need for Selected Service Types

State	MD	MDM	S	SM	All Medicaid	All non-Medicaid
AL	406	714	524	2494	3208	930
AR	172	960	153	1647	2607	326
GA	133	1309	182	3788	5097	315
LA	107	474	380	2164	2638	488
MS	312	134	831	670	804	1142
NC	365	953	433	3088	4041	798
TN	118	398	334	1640	2038	453

TABLE 2.5 Unmet Need in Each State Reported as the Number and percent of Visits that cannot be Assigned to a Provider within the 30 and 45 miles for Children Living in Rural and Urban Communities, Respectively

State	Rural non-Medicaid		Rural Medicaid		Urban non-Medicaid		Urban Medicaid	
	No.	%	No.	%	No.	%	No.	%
AL	244	5.5	181	8.5	1283	1.8	2629	7.8
AR	225	4.8	275	5.2	341	2.1	1825	10.3
GA	44	0.7	360	4.9	206	0.1	3514	3.2
LA	56	5.4	88	5.6	648	1.9	2711	4.6
MS	141	2.8	73	2.7	1056	2.1	757	3.1
NC	327	5.5	394	8.6	844	1.0	3256	5.2
TN	30	1.7	191	10.3	517	0.8	1648	3.3

need is also worse for the Medicaid population in urban areas, reaching 10.3% in Arkansas. For both urban and rural areas, Georgia has the lowest unmet need for non-Medicaid children, and is second lowest for unmet need for Medicaid visits.

Discussion   Some significant findings from this study are as follows:

- There are more variations in the healthcare supply by specialists, highlighting that the asthma specialist caseload is not dependent on the provider type or number of specialists in a state.
- There are not significant seasonal differences in spatial access to care despite the seasonal variations in demand. This means that where there is access to care, the caseload is large enough to handle the seasonal demand. In areas with unmet need, even during the lower demand seasons, the lower access is primarily driven by the lack of providers rather than the lack of provider availability. These results suggest that seasonal interventions, such as school-based programs, may not be sufficient to provide access to asthma care, and more permanent interventions, such as adding additional asthma specialists to the care network, should be considered.
- The distance traveled for Medicaid specialist visits is significantly higher than the distance for other visits. In some of the states, the average distance to receive Medicaid specialist care is 10+ miles greater than the distance to receive either non-Medicaid specialist care or Medicaid primary care. For the Medicaid population, traveling an additional 10 miles for care may be a greater barrier to receive care than it would be for some of the non-Medicaid population.
- For the non-Medicaid population, the percent unmet need is greater in rural than urban areas. For the Medicaid population, Mississippi has the lowest percent of unmet need in both rural and urban areas, with similar values in Georgia and Tennessee's urban areas. Except for Arkansas and Mississippi, the percent unmet need is greater in rural than urban areas.
- For children in rural areas, the percent unmet need is greater in the Medicaid population than the non-Medicaid population for every state except Mississippi. Because the unmet need for non-Medicaid visits is low, increasing the percent of providers accepting Medicaid in rural areas may be sufficient to reduce unmet need.
- Because the availability of primary care is consistently higher than that of specialist care for both Medicaid and non-Medicaid patients, increasing asthma specific training among primary care providers may be another way to improve health outcomes among children with more severe or uncontrolled asthma. This type of intervention would provide better asthma care for patients without requiring the location of a new provider in the system.
- While the percent unmet need is similar across the seasons, the number of visits that are unmet varies because the number of visits needed in the fall is higher than in other seasons. This inconsistency may interfere with the overall control of a child's asthma. Inadequate care is known to result in worse asthma

outcomes, and in some cases these outcomes may be severe or require more expensive care (The American College of Allergy Asthma and Immunology 2015).

CONCLUSIONS

This chapter has reviewed concepts and methods for measuring healthcare access. There are several take home points:

- I concurred with the existing literature in that defining and measuring access is challenging. Access to care is a multidimensional construct. This warrants policy makers to refer and address access by considering multiple dimensions, for example, going beyond the most commonly cited dimensions in public policy, the financial access.
- I highlighted that we can only obtain estimated access not the "true" access. Multiple data sources need to be used to estimate access; they come with various levels of uncertainty resulting in estimation error in the access estimates.
- I illustrated modeling and estimation of access for two of the dimensions of access, accessibility, and availability referred together as spatial access. I presented several modeling approaches, pointing to limitations of those models. Because access is estimated based on a model, we also have another source of error in its estimation, particularly the modeling error. It is important to understand this error since it can result in biased estimates; for example, gravity-based modeling approaches tend to overestimate access.
- The case study used to illustrate access estimation using a mathematical model also pointed out the complexity of studying access. The modeling approach incorporated many aspects about the system of care that needs to be accessed, including constraints of the system and of the providers as well as preferences of those accessing the system. The modeling approach also made several assumptions; a sensitivity analysis of the model to these assumptions is warranted. Last, there are many data sources used to inform the model toward getting more accurate estimates. For example, we found wide variations in the provider caseload for multiple provider types providing asthma care and across the states considered in the study; appropriately accounting for these variations best inform the level of access estimated at the community level.

ACKNOWLEDGMENTS

The author is thankful to Paul Griffin who reviewed this chapter, providing very useful suggestions to improve the presentation. This chapter draws substantially upon the recent research presented in a doctoral thesis. In this regard, the author gratefully acknowledges the contributions of Erin Garcia and Anne Fitzpatrick who have given their permission to illustrate the concepts and methodologies presented in this chapter using the study from our collaborative work. I also acknowledge the support from the National Heart, Lung, and Blood Institute of the National Institutes of Health under Award Number R56HL126761. The content is solely the responsibility of the authors and does not necessarily represent the official views of the National Institutes of Health. The funding agreements ensured the authors' independence in designing the study, interpreting the data, writing, and publishing the work.

REFERENCES

Academy for Health Services Research and Health Policy (2004). Glossary of Terms Commonly used in Health Care.

Aday, L.A. and Andersen, R.M. (1974). A framework for the study of access to medical care. *Health Services Research* 9: 208–220.

Ahmed, A. and Fincham, J.E. (2010). Physician office vs retail clinic: patient preferences in care seeking for minor illnesses. *Annals of Family Medicine* 8(2): 117–123.

Akinbami, L.J., Moorman, J.E., and Liu, X. (2011). *Asthma Prevalence, Healthcare Use, and Mortality: United States, 2005–2009*. National Center for Health Statistics: Hyattsville, MD.

Altschuler, J., Margolius, D., Bodenheimer, T., and Grumbach, K. (2012). Estimating a reasonable patient panel size for primary care physicians with team-based task delegation. *The Annals of Family Medicine* 10(5): 396–400.

Andersen, R.M. (1968). *Behavioral Model of Families' Use of Health Services*. Chicago, IL: Center for Health Administration Studies, University of Chicago.

Andersen, R.M. (1995). Revisiting the behavioral model and access to medical care: does it matter? *Journal of Health and Social Behavior* 36: 1, 10.

Andersen, R. and Davidson, P. (2007). Improving access to care in America: individual and contextual indicators. In: *Changing the US Healthcare System: Key Issues in Health Services, Policy and Management* (eds. R. Andersen, T. Rice and G. Kominski), 3–32. San Francisco, CA: Wiley.

Ansari, Z. (2007). A review of literature on access to primary health care. *Australian Journal of Primary Health* 13(2): 80–95.

Apparicio, P., Cloutier, M.S., and Shearmur, R. (2007). The case of Montreal's missing food deserts: evaluation of accessibility to food supermarkets. *International Journal of Health Geographics* 6: 4.

Bacharier, L.B., Strunk, R.C., Mauger, D. et al. (2004). Classifying asthma severity in children: mismatch between symptoms, medication use, and lung function. *American Journal of Respiratory and Critical Care Medicine* 170(4): 426–432.

Ball, M.O. and Lin, F.L. (1993). A reliability model applied to emergency service vehicle location. *Operations Research* 41(1): 18–36.

Barnhart, C. and Laporte, G. (eds.) (2007). *Handbooks in Operations Research and Management Science: Transportation*. North Holland.

Barton, M.B., Dayhoff, D.A., Soumerai, S.B. et al. (2001). Measuring access to effective care among elderly medicare enrollees in managed and fee-for-service care: a retrospective cohort study. *BMC Health Services Research* 1: 11.

Begur, S.V., Miller, D.M., and Weaver, J.R. (1997). An integrated spatial DSS for scheduling and routing home-health-care nurses. *Interfaces* **27**(4): 35–48.

de Bekker-Grob, E.W., Ryan, M., and Gerard, K. (2012). Discrete choice experiments in health economics: a review of the literature. *Health Economics* **21**(2): 145–172.

Ben-akiva, M. and Lerman, S.R. (1985). *Discrete Choice Analysis: Theory and Application to Travel Demand*. The MIT Press.

Berman, S., Wasserman, S., and Grimm, S. (1991). Participation of Colorado pediatricians and family physicians in the Medicaid program. *Western Journal of Medicine* **155**(6): 649–652.

Berman, S., Doilns, J., Tang, S.F., and Yudkowsky, B. (2002). Factors that influence the willingness of private primary care pediatricians to accept more Medicaid patients. *Pediatrics* **110**(2): 239–248.

Blackwell, A.G. and Treuhaft, S. (2008). *Regional Equity and the Quest for Full Inclusion*. PolicyLink.

Brotcorne, L., Laporte, G., and Semet, F. (2003). Ambulance location and relocation models. *European Journal of Operational Research* **147**(3): 451–463.

Cao, S., Gentili, M., Griffin, P.M. et al. (2017). Disparities in preventive dental care among children in Georgia. *Preventing Chronic Disease* **14**: 170176.

Centers for Disease Control and Prevention (2010). 2010 Child Asthma Data: Prevalence Tables. http://www.cdc.gov/asthma/brfss/2010/child/current/tableC3.htm (accessed February 2019).

Centers for Disease Control and Prevention (2014). Uncontrolled Asthma among Persons with Current Asthma. https://www.cdc.gov/asthma/asthma_stats/uncontrolled_asthma .htm (accessed February 2019).

Centers for Disease Control and Prevention (2015). The 6|18 Initiative: Accelerating Evidence into Action https://www.cdc.gov/sixeighteen/ (accessed June 2019).

Chang, R.K. and Halfon, N. (1997). Geographic distribution of pediatricians in the United States: an analysis of the fifty states and Washington, DC. *Pediatrics* **100**(2 Pt 1): 172–179.

Chang, J., Freed, G.L., Prosser, L.A. et al. (2014). Comparisons of health care utilization outcomes in children with asthma enrolled in private insurance plans versus Medicaid. *Journal of Pediatric Health Care* **28**(2): 185.

Community Preventive Services Task Force (2008). Asthma Control: Home-Based Multi-Trigger, Multicomponent Environmental Interventions: Task Force Finding and Rationale Statement Interventions for Children and Adolescents with Asthma.

Crocker, D.D., Kinyota, S., Dumitru, G. et al. (2011). Effectiveness of home-based, multi-trigger, multicomponent interventions with an environmental focus for reducing asthma morbidity a community guide systematic review. *American Journal of Preventive Medicine* **41**(2S1): S5–S32.

Daskin, M.S. and Dean, L.K. (2004). Location of health care facilities. In: *Handbook of OR/MS in Health Care: A Handbook of Methods and Applications* (eds. M.B.F. Sainfort and W. Pierskalla). Springer 43–76.

Delamater, P.L. (2013). Spatial accessibility in suboptimally configured health care systems: a modified two-step floating catchment area (M2SFCA) metric. *Health & Place* **24**: 30–43.

Dempe, S. (2013). Wiley encyclopedia of operations research and management science. *Optimization* **62**(1): 167–168.

Dill, M.J., Pankow, S., Erikson, C., and Shipman, S. (2013). Survey shows consumers open to a greater role for physician assistants and nurse practitioners. *Health Affairs (Millwood)* **32** (6): 1135–1142.

Dunkley, B., Helling, A., and Sawicki, D.S. (2004). Accessibility versus scale – examining the tradeoffs in grocery stores. *Journal of Planning Education and Research* **23**(4): 387–401.

Ekici, A., Keskinocak, P., and Swann, J.L. (2013). Modeling influenza pandemic and planning food distribution. *Manufacturing & Service Operations Management* **16**(1).

Felder, S. and Brinkmann, H. (2002). Spatial allocation of emergency medical services: minimising the death rate or providing equal access? *Regional Science and Urban Economics* **32**: 27–45.

Flournoy, R. and Treuhaft, S. (2005). *Healthy Food, Healthy Communities: Improving Access and Opportunities Through Food Retailing*. PolicyLink.

Freed, G.L., Dunham, K.M., Clark, S.J. et al. (2010). Perspectives and preferences among the general public regarding physician selection and board certification. *The Journal of Pediatrics* **156**(5): 841–845, 845.e841.

Frumkin, H., Frank, L., and Jackson, R. (2004). *Urban Sprawl and Public Health Designing, Planning, and Building for Healthy Communities*. Island Press.

Garcia, E. (2017). Evaluating access to care and utilization for chronic pediatric conditions. school of industrial and system engineering. PhD thesis. Georgia Institute of Technology, Atlanta.

Garcia, E., Serban, N., Swann, J. et al. (2015). The effect of geographic access on severe health outcomes for pediatric asthma. *Journal of Allergy and Clinical Immunology* **136** (3): 610–618.

Gentili, M., Isett, K., Serban, N. et al. (2015). Small-area estimation of spatial access to pediatric primary care and its implications for policy. *Journal of Urban Health* **92**(5): 864–909.

Gentili, M., Serban, N., Harati, P. et al. (2018). Quantifying disparities in accessibility and availability of pediatric primary care with implications for policy. *Health Services Research* **53**(3): 1458–1477.

Gerard, K., Lattimer, V., Turnbull, J. et al. (2004). Reviewing emergency care systems 2: measuring patient preferences using a discrete choice experiment. *Emergency Medicine Journal* **21**(6): 692–697.

Griffin, P.M., Scherrer, C.R., and Swann, J.L. (2008). Optimization of community health center locations and service offerings with statistical need estimation. *IIE Transactions* **40**(9): 880–892.

Guagliardo, M.F. (2004). Spatial accessibility of primary care: concepts, methods and challenges. *International Journal of Health Geographics* **3**(3): 1–13.

Guagliardo, M.F., Ronzio, C.R., Cheung, I. et al. (2004). Physician accessibility: an urban case study of pediatric providers. *Health & Place* **10**(3): 273–283.

Harati, P., Gentili, M., and Serban, N. (2016). Projecting the impact of the affordable care act provisions on accessibility and availability of primary care for the adult population in Georgia. *American Journal of Public Health* **106**(8): 1470–1476.

Health Policy Institute (2015). *The Oral Health Care System: A State by State Analysis*. American Dental Association.

Health Resources and Services Administration (2013a). Projecting the Supply and Demand for Primary Care Practitioners Through 2020. Health Resources and Services Administration Bureau of Health Workforce, National Center for Health Workforce Analysis.

Health Resources and Services Administration 2013b). Compendium of Federal Data Sources to Support Health Workforce Analysis, April 2013. Health Resources and Services Administration Bureau of Health Workforce, National Center for Health Workforce Analysis.

Heier Stamm, J. (2010). Design and analysis of humanitarian and public health logistics systems. PhD thesis. Georgia Institute of Technology, Atlanta.

Heir Stamm, J.H., Serban, N., Swann, J.L. et al. (2017). Quantifying and explaining accessibility with application to the 2009 H1N1 vaccination campaign. *Health Care Management Science* **20**(1): 76–93.

Institute of Medicine (1993). *Access to Health Care in America*. Washington, DC: National Academy Press.

Jackson, R. J. and C. Kochtitzky (2002). Creating A Healthy Environment: The Impact of the Built Environment on Public Health. Sprawl Watch Clearinghouse, Centers for Disease Control and Prevention.

Jeffers, J.R., Boganno, M.F., and Bartlett, J.C. (1971). On the demand versus need for medical services and the concept of "shortage". *American Journal of Public Health* **61**(1): 46–63.

Joseph, A.E. and Phillips, D.R. (1984). *Accessibility & Utilization: Geographical Perspectives on Health Care Delivery*. New York, NY: Harper & Row.

Khan, A.A. (1992). An integrated approach to measuring potential spatial access to health care services. *Socio-Economic Planning Sciences* **26**(4): 275–287.

Lancsar, E. and Louviere, J. (2008). Conducting discrete choice experiments to inform health-care decision making. *Pharmacoeconomics* **26**(8): 661–677.

Lee, M. and Rubin, V. (2007). *The Impact of the Built Environment on Community Health: The State of Current Practice and Next Steps for a Growing Movement*. PolicyLink.

Li, Z., Serban, N., and Swann, J.L. (2015). An optimization framework for measuring spatial access over healthcare networks. *BMC Health Services Research* **15**: 273.

Luo, W. and Qi, Y. (2009). An enhanced two-step floating catchment area (E2SFCA) method for measuring spatial accessibility to primary care physicians. *Health & Place* **15**(4): 1100–1107.

MacKinney, A. C., Coburn, A.F., Lundblad, J.F. et al. (2014). Access to Rural Health Care – A Literature Review and New Synthesis, Rural Policy Research Institute.

Mao, L. and Nekorchuk, D. (2013). Measuring spatial accessibility to healthcare for populations with multiple transportation modes. *Health & Place* **24**: 115–122.

Mayer, M.L. (2006). Are we there yet? Distance to care and relative supply among pediatric medical subspecialties. *Pediatrics* **118**(6): 2313–2321.

Mayer, M.L., Skinner, A.C., and Slifkin, R.T. (2004). Unmet need for routine and specialty care: data from the National Survey of Children with Special Health Care Needs. *Pediatrics* **113**(2): e109–e115.

Mayer, M.L., Beil, H.A., and von Allmen, D. (2009). Distance to care and relative supply among pediatric surgical subspecialties. *Journal of Pediatric Surgery* **44**(3): 483–495.

McGrady, M.E. and Hommel, K.A. (2013). Medication adherence and health care utilization in pediatric chronic illness: a systematic review. *Pediatrics* **132**(4): 730–740.

McGrail, M. and Humphreys, J. (2009). Measuring spatial accessibility to primary care in rural areas: improving the effectiveness of the two-step floating catchment area method. *Applied Geography* **29**(4): 533–541.

Murrin, S. (2014). State Standards for Access to Care in Medicaid Managed Care. United States Department of Health and Human Services.

National Asthma Education and Prevention Program (2007). *Expert Panel Report 3: Guidelines for the Diagnosis and Management of Asthma*. Bethesda, MD: National Heart, Lung, and Blood Institute.

National Center for Health Statistics (2015). Ambulatory Health Care Data. Centers for Disease Control and Prevention.

National Center for Health Statistics (2016). Health Insurance Coverage. Centers for Disease Control and Prevention.

Nobles, M., Serban, N., and Swann, J.L. (2014). Measurement and inference on pediatric healthcare accessibility. *Annals of Applied Statistics* **8**(4): 1922–1946.

Odoki, J.B., Kerali, H.R., and Santorini, F. (2001). An integrated model for quantifying accessibility-benefits in developing countries. *Transportation Research Part A* **35**: 601–623.

Pearson, W.S., Goates, S.A., Harrykissoon, S.D., and Miller, S.A. (2014). State-based Medicaid costs for pediatric asthma emergency department visits. *Preventing Chronic Disease* **11**: 140139.

Penchansky, R. and Thomas, J.W. (1981). The concept of access: definition and relationship to consumer satisfaction. *Medical Care* **19**(2): 127–140.

Perloff, J.D., Kletke, P., and Fossett, J.W. (1995). Which physicians limit their Medicaid participation, and why. *Health Services Research* **30**(1 Pt 1): 7.

Philips, H., Remmen, R., Van Rouyen, P. et al. (2012). Predicting the place of out-of-hours care-a market simulation based on discrete choice analysis. *Health Policy* **106**(3): 284–290.

Piecoro, L.T., Potoski, M., Talbert, J.C. et al. (2001). Asthma prevalence, cost, and adherence with expert guidelines on the utilization of health care services and costs in a state Medicaid population. *Health Services Research* **36**(2): 357–371.

Porteous, T., Ryan, M., Bond, C.M., and Hannaford, P. (2006). Preferences for self-care or professional advice for minor illness: a discrete choice experiment. *British Journal of General Practice* **56**(533): 911–917.

Pylypchuk, Y. and Sarpong, E.M. (2012). Comparison of health care utilization: United States versus Canada. *Health Services Research* **48**(2): 560–581.

Raffoul, M., Moore, M., Kamerow, D., and Bazemore, A. (2016). A primary care panel size of 2500 is neither accurate nor reasonable. *Journal of the American Board of Family Medicine* **29**(4): 496–499.

Rardin, R. (1997). *Optimization in Operations Research*. Lebanon, IN: Prentice Hall.

Rouse, W.B. and Cortese, D.A. (2010). Introduction. In: *Engineering the System of Healthcare Delivery* (eds. W.B. Rouse and D.A. Cortese), 3–14. Amsterdam: IOS Press.

Rouse, W.B. and Serban, N. (2015). *Understanding and Managing the Complexity of Healthcare*. Cambridge, MA: MIT Press.

Ryan, M. and Farrar, S. (2000). Using conjoint analysis to elicit preferences for health care. *British Medical Journal* **320**(7248): 1530–1533.

Schweikhart, S.B. and Smithdaniels, V.L. (1993). Location and service mix decisions for a managed health-care network. *Socio-Economic Planning Sciences* **27**(4): 289–302.

Sebelius, K. (2011). HHS Secretary's Efforts to Improve Children's Health Care Quality in Medicaid and CHIP. Department of Health and Human Services.

Serban, N. and Tomar, S. (2018). ADA Health Policy Institute's methodology overestimates spatial access to dental care for publicly insured children. *Journal of Public Health Dentistry* **78**(4): 291–295.

Serban, N., Bush, C., and Tomar, S. (2019). Medicaid capacity for pediatric dental care. *Journal of the American Dental Association* **150**(4): 294–304.

Talen, E. (2001). School, community, and spatial equity: an empirical investigation of access to elementary schools in West Virginia. *Annals of the Association of American Geographers* **91**(3): 465–486.

Talen, E. and Anselin, L. (1998). Assessing spatial equity: an evaluation of measures of accessibility to public playgrounds. *Environment and Planning A* **33**: 595–613.

The American College of Allergy Asthma and Immunology (2015). Asthma Management and the Allergist: Better Outcomes at Lower Cost. http://college.acaai.org/practice-management-information-related-health-care-providers/asthma-management-and-allergist-better (accessed February 2019).

Train, K.E. (2009). *Discrete Choice Models with Simulation*. Cambridge University Press.

U.S. Census Bureau (2010). American Community Survey 1-Year Estimates, Tables B09001, B09010, B19125, B23006. American FactFinder.

Wan, N., Zou, B., and Sternberg, T. (2012). A three-step floating catchment area method for analyzing spatial access to health services. *International Journal of Geographical Information Science* **26**(6): 1073–1089.

Wang, F.H. (2012). Measurement, optimization, and impact of health care accessibility: a methodological review. *Annals of the Association of American Geographers* **102**(5): 1104–1112.

Wang, F. and Luo, W. (2005). Assessing spatial and nonspatial factors for healthcare access: towards an integrated approach to defining health professional shortage areas. *Health & Place* **11**: 131–146.

Weiner, J.P. (2004). Prepaid group practice staffing and US physician supply: lessons for workforce policy. *Health Affairs* **23**(2): W43–W59.

World Health Organization (1978). Primary Health Care. Alma-Ata, USSR.

World Health Organization (2008). Primary Health Care: Now More Than Ever. The World Health Report. Geneva.

Zheng, Y., Lee, I., and Serban, N. (2018). Regularized optimization with spatial coupling for robust decision making. *European Journal of Operational Research* **270**(3): 898–906.

3

DISPARITIES IN HEALTHCARE ACCESS

To "achieve health equity, eliminate disparities, and improve the health of all population groups" are the main goals in Healthy People 2020 (n.d.).

The term *disparity* is often used to describe any difference in some fundamental need between groups or individuals, where a fundamental need includes economic opportunity, education, or health. When referring to health, it is common to distinguish between *health disparities* and *healthcare disparities*, where the former refers to differences in health outcomes and the latter refers to differences attributed to the healthcare delivery. This chapter primarily focuses on healthcare disparities, particularly in healthcare access.

Disparities are not the same as variations in health or healthcare of individuals. Some variation in health among individuals is expected and may be due to basic biology and genetics, or random chance. Some variation in healthcare is also expected and may be due to specific preferences in the selection of services. Moreover, disparities are also not the same as inequities; not all disparities observed at the population level necessarily reflect inequity (US Department of Health and Human Services 2003). Braveman and Gruskin (2003) defined *inequity* in health as the presence of systematic disparities in health (or in major social determinants of health) between population groups with different levels of social advantage/disadvantage. Two distinctive facets of disparities are implied in health inequity as introduced by this definition. First, differences are *systematic* not at random. Secondly, the *comparison across population groups* is needed to infer who is benefiting the most or the least from policies affecting health, and therefore, how best to target interventions.

Therefore, a health disparity between more and less disadvantaged population groups constitutes an inequity not because we know the proximate causes of that disparity and judge them to be unjust, but rather because the disparity is *systematically associated* with unjust social and economic structures (Morrison 2009). However, systematic association does not imply causation. For example, the underlying causality of a health disparity could be in factors associated with income rather than in

Healthcare System Access: Measurement, Inference, and Intervention, Nicoleta Serban.
© 2020 John Wiley & Sons, Inc. Published 2020 by John Wiley & Sons, Inc.

income itself; equalizing income would not necessarily be effective in reducing that particular disparity.

Because the overarching objective is to reduce inequities, both distinctive facets of disparities need to be rigorously incorporated in measuring and making inference on healthcare access. In this chapter, I will overview the concepts of systematic disparities between sub-populations by highlighting the need for rigorous methodology. Raghunathan (2006) differentiated between three different perspectives when measuring and understanding disparities:

- *Social Equity*: This perspective focuses on the health disparities between various groups differentiated by race/ethnicity, socioeconomic status, rural/urban living conditions, health insurance status, or access to healthcare.
- *Public Health*: This perspective focuses on the health status of all groups through preventive care, access to care, and treatment of disease within a given target outcome level.
- *Disease Burden*: This perspective focuses on identifying population subgroups with relatively high rates of a disease burden, particularly evaluating the extent to which the burden of disease or a particular condition is unevenly distributed.

This chapter focuses on the first two perspectives, a public health view on social equity, where the end point is to reduce disease burden and to improve health overall. The first perspective is often the stepping stone in decision making for public health, addressing questions such as: *Are there disparities with respect to health and/or healthcare outcomes? How severe are the disparities? Have disparities decreased or increased over years?* Once disparities are established, public health questions need to be addressed: *What sub-populations are in most need of intervention? What communities to target? How to intervene?* Depending on the focus or perspective, different methodology is to be considered as further developed in this chapter.

OVERVIEW OF SYSTEMATIC DISPARITY MEASURES

The existing literature and research on disparities covers a wide spectrum of health(care) areas, including mortality (Laporte 2002; Chen et al. 2006; Sergeant and Firth 2006; Tassone et al. 2009), life expectancy (Regidor et al. 2003; Singh and Siahpush 2006), mobility and poverty (Biewen 2002), child cognitive function (Maika et al. 2013), health and pollution (Levy et al. 2006), preterm birth (Kramer et al. 2010), environmental justice (Waller et al. 1999), health and built environment (Gordon-Larsen et al. 2006), among other studies.

There are also many studies introducing and reviewing approaches to evaluating (systematic) disparities in health and healthcare (Wagstaff et al. 1991; Mackenbach and Kunst 1997; Hayward et al. 2008; Harper and Lynch 2012; Talih 2013), without a consensus on the most appropriate methods for identifying and monitoring changes in health disparities. The overarching learning lesson across all studies is that the choice of disparity measures involves implicit value judgments about many facets of what disparity means to those seeing fairness in health(care) (Harper et al. 2010).

In this section, I will overview most common measures of disparities used in quantifying or measuring health disparities. However, such measures are only addressing social equity questions: "Are there disparities?" Identifying disparities is not sufficient to address public health questions: "Are the disparities systematic and significant? How and where to intervene?" To establish interventions for addressing systematic disparities, the development and implementation of statistical modeling and inference is further needed, as illustrated in the case studies presented in this chapter.

Fundamentals

When measuring disparities, the population groups that are to be targeted for comparison need to be first established. In the simplest disparity studies, only two groups are compared; however, it may be more informative to evaluate disparities in a given outcome across more than two groups. The decomposition of the population into groups along with the number of groups can highly impact the level of disparities identified. Most common decompositions are by gender, social class, race and/or ethnicity, disability, geographic location (e.g. urban vs rural), by education, sexual orientation, or healthcare insurance type (public vs commercial). Each decomposition generally captures different types of disparities (if any are identified) with respect to the outcome of interest.

Harper and Lynch (2012) outlined several considerations in selecting a measure, including the choice between an absolute or relative measure, a measure that weights each group according to the group's size, and the choice of a reference group, briefly introduced below:

1. *Distinguishing between an absolute measure and a relative measure.* Relative measures, for example ratios of rates, are scale invariant in contrast to absolute measures (e.g. difference in rates), which are not. That is, the measure does not change with uniform proportional changes in the rates (i.e. if all rates decreased by 50%, the measure would not change). The use of absolute and relative measures can lead to different conclusions in terms of the level of disparities (Harper and Lynch 2009).

2. *Applying the same weights or different size-adjusted weights to each group.* When the weights are size adjusted, each individual gets equal weight in the calculation of disparity. Measures that do not use size-adjusted weighting give more weight to individuals in minority groups.

3. *Selecting a reference group.* The *reference group* defines a baseline from which the magnitude of disparities is judged. Common reference groups are the overall population rate, the best group rate, and a target/goal rate.

Levy et al. (2006) argued that measures of health disparities should satisfy certain properties, including the Pigou–Dalton transfer principle and subgroup decomposability. The *Pigou–Dalton principle* requires that the measure does not decrease when health is transferred from a person in a less advantaged group to a person in a more advantaged group, or vice versa. While the transfer of health may not seem like a practical consideration, when policymakers make decisions regarding issues such as pollution, it may affect exposure to potential health hazards and thus, health. *Subgroup decomposability* allows the measure of total disparity in the population to be broken into between group and within group components.

Levy et al. (2006) also suggested other properties such as *anonymity*, which requires that a measure does not include any characteristics of individuals other than their health, as a desirable property, while Wagstaff et al. (1991) contended that the socioeconomic dimension should be included in any measure of inequities in health. These considerations and their implication in studying disparities are discussed by Harper et al. (2010). Because of the different properties of various measures, Harper et al. (2010) recommended using a variety of measures because of the implicit value judgments that exist when relying on one measure only.

In what follows, I will discuss several commonly used measures of *health disparities*. I will focus on two primary sets of measures as defined by Harper and Lynch (2012):

1. *Social-Group Disparity* measures quantify disparities *between* sub-populations or groups differentiated by social and/or economic characteristics.

2. *Disproportionality* measures quantify disparities *between* and *within* groups of populations differentiated by social and/or economic characteristics.

Before introducing common measures in the two categories, I will describe the input data and specifications needed in the derivation of the disparities measured:

- *Division of the study population* into sub-populations or groups, indexing with $g = 1, \ldots, G$ where G is the number of groups.
- *Group or sub-population size*: n_g for $g = 1, \ldots, G$ with the total population $N = n_1 + \ldots + n_G$.
- *Outcome data*: $Y_{gi}, i = 1, \ldots, n_g$, for the gth group for $g = 1, \ldots, G$.
- *Reference group* represented by the rth group among the G groups or the overall population.

The outcomes of interest can be observed for all individuals or for a sample of individuals in the gth group across all $g = 1, \ldots, G$ groups. However, such data may not be available due to privacy data constraints (e.g. individuals can be identified) or due to lack of resources to collect and maintain individual outcome data. Thus, it may be the case that only group aggregated outcome data is available, $Y_g, g = 1, \ldots, G$.

Another important consideration for the outcome data is the type of data to be observed:

- If the individual outcome is *binary*, then the individual outcome Y_{gi} takes only two possible outcomes for all individuals, with the aggregated outcome Y_g

being the number of cases within the gth group. Examples of binary individual outcomes include whether an individual has a condition or not, whether with unmet need for a given healthcare service, whether having a severe outcome (e.g. hospitalization), among many others.

- If the individual outcome is a (discrete) *count*, then the individual outcome Y_{gi} takes only discrete values reflecting the number of events, with the aggregated outcome Y_g being the average count or the total count of events across all individuals in the gth group. Examples of count outcomes include the number of emergency department visits, the number of opioid prescriptions, among others.

- If the individual outcome is a (continuous) *numeric* value, then the individual outcome Y_{gi} takes numeric values with the aggregated outcome Y_g being the average, median or some other summary of the outcomes of all individuals in the gth group. Examples of numeric outcomes are income, travel distance to a provider, wait time for an appointment, among others.

The *outcome data* consist of the random variables Y_g, $g = 1, \dots, G$ where $Y_g \sim F_g = F(\mu_g, \sigma_g)$ is the distribution of the outcome variable for the gth group with mean μ_g and standard deviation σ_g. The *observed outcome data* consist of realizations from the distributions $F(\mu_g, \sigma_g)$, $g = 1, \dots, G$ and they will be defined as y_g, $g = 1, \dots, G$. It is common in statistics to define the random data with capital letters and their observations with lower-case letters; I will be using this notation throughout this chapter consistently.

To the extent possible, I will define the disparity measures in this section based on these specifications. Some measures are defined as estimates given the observed or realized group outcome data while others are defined based on the summaries of the distribution of the group outcome data. When disparity measures are defined based on the summaries of the distribution of the outcome data, more granular observations of the outcome data are needed to be able to estimate the distribution summaries.

Social-Group Disparity Measures

While, in principle, most social-group disparity measures could be modified to study individual level disparities, they are most commonly used for quantifying between-group disparities. Some measures, such as absolute/relative risk and the slope/relative index of inequality (RII), capture the difference between ill-health outcomes for groups within a population of interest. Others, such as the index of disparity(ID) and the between-group variance (BGV), measure the variability with respect to a reference group outcome. The reference can be chosen to represent the equally distributed outcome (e.g. population mean) or some idealized outcome (e.g. best group mean). The measures provided in this sub-section ignore individual-level and within-group outcome disparities. However, these measures allow the study of systematic disparities between social groups, which has been an issue of concern for policymakers (Luo and Qi 2009). These measures do not satisfy the principle of transfers, as a transfer among individuals within the same group is not considered.

Absolute and Relative Disparity The simplest measures of disparity are the relative and absolute disparity. *Absolute disparity* is the range of the group averages, given by the difference in an indicator of health between the groups. *Relative disparity* is the ratio of health outcomes for two groups. Often, the two groups being compared are the groups with the most extreme outcomes.

$$\text{Absolute Disparity} = \text{outcome of ill health for worst} - \text{off group}$$
$$- \text{outcome of ill health for best} - \text{off group}$$

$$\text{Relative Disparity} = \frac{\text{outcome for worst} - \text{off group}}{\text{outcome for best} - \text{off group}}$$

If Y_g measures ill-health (or the larger the value, the more ill-health in the population) for the gth group with $g = 1, \ldots, G$, then the two disparity measures can be derived from the realized outcome data $y_g\ g = 1, \ldots, G$ as follows:

$$\text{Absolute Disparity} = \max_{g=1,\ldots,G} y_g - \min_{g=1,\ldots,G} y_g$$

$$\text{Relative Disparity} = \frac{\max\limits_{g=1,\ldots,G} y_g}{\min\limits_{g=1,\ldots,G} y_g}$$

Absolute/relative disparity measures are also easy to interpret; the absolute risk is on the same scale as the health outcome and the relative risk is on a 0–1 scale. These measures can be too simple when summarizing disparities across multiple groups because they only include information from the two groups with the most extreme rates. Because of these concerns, these measures are only appropriate when comparing two groups. Absolute and relative disparity measures are also best used together in order to give a measure of disparity from both an absolute and a relative perspective.

Index of Dissimilarity The index of dissimilarity, in the context of health disparities, measures the difference between the observed and the expected ill-health outcome for each group, under the assumption of equality. There is both an absolute and a relative version of the index.

$$\text{Absolute Index of Dissimilarity} = \frac{1}{2} \sum_{g=1}^{G} |y_g - n_g \mu|$$

$$\text{Relative Index of Dissimilarity} = \frac{1}{2} \sum_{g=1}^{G} |s_{gh} - s_{gp}|$$

For the absolute version, the absolute difference is taken between the observed and the expected outcome measure for group g, where the expected number is based on the group's size and the mean outcome of the total population (μ). The expected outcome is the expectation of the distribution of Y_g under the assumption that each group's ill-health outcome mean is equal to the population outcome mean. If this assumption is true, then the index should be close to zero. The differences for all G groups are added and divided by 2. Dividing by 2 allows the index to be interpreted as the amount of ill health in the sample that would need to be redistributed in order for all groups to experience equal rates of ill-health outcomes.

The relative version uses the absolute difference in the proportion of the ill-health outcome that is in each group g (s_{gh}) and that group's proportion of the total population (s_{gp}). Here, s_{gp} is the expected proportion of ill health experienced by group g, under the assumption that each group's share of ill health is equal to its share of the population. The relative version can be interpreted as the proportion of ill health that would need to be redistributed in order for all groups to experience the same ill-health outcome. Note that these measures are commonly defined for binary or count outcome disparity measures.

An important aspect in the definition of the two measures is that they consider the absolute difference or the so called L_1-norm to summarize the disparity between the observed and expected distributions. By using the L_1-norm, these measures are less sensitive to extreme differences than measures using the L_2-norm or the squared difference.

While the index of dissimilarity includes information on all groups, it only includes information about the distribution of health outcomes between groups. It does not include any information about how health is distributed within each group, which may be an important aspect in quantifying disparities.

Index of Disparity   The ID, introduced by Pearcy and Keppel (2002), is the relative mean deviation from the reference group mean outcome (μ_r) for the G group mean outcome responses (μ_g). It is similar to the coefficient of variation, using the L_1-norm instead of the L_2-norm, making it less sensitive to extreme differences from the reference distribution. The general formulation is as follows:

$$ID = \frac{1}{\mu_r} \sum_{g=1}^{G} \frac{|\mu_g - \mu_r|}{G}$$

Given the notation of the outcome measures as a random variable, then we can rewrite the ID as follows:

$$ID = \frac{1}{E[Y_r]} \sum_{g=1}^{G} \frac{|E[Y_g] - E[Y_r]|}{G}$$

The advantages/disadvantages of the ID are similar to the relative index of dissimilarity, with some important differences. The ID does not account for the sizes of the groups, as each group is given equal weight. Thus, the measure places more weight on individuals within the minority group, whereas the index of dissimilarity places equal weight on each individual by accounting for group sizes. It also does not account for the distribution of health within groups.

Between-Group Variance   The BGV is the sum of squared differences between each of the G group mean outcomes (μ_g) and the overall population mean outcome (μ), weighted by the size of the group (n_g). This index can be interpreted as the amount of variance that would exist in the population if every individual experienced the health outcome of their respective group (Harper et al. 2008) and it is defined as follows:

$$BGV = \frac{1}{N} \sum_{g=1}^{G} n_g (\mu_g - \mu_r)^2$$

Its equivalent in terms of statistical formulation is as follows:

$$BGV = \frac{1}{N} \sum_{g=1}^{G} n_g (E[Y_g] - E[Y_r])^2$$

BGV can be interpreted as the population weighted absolute version of the ID. Like the ID, BGV is easy to calculate, uses information on all groups under consideration, and does not require the groups to be ordered. Unlike the ID, however, it uses L_2-norm, rather than L_1-norm, to measure the difference between each group outcome and the reference outcome. This makes BGV more sensitive to outcomes further from the reference outcome.

Slope/Relative Index of Inequality   The slope index of inequality (SII) and RII represent an absolute and relative, respectively, measure of disparity derived from weighted least squares linear regression. This measure requires that the social groups have some natural ordering, such as provided by the median socioeconomic status. The weights are the square root of each group size (Wagstaff et al. 1991). The linear model is:

$$n_g^{-1/2} Y_g = n_g^{-1/2} \beta_0 + \beta_1 n_g^{-1/2} x_g + \varepsilon_g$$

with a health outcome as the response (Y_g) and the midpoint of the socioeconomic indicator for each group as the predictor (x_g). The SII is simply the estimated coefficient associated with the midpoint, or the slope of the regression line $(\hat{\beta}_1)$. The RII is equal to the SII divided by the population average (μ) for the health indicator $(\hat{\beta}_1/\mu)$. Since these indices are based on the linear regression model, they require ordering the groups of interest and the assumption of a linear relationship between the socioeconomic status of each group and the health outcome.

The key difference between the SII or RII and other social group disparity measures is the inclusion of information about the socioeconomic status of each group, providing an order on the weighing of disparities. Moreover, these measures can also be accompanied by confidence intervals derived from the regression model, providing insights on the variability in the disparity measures for the observed outcome data. Along with the health concentration index, the SII and RII are two of the most commonly used indices for examining socioeconomic health disparities.

Disproportionality Measures

Disproportionality measures are relative measures that compare shares or proportions of health outcomes to shares of population outcomes (Harper and Lynch 2009). As measures of total disparity, these measures consider disparities between individuals, and most of them can be decomposed into between-group and within-group disparities, similar to how the total sum of squares is decomposed into between-group and within-group sums of squares in ANOVA. Each of the measures provided in this sub-section satisfies the Pigou–Dalton principle of transfers.

Lorenz Curve and Gini Coefficient A Lorenz curve is constructed by plotting the cumulative burden of disease or other health outcome against the cumulative population, ranked by health status. When the burden is evenly distributed throughout the population, the Lorenz curve will be diagonal between the two axes, called the line of equality. The Gini coefficient is proportional to the total area below the line of equality, that is between the diagonal and the Lorenz curve:

$$GC = \frac{\sum_{l=1}^{G}\sum_{j=1}^{G}|y_l - y_j|}{2\bar{y}G^2}$$

where $\bar{y}$ is the average outcome across all groups. Since the area below the line of equality is equal to 0.5, the Gini coefficient is equal to twice the area between the line of equality and the Lorenz curve. Thus, values close to 0 indicate an equal distribution of the outcome across the populations; values close to 1 indicate an unequal distribution. The Gini coefficient has several desirable properties: mean independence (if the outcome across all groups doubles, the coefficient would not change), population size independence, and Pigou–Dalton transfer sensitivity (Haughton and Khandker 2009). The graphic representation of the Lorenz curve is another advantage of the Gini coefficient. However, it is not decomposable into within-group/between-group components, unless the groups can be ordered without overlapping (Cowell and Mehta 1982).

Health Concentration Curve and Concentration Index The health concentration curve is similar to the Lorenz curve, except that the population is ranked by socioeconomic status, instead of health status. The analogue of the Gini coefficient, in this setting, is the concentration index, defined as the proportion of area above (or below) the line of equality, that is between the line of equality and the health concentration curve. Thus, the health concentration index is a socioeconomic-related health inequality measure, while the Gini index is purely a health inequality measure. For G groups ranked by socioeconomic status, with average level of health, $\bar{y}$, and letting the relative rank be denoted r_g, the relative concentration index (RCI) and absolute concentration index (ACI) are calculated as follows:

$$RCI = \frac{2}{G\bar{y}}\sum_{g=1}^{G}y_g r_g - 1$$

$$ACI = \bar{y} \times RCI$$

When the cumulative share of the population is plotted against cumulative share of ill health population, the resulting concentration index is referred to as the ACI. However, an RCI can be calculated by plotting the cumulative population against each group's share of ill health (Harper and Lynch 2012). The added element, including information about the socioeconomic status of the groups, can be a desirable property, as noted by Wagstaff et al. (1991). While the RCI is not subgroup decomposable, a decomposition analysis can be performed by taking advantage of the index's relationship with the RII (Maika et al. 2013). Additionally, the ACI can be extended to include an inequality aversion parameter, similar to the other disproportionality measures (Wagstaff 2002; O'Donnell et al. 2008).

Generalized Entropy Measures I will first introduce the concept of generalized entropy (GE), the divergence between the distributions of the (health) outcomes of two populations. Generally, divergence seeks to measure the dissimilarity between the probability density/mass functions representing the distributions of the outcomes of two populations. The GE measure is calculated as the difference or divergence between the outcome probability functions for population and health. Suppose p_g and q_g are the distributions of a population and its ill-health outcome for the gth group, respectively. Defining $r_g = q_g/p_g$, for $\alpha \neq 0, 1$ we can write the GE measure as

$$D_\alpha(p \parallel q) = GE_\alpha := \frac{-1}{\alpha(1-\alpha)}\left(1 - \sum_{g=1}^{G} p_g r_g^{1-\alpha}\right) = \frac{-1}{\alpha(1-\alpha)}\left(1 - \frac{E[Y^{1-\alpha}]}{E[Y]^{1-\alpha}}\right)$$

where $E[Y]$ is the expectation of the distribution of Y, which is a random variable representing the health of an individual in the population. The Theil index (TI) (GE_0) and mean log deviation (MLD) (GE_1), referred to collectively as Theil's measures, are limiting cases of GE_α (Theil 1967). Their formulations are as follows:

$$TI = GE_0 = \sum_{g=1}^{G} p_g r_g \log r_g = \frac{E[Y \log Y]}{E[Y]} - \log E[Y]$$

$$MLD = GE_1 = - \sum_{g=1}^{G} p_g \log r_g = \log E[Y] - E[\log Y]$$

Since each individual accounts for the same share of the population, in effect, the indices provided above are measuring the difference between the observed distribution of ill health and a uniform distribution where each individual bears an equal burden of ill health.

For those familiar with more advanced statistical hypothesis testing, the TI defined above can be seen as the log-likelihood ratio test statistic, testing the null hypothesis that the shares of the population have been distributed according to the shares of adverse health that each group experiences (Talih 2013). Thus, the TI can be more influenced by groups with large shares of ill health. The MLD defined above can be seen as the log-likelihood ratio test statistic, testing the null hypothesis that shares of adverse health are distributed according to each group's population share. This causes the MLD to be more influenced by groups with large population shares. To avoid this value judgment inherent in these two measures, the symmetrized Theil index (STI) was proposed by Borrell and Talih (2011) as the average of the TI and MLD:

$$STI = \frac{1}{2}(TI + MLD) = \frac{1}{2}\sum_g (r_g - 1)p_g \ln r_g$$

The symmetric property allows STI to avoid the value judgment mentioned as one important consideration of disparity measures, while keeping the decomposability possessed by the TI and MLD. A symmetric version of the GE class of measures has also been proposed (Talih 2013). A key attribute of the GE class of disparity measures is that they are decomposable into within-group and between-group components.

For a sample of observed G groups' ill health realized outcomes, $y_1, y_2, \ldots, y_g$, an estimate of these entropy measures can be obtained by replacing each component with its sample counterpart, with $\hat{p}_g = \frac{n_g}{N}$ being the proportion of the sample represented by one group, $\hat{q}_g = \frac{y_g}{\sum_{g=1}^{G} y_g}$ being the proportion of the total ill health borne by the gth individual/group, and

$$\hat{r}_g = \frac{\hat{q}_g}{\hat{p}_g}$$

being the relative burden of ill health for the gth group. We also can give equal weight to each group by considering $\hat{p}_g = \frac{1}{G}$.

If we consider the general case when we observe a sample of individuals' ill health within each group $(y_{gj}: i = 1, \ldots, n_g, g = 1, \ldots, G)$, GE_α^B can be estimated by replacing the population parameters with their sample estimates for each group, where the only difference is in

$$\hat{q}_g = \frac{\sum_{i=1}^{n_g} y_{ig}}{\sum_{j=1}^{G} \sum_{i=1}^{n_j} y_{ij}}$$

which is the proportion of the total ill health borne by individuals in group g.

When the individual outcome takes zero values, such as for binary outcomes, the TI and MLD are undefined. However, even in these particular cases, the between group components of the TI and MLD can still be used as stand-alone measures of between-group inequality. In fact, since between-group inequalities are often of primary interest in the study of healthcare disparities, the TI and MLD used in disparities research are actually the between-group component of the indices.

Because both measures use natural logarithm of r_g, they are sensitive to group outcome means further from the population mean. Drawbacks of this class of indices include its incompatibility with non-positive outcome data and its difficulty in interpretation relative to other disparity indices.

Atkinson Index   The Atkinson index (A_ε) is an inequality measure developed by Atkinson (1970). The index ranges between 0 and 1, with higher values indicating higher levels of inequality. Originally developed to measure income inequality, this measure involves the calculation of the equally distributed equivalent level of the outcome of interest, the level of income, which would result in the same level of societal welfare experienced under the actual distribution of income if the income is evenly distributed across the study population. We can generalize to replace income with a health outcome of interest; in this context, the 1 minus the Atkinson index can be interpreted as the percentage by which an outcome could be improved while maintaining the same level of utility. Mathematically, given the distribution of the outcome $Y \sim f(y)$ and a utility function $u(y)$, y_{OUT} is the level of an outcome such that

$$u(y_{OUT}) \int f(y)\,dy = E[u(Y)] = \int u(y)f(y)\,dy$$

For the utility function of the form $u(y) = y^{1-\varepsilon}/(1-\varepsilon)$, y_{OUT} is derived as follows:

$$y_{OUT} = u^{-1}\left(E\left[\frac{Y^{1-\varepsilon}}{1-\varepsilon} \right] \right) = (E[Y^{1-\varepsilon}])^{\frac{1}{1-\varepsilon}}$$

Drawing from this idea, and using the same notation as above, the Atkinson index is defined as:

$$A_\varepsilon(p \parallel q) := 1 - \frac{y_{OUT}}{\mu} = 1 - \left(\sum_g p_g r_g^{1-\varepsilon} \right)^{\frac{1}{1-\varepsilon}} = 1 - \left(\frac{E[Y^{1-\varepsilon}]}{E[Y]^{1-\varepsilon}} \right)^{\frac{1}{1-\varepsilon}}, 1 \neq \varepsilon > 0.$$

The concavity of the utility function insures y_{OUT} does not exceed the average so that the index only takes on values between 0 and 1, with higher values representing higher levels of inequality with respect to the outcome of interest. This index includes a parameter, ε, which specifies the utility function and can be interpreted as society's aversion to inequality. Larger values of this parameter increase the index's sensitivity to outcomes for the least advantaged groups (Harper and Lynch 2012). For $\varepsilon = 0$, $A_0 = 0$, indicating societal indifference to inequality.

Levy et al. (2006) found that the Atkinson index satisfies their axioms for health inequality indices, including the Pigou–Dalton transfer principle and scale invariance. A drawback, however, is that it is not additively decomposable.

Renyi Index   A more recently developed class of indices for measuring health disparities are the Renyi indices, introduced by Talih (2013). The Renyi indices have many of the same properties as the GE class. Like the GE class of measures, the Renyi index is an entropy measure based on the Renyi divergence between two distributions. The Renyi index measures the discrepancy between the distribution of the population of interest and the distribution of ill health between individuals/groups. The index is defined as follows:

$$RI_\alpha(p \parallel q) = \frac{-1}{\alpha(1-\alpha)} \log\left(\sum_g p_g r_g^{1-\alpha}\right) = \frac{-1}{\alpha(1-\alpha)} \log\left(\frac{E[Y^{1-\alpha}]}{E[Y]^{1-\alpha}}\right), \quad \alpha \geq 0$$

Similar to the GE class of indices, the TI and MLD are limiting cases of the Renyi index ($\alpha \to 0$ and $\alpha \to 1$, respectively) and the Atkinson index is the exponential transformation of the Renyi index ($A = 1 - e^{-\alpha RI_\alpha}$). Like the GE and Atkinson indices, the Renyi index includes an aversion parameter that allows to incorporate societal aversion to disparities into the measure. This class satisfies the principle of transfers and is subgroup decomposable (Talih 2013). The Renyi index class is also asymmetric and thus, places a value judgment depending on whether the distribution of ill health is being compared with the distribution of population, or vice versa. To address this issue, the symmetrized Renyi index (SRI) is proposed by Talih (2013).

A key advantage of the Renyi index is that it is reference indifferent. That is, while the Renyi index is calculated here using the population average as the reference group, this choice of reference group does not matter, as the Renyi index is scale invariant, thus not requiring to set a reference group, or a choice with implicit value judgments about which distribution of health is fair or just (Harper et al. 2010). While a symmetric and reference indifferent version of the GE index can be constructed, Talih argues that the SRI is preferable because it is more robust to small changes in the distribution of ill health (Talih 2013).

A disadvantage of the Renyi index is that it is incompatible with binary outcomes. However, even when this is the case, the between group component of the Renyi index can be used to measure between group disparities.

Overall, the disproportionality measures are more difficult to implement than the social-group disparity measures; the latter set of measures are simple plug-ins of outcome summaries such as means. Fortunately, Talih and collaborators have developed and implemented many versions of the disproportionality measures, particularly those based on the GE measure. A recent implementation in the R statistical software is given by Talih (2013), including most of the measures presented in this section.

GEOGRAPHIC DISPARITIES AND HEALTHCARE ACCESS

One limitation of the disparity measures in the previous section is that they assume that the outcomes are independent across individuals or groups. However, when spatial correlation is present, this assumption is invalid. Spatial autocorrelation is any systematic pattern in the distribution of a variable through space or geography. As noted by Dubin (1998), "spatial autocorrelation is likely to be present in any situation in which location matters." In the study of health inequality, geography often plays an important role in defining the way in which disparities are defined. Disparities in an outcome variable due to geographical variations are often studied. For example, Krieger et al. (2002) explored how the choice of geographical level affects conclusions about socioeconomic disparities in mortality and cancer incidence using the RII and relative/absolute disparity measures.

For outcome variables such as healthcare access, the distribution of the outcome variable is inherently related to geography. In other cases, geography can play an important role, even when disparities among geographical units are not specifically of interest. For example, interactions between geography and race may lead to mistaken geographical variations for racial inequality, and vice versa. Populations in the minority in the United States, specifically African American populations, tend to live in areas with a lower quality of care (Chandra and Skinner 2003; Baicker et al. 2005) and with poorer access to care (Chandra and Skinner 2003; Dai 2010). Geography has been shown to play an important role in cardiovascular disease (Brown et al. 2011), low birth weight (Grady 2006), self-rated health (Browning et al. 2003), and knee arthroplasty (Skinner et al. 2003), among many others.

Because the healthcare access measures, simple or more advanced mathematically, vary geographically, from one community to another, it is appropriate to consider spatial models to identify disparities in access between sub-populations and across geography as described in the next section. More generally, the statistical models described in the next section can be applied to disparities in health outcomes, not only access measures, if varying by geography.

Statistical Models for Identifying Geographic Disparities in Healthcare Access

If an access measure is derived for different population groups but also varying over geography, we can write these measures as spatially varying $Y_{s,g} = Y_g(s)$, for $g = 1, \ldots, G$ where "s" indicates the functionality with respect to geography or spatial distribution, for example, "s" can be the (population) centroid of neighborhoods within a geographic space (e.g. state or national) or other location information about the geographic units within a region.

To evaluate the equity of access measures, we differentiate two objectives:

1. Compare geographically varying outcomes across groups.
2. Estimate a *geographically varying association map* with respect to potential contributors to disparities in healthcare access.

Addressing the two objectives requires using spatial statistical modeling, called *geostatistics* (Cressie 1993). In geostatistics, the objective is to make inference on a *spatial process* $\{Y(s), s \in \mathcal{R}\}$ where $\mathcal{R}$ is the geographic region over which we observe the process at M discrete spatial units, $s_1, \ldots, s_M$. Such measurements are often referred to as *geostatistical data*. Typical data analysis problems to be addressed in geostatistics are estimating the mean of the spatial process, testing whether the spatially varying mean is statistically different from zero, regression analysis concerning Y, and prediction of values of Y at unobserved locations.

A straightforward approach to comparing geographically varying measures across population groups is by means of visualization, i.e. map their geographic patterns.

Mapping such spatial processes is the most common approach in existing studies; the maps could provide some initial insights on variations across space and across populations. While the maps can reveal geographical patterns for each population, they do not provide statistically significant insights into how the measures differ between groups. To meaningfully compare geographically varying outcomes, a more rigorous approach is to use statistical inference. For this, I distinguish between three questions as shown below.

Are the disparities between two groups statistically significant? To address this first question, we can test the following statistical hypotheses:

$$H_{0,(g,g')} : Y_g(s) = Y_{g'}(s) \text{ for all } s \text{ vs } H_{1,(g,g')} : Y_g(s) \neq Y_{g'}(s) \text{ for some } s.$$

In this hypothesis testing procedure, the null hypothesis means that the spatially varying access measure for groups g and g', Y_g and $Y_{g'}$, are equal across all spatial locations and the alternative hypothesis means that there are locations where the measures for the two groups are statistically significant different. If the null hypothesis is rejected, then there are regions where the access measure is different for two groups, g and g', hence indicating the presence of systematic disparities. A note of caution! When testing multiple hypothesis tests, here $G(G-1)/2$ pairwise tests consisting of all possible combinations of pair groups among the G groups, we need to correct for the multiplicity in hypothesis testing. Generally, this is not a straightforward statistical problem because the hypothesis tests are not independent in pairwise comparisons.

More generally, when rejecting the null hypothesis, we can further identify specific locations where the difference is statistically different from zero. Mapping these locations will reveal systematic patterns in disparities in the access measure of interest among sub-populations or communities. This framework thus can be used to identify inequities, being in line with the definition of equity by Braveman and Gruskin (2003): *equity is the absence of systematic disparities between different groups of people, distinguished by different levels of social advantage/disadvantage.* In the context of geographic variations, systematic disparities are statistically significant differences in the access measure across a large number of communities within a given region.

One approach to identify locations with a significant difference in the access measure between two groups is to estimate confidence bands around the space-varying difference and then check for locations where the confidence band is above or below the zero plane. Specifically, consider the difference process $Z(s) = Y_g(s) - Y_{g'}(s)$ for each spatial unit s within a geographic domain for two groups, g and g'. Furthermore, decompose $Z(s) = f(s) + \varepsilon_s$, with $f(s)$ the regression function assumed unknown and estimated using nonparametric regression. Existing methods can be used to estimate simultaneous confidence bands $[l(s), u(s)]$ for the regression function $f(s)$ (Krivobokova et al. 2010; Serban 2011). For the spatial units s or regions such that $u(s) < 0$, the difference is *significantly negative*, while for the spatial units s such that $l(s) > 0$, the difference is *significantly positive*. The results are displayed as point maps, where the points correspond to the centroids of the spatial units where the difference process $Z(s)$ is significantly negative or positive, defined as *significance maps* (Nobles et al. 2014; Cao et al. 2017; Gentili et al. 2018).

Are the disparities localized in specific regions within the geographic space under study? The approach described above using simultaneous confidence bands can not only be used to identify systematic disparities between population groups but also geographic disparities. Instead of considering the access measure of two populations groups, we can consider the geographically varying access measure of the overall population, $Y(s), s \in \mathcal{R}$, and test the following hypothesis:

$$H_0 : Y(s) = T \text{ for all } s \text{ vs } H_1 : Y(s) > T \text{ for some } s.$$

This test specifies that the access measure is equal to (or smaller than) an access standard T against the alternative hypothesis that there are communities where it is larger than the access standard if the access measure is higher for worse access. In order to carry out the test, once we obtain the simultaneous confidence bands we check whether the plane corresponding to the constant T is contained within the confidence band; if it is, we do not reject the null hypothesis concluding that it is plausible that the communities within the region of interest have access to the service of interest according to the access standard. If we reject the null hypothesis hence geographic disparities are identified, we will further obtain a set of communities which can be targeted for interventions since access is statistically significantly higher than the access standard. I will call the point maps indicating communities with a statistically significantly higher access measure than the access standard as *threshold maps*.

Are the disparities due to variations in other factors influencing access? To address this second question, we seek to understand the level of disparities as they relate to geographic, socioeconomic, and service infrastructure factors, known to drive disparities. More specifically, *equity is achieved when the expectation of the outcome of interest given potential contributing factors to inequities is (approximately) equal to the expectation of the outcome unconditional of any contributing factor* (Fleurbaey and Schokkaert 2009). Statistically speaking, if $Y(s)$ is the access measure, and $X(s)$ is the set of contributing factors, equity is achieved when the expectation of the conditional distribution $Y(s)|X(s)$ is equal to the expectation of the marginal distribution of $Y(s)$. Practically speaking, in an equitable system, no systematic association will be found between the measure and the independent factors. This idea is an extension of the definition of the *Slope/RII* described in the previous section, except that now I consider a spatially varying relationship, defining the *geographically varying association map*.

The statistical model estimates the relationships between the dependent variable (Y), spatial accessibility, and the contributing factors (X), then test whether this association is statistically significant. The difficulty lies in that both the accessibility metrics and the predictive factors are geographically varying; that is, we can write $Y(s)$ and $X(s)$ for s varying within a geographic space. Therefore, to examine the relationship between $Y(s)$ and $X(s)$, we suggest using spatial regression modeling, which will return association maps between accessibility and various contributing factors.

That is, given a set of factors, $X_1(s), \ldots, X_r(s)$, we seek to estimate the conditional mean

$$E\{Y(s) \mid X_1(s), \ldots, X_r(s)\} = H\{X_1(s), \ldots, X_r(s)\}$$

where $H\{.\}$ is a known function. The explanatory factors can vary over the spatial domain $\mathcal{R}$ or can be constant. Moreover, they can be numerically (e.g. income level) or categorically (rural vs non-rural community) observed.

The simplest version of the model is an extension from the linear regression model to the space-varying coefficient model (Assuncao 2003; Gelfand et al. 2003; Waller et al. 2007; Serban 2011). This model assumes that the contributing factors are linearly associated with the response variable, but the association varies over the geographic space. Specifically,

$$H\{X_1(s), \ldots, X_r(s)\} = \alpha_1(s)X_1(s) + \ldots + \alpha_r(s)X_r(s)$$

where $\alpha_1(s), \ldots, \alpha_r(s)$ are unknown functions varying over the space domain $\mathcal{R}$, defined herein as *spatial association maps*. This model is simple enough to be implementable with standard statistical software and make inferences on the association coefficients while capturing the spatial variations in the association between accessibility and the explanatory factors. Under this model, a spatially varying association coefficient between a particular factor and the response measure indicates potential inequities with respect to that factor.

In my research, I employed the approach introduced in Serban (2011) and Heir Stamm et al. (2017) to estimate the model introduced above, considering nonparametric regression instead of a Bayesian approach to reduce the computational effort, especially when the association maps are estimated for large geographic regions. In particular, I used the penalized splines regression for estimating the association maps using the *mgcv* library in the R statistical software. However, it is important to underline that Bayesian modeling approaches can be quite useful in this context because of the potential non-identifiability in the estimation of the association maps; there may be strong spatial correlation between the predicting variables that may result in unstable estimates for the spatially varying coefficients.

While the statistical models presented in this section are more advanced than those employed in the existing literature, I will highlight that we need to make statistical statements on whether systematic disparities exist in an access measure to make informed decisions on how to reduce disparities. It is not only important to estimate the regression coefficients or the association maps but also to evaluate whether they are statistically significant, constant, or varying over geography. In my research, I introduced inference on the shape of the coefficients using simultaneous confidence bands. Specifically, if CB_α is a $1 - \alpha$ confidence band for the coefficient $\alpha_k(s)$, then

$$P\{\alpha_k(s) \in CB_\alpha, s \in \mathcal{R}\} \geq 1 - \alpha$$

where $\mathcal{R}$ is the space domain. Because we are interested in the shape of the function over the entire space domain, we employ simultaneous confidence bands. For example, the procedure introduced in Serban (2011).

The simultaneous confidence bands can be used to examine the statistical significance of constant coefficients and construct positive and negative *significance maps*. A positive (negative) significance map consists of point locations that have a statistically significant positive (negative) association between an access measure and the corresponding explanatory variable. The presence of a large number of points in a significance map is an indication of potential inequities with respect to the corresponding explanatory variable. Such inference can not only point to the presence of disparities but also to address "where" such systematic disparities exist.

Evaluating Systematic Disparities in Healthcare Access: Specifications

In deriving systematic disparities in healthcare access, the groups can be selected a priori, depending on what sub-populations have been known to have lower or higher access, for example, a comparison between Medicaid and non-Medicaid insured populations. In this specific comparison, the pairwise difference in access between the two groups can be analyzed using the hypothesis testing procedure provided in the previous section to identify systematic disparities.

The groups with different levels of access can also be identified by selecting a series of population attributes known to be potentially related to health disparities and integrated into a spatial regression model, in which factors identified to be associated with variations in healthcare access could pinpoint systematic disparities. Attributes can include demographics and socio-economic factors, for example. Under this modeling setting, the disparity measurement approach consists of the spatial association maps that reveal spatially varying associations of contributing factors to spatial access. In the case study included in this section, I will illustrate both approaches and show how the two approaches complement each other, allowing for a more rigorous understanding of the level of disparities in healthcare access.

Does insurance status impact access to healthcare? Caring for disadvantaged populations, particularly the Medicaid-insured population, has been a priority for public health policies. Because of variations in care provisions and because of low reimbursement rates and/or the involved administration of Medicaid claims (Perloff et al. 1995; Berman et al. 2002), this population has historically had lower access to the care system. Understanding and quantifying the disparity in healthcare access for this sub-population versus those on commercial health insurance will suggest which geographic areas need to be improved in terms of access dimensions of interest and it will make it possible to assess the impact of health policies.

Is the level of access to care significantly larger than a state access standard? While for some services, for example, primary care or preventive dental care, there may be enough caseload in the system to serve both the commercial and publicly insured population, for other services, for example obstetrics/gynecology or more specialized services, there may be communities with poor access over the entire population, particularly in rural communities. To identify communities in high need for specific healthcare services, where need can be specified by any of the healthcare access dimensions, one approach is to set a specific geographic threshold for access then compare the access measure with that threshold using statistical inference.

What are the factors associated with disparities in healthcare access? The analysis of healthcare access without consideration of factors influencing access can only provide insights on geographic disparities and what communities are subject to such disparities. It is also important to establish the factors that are associated with healthcare access and whether the association varies geographically, or whether it is statistically significant overall. To this end, the space-varying models as introduced in the previous section can be used to address such association analyses.

In the implementation of the space-varying model to identify association patterns with factors influencing access, it is important to begin with an understanding of what factors are to be included in the analysis, focusing on those most relevant since a space-varying model with too many predicting factors can be challenging to estimate (Serban 2011). First, it can be computationally expensive especially when considering large geographic spaces. Secondly, the potential spatial correlation among the predicting factors can result in so called non-identifiability of the association patterns due to the complexity of the spatial correlation with the response or access measure and the spatial correlation among the predicting factors. Thirdly, not all factors may be observed on the same geographic granularity as the access measures; for example, if observed at higher geographic resolution (e.g. census tract), then the predicting factors need to be aggregated into the lower geographic resolution (e.g. county) with consideration of the challenges of combining incompatible spatial data, particularly the modifiable areal unit problem (Gotway and Young 2002).

Case Study: Access to Pediatric Primary Care

Healthcare systems have the best health outcomes when based in primary and preventive healthcare. The first case study in this chapter focuses on evaluating disparities in healthcare access to primary care with an emphasis on disparities between children with public insurance (Medicaid/CHIP) and those with other forms of health insurance. Specifically, the aim of this study is to assess systematic disparities across two substantive dimensions of access for pediatric primary care, accessibility, and availability, together referred to as spatial access, defined in earlier chapters.

The implementation of the optimization model for estimating spatial access to pediatric primary care is introduced and described to a great extent in a collaborative paper (Gentili et al. 2018). Low geographic granularity estimates are needed to evaluate geographic disparities and capture the nuances of healthcare access, important for targeting interventions (Gentili et al. 2015). Thus, we estimated access at the census tract level, where census tracts are delineated to be proxies of communities. This can aid in the design of public policies having the highest impact at the community level, or facilitate more appropriate actions by local agents.

Accessibility and availability measures of primary care at the census tract level are derived from the optimization model for all children, children eligible for public insurance, and children likely to be privately insured. *Accessibility* is quantified as the *average distance* a child in a census tract must travel for each visit to his/her matched provider; thus, smaller values of the measure indicate better accessibility. *Availability* is quantified by the *congestion* a child experiences for each visit at his/her matched provider, where patient congestion is measured as the ratio between all assigned visits to a provider and the provider's maximum caseload; thus, smaller values indicate better availability. Children experiencing a distance of 25 miles or greater are assumed to be *unserved* by the existing network following the recommendations of the US Department of Health and Human Services defining Medically Underserved Area (MUA) as regions with no primary care providers within 25 miles.

In this sub-section, I will only provide insights on quantifying geographic disparities with inference on where to intervene to improve access given the access estimates developed in a collaborative journal article (Gentili et al. 2018). I will also compare the access measures for the two groups of children differentiated by healthcare insurance type and by urbanicity level provided by the rural-urban commuting area (RUCA) codes (Morrill et al. 1999; Bayoumi 2009). In the collaborative research (Gentili et al. 2018), we differentiated the child population by healthcare insurance type assuming the Medicaid/CHIP eligibility criteria for children under the Patient Protection and Affordable Care Act (PPACA). We further classified the census tracts as urban (RUCA code = 1.0, 1.1, 2.0, 2.1, 3.0, 4.1, 5.1, 7.1, 8.1, 10.1), large rural (RUCA code = 4.0, 5.0, 6.0), and small rural (RUCA code = 7.0, 7.2, 8.0, 8.2, 9.0). The analysis was across seven states (California, Georgia, Louisiana, Minnesota, Mississippi, North Carolina, and Tennessee).

Data Sources Providers' practice location addresses were obtained from the 2013 National Plan and Provider Enumeration System (NPPES). Specific information on the caseload dedicated to children by different types of healthcare providers was obtained from the National Ambulatory Medical Care Survey. The 2009 MAX Medicaid claims data obtained from the Centers for Medicare and Medicaid Services were used to determine what percentage of providers have seen Medicaid patients.

The patient population was aggregated at the census tract level, using the 2010 SF2 100% census data and the 2012 American Community Survey data to compute the number of children in each census tract by age class along with information on poverty and ownership of cars, to estimate access to private transportation means.

Access Estimates: Exploratory Analysis To begin, I will first present a brief exploratory analysis of the estimates for accessibility, measured by distance, and availability, measured by congestion, defined above.

Figure 3.1 illustrates the access maps derived for one state, California. Maps for the other six states along with access measures are available from the Health Analytics Group at Georgia Tech (https://www.healthanalytics.gatech.edu/data/data-descriptors). The maps are differentiated by the two access measures and also by the population of interest, including the Medicaid-eligible population or the non-Medicaid population. Some important observations from the access maps are that where the travel distance is large, the congestion is high also. When comparing the access maps across the three population groups, there is little difference that can be distinguished from the maps. Thus, based on the maps themselves, I can only pinpoint that there are geographic disparities, particularly when comparing urban areas (on the west side of California) over more rural areas but I cannot identify

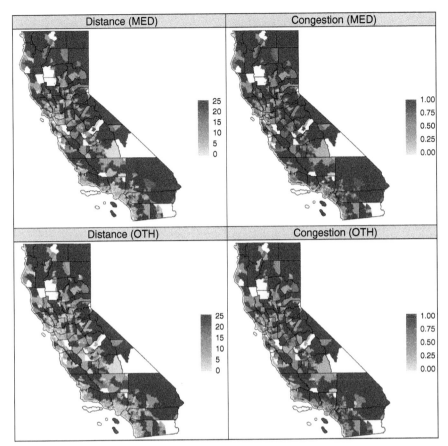

FIGURE 3.1 Maps of the access measures, distance traveled (accessibility) and congestion (availability), estimated and visualized at the census tract level for the state of *California*. The access maps are provided for each population group, including children eligible for public insurance (MED), and children likely to be privately insured (OTH).

systematic disparities between Medicaid and non-Medicaid population. Maps alone can only provide a first exploratory perspective onto differences among population groups or geography, but for rigorously identifying systematic disparities, statistical modeling and inference are needed.

Table 3.1 presents the state median access estimates for all seven states. The estimates are differentiated by urbanicity level as well as by the population of interest, including all child population, only Medicaid-eligible population, or only non-Medicaid population. Across all states, the state-level median of travel distance is less than 10 miles for all population groups. California has a state median travel distance larger than 15 miles for rural communities, primarily because of large travel distances for the Medicaid population. Congestion at the provider (proxy of wait time) as a measure of availability has an increasing trend from urban to rural

TABLE 3.1 State-level Median Values of the Distance (Accessibility) and Congestion (Availability) for the Seven States, for each Urbanicity Level and for Each Population Group, Including all Children (ALL), Children Eligible for Public Insurance(MED), and Children Likely to be Privately-insured (OTH)

			California	Georgia	Louisiana	Minnesota	Mississippi	North Carolina	Tennessee
Distance: Average (10th, 90th)	ALL	State	6.66 [0.33, 12.97]	8.12 [0.61, 17.32]	7.15 [0.51, 17.75]	7.85 [0.35, 18.33]	9.45 [0.90, 17.31]	8.82 [1.04, 17.91]	8.33 [0.63, 17.45]
		Large Urban	6.25 [0.31, 11.48]	7.29 [0.55, 15.93]	6.47 [0.49, 14.79]	6.04 [0.27, 11.59]	8.40 [0.86, 16.20]	8.08 [0.97, 16.90]	7.21 [0.52, 15.52]
		Small Urban	10.17 [0.51, 22.35]	10.93 [0.91, 22.06]	8.15 [0.41, 18.42]	9.31 [0.60, 19.57]	9.89 [0.84, 16.57]	9.97 [1.19, 18.09]	10.81 [0.72, 19.61]
		Rural	16.61 [5.44, 25.00]	12.98 [6.57, 25.00]	12.11 [0.98, 25.00]	13.45 [0.60, 25.00]	10.94 [1.35, 19.50]	13.16 [5.12, 25.00]	12.34 [5.06, 24.17]
	MED	State	7.54 [0.36, 14.97]	8.61 [0.59, 18.02]	7.58 [0.51, 18.38]	8.00 [0.33, 19.02]	9.79 [0.87, 18.63]	9.01 [0.98, 18.55]	8.82 [0.61, 18.52]
		Large Urban	7.11 [0.35, 13.63]	7.81 [0.54, 16.87]	6.89 [0.50, 16.10]	6.13 [0.26, 12.19]	8.92 [0.85, 18.34]	8.26 [0.95, 17.57]	7.66 [0.50, 16.11]
		Small Urban	11.23 [0.45, 25.00]	11.31 [0.90, 25.00]	8.34 [0.41, 18.58]	9.51 [0.60, 20.02]	10.03 [0.85, 17.48]	10.14 [1.19, 19.15]	11.36 [0.72, 22.89]
		Rual	17.91 [6.15, 25.00]	13.24 [6.16, 25.00]	12.77 [0.98, 25.00]	13.81 [0.60, 25.00]	11.19 [1.35, 19.94]	13.37 [2.58, 25.00]	13.09 [5.69, 25.00]
	OTH	State	4.78 [0.16, 10.02]	7.04 [0.42, 16.10]	6.29 [0.34, 16.41]	7.41 [0.28, 17.36]	8.50 [0.76, 15.47]	8.27 [0.91, 17.35]	7.17 [0.43, 15.95]
		Large Urban	4.44 [0.15, 9.62]	6.26 [0.39, 14.57]	5.63 [0.31, 13.23]	5.66 [0.21, 11.77]	7.31 [0.54, 13.94]	7.63 [0.85, 16.55]	6.18 [0.34, 13.66]
		Small Urban	7.40 [0.29, 15.91]	9.89 [0.90, 18.97]	7.62 [0.41, 17.66]	8.99 [0.60, 20.08]	9.19 [0.82, 15.93]	9.29 [1.08, 17.93]	9.50 [0.65, 18.14]

Congestion: Average (10th, 90th)	Rural	13.49 [0.77, 25.00]	11.32 [2.94, 25.00]	10.69 [0.82, 25.00]	12.73 [0.60, 25.00]	9.86 [0.95, 18.88]	12.03 [3.00, 25.00]	10.49 [1.24, 19.78]
ALL	State	0.54 [0.18, 0.92]	0.50 [0.10, 0.94]	0.45 [0.10, 0.93]	0.63 [0.23, 1.00]	0.73 [0.39, 1.00]	0.40 [0.15, 0.86]	0.48 [0.10, 0.94]
	Large Urban	0.54 [0.18, 0.91]	0.47 [0.10, 0.93]	0.40 [0.10, 0.92]	0.61 [0.20, 1.00]	0.75 [0.34, 0.99]	0.36 [0.15, 0.81]	0.42 [0.10, 0.91]
	Small Urban	0.60 [0.29, 0.98]	0.59 [0.26, 0.99]	0.60 [0.24, 0.89]	0.59 [0.26, 1.00]	0.67 [0.37, 0.99]	0.49 [0.15, 0.89]	0.60 [0.27, 1.00]
	Rural	0.74 [0.37, 1.00]	0.69 [0.40, 1.00]	0.70 [0.39, 1.00]	0.70 [0.36, 1.00]	0.79 [0.51, 1.00]	0.61 [0.19, 1.00]	0.70 [0.42, 1.00]
MED	State	0.53 [0.15, 1.00]	0.50 [0.10, 1.00]	0.45 [0.10, 0.95]	0.63 [0.22, 1.00]	0.74 [0.38, 1.00]	0.40 [0.15, 0.88]	0.48 [0.10, 0.98]
	Large Urban	0.52 [0.14, 0.96]	0.47 [0.10, 0.99]	0.41 [0.10, 0.92]	0.61 [0.20, 1.00]	0.75 [0.34, 1.00]	0.35 [0.15, 0.80]	0.42 [0.10, 0.93]
	Small Urban	0.62 [0.29, 1.00]	0.61 [0.27, 1.00]	0.61 [0.23, 0.91]	0.60 [0.26, 1.00]	0.68 [0.37, 1.00]	0.50 [0.15, 0.89]	0.62 [0.28, 1.00]
	Rural	0.79 [0.40, 1.00]	0.70 [0.39, 1.00]	0.72 [0.40, 1.00]	0.71 [0.37, 1.00]	0.80 [0.52, 1.00]	0.61 [0.17, 1.00]	0.72 [0.46, 1.00]
OTH	State	0.52 [0.13, 0.99]	0.47 [0.10, 0.98]	0.43 [0.10, 0.98]	0.62 [0.23, 1.00]	0.70 [0.34, 1.00]	0.39 [0.15, 0.87]	0.45 [0.10, 0.96]
	Large Urban	0.51 [0.13, 0.98]	0.45 [0.10, 0.97]	0.39 [0.10, 0.95]	0.62 [0.20, 1.00]	0.73 [0.32, 1.00]	0.35 [0.15, 0.81]	0.40 [0.10, 0.94]
	Small Urban	0.53 [0.18, 0.97]	0.56 [0.16, 0.99]	0.57 [0.16, 0.89]	0.57 [0.23, 1.00]	0.63 [0.29, 0.99]	0.47 [0.15, 0.90]	0.54 [0.18, 0.98]
	Rural	0.64 [0.17, 1.00]	0.62 [0.26, 1.00]	0.66 [0.35, 1.00]	0.68 [0.35, 1.00]	0.77 [0.47, 1.00]	0.57 [0.15, 1.00]	0.64 [0.31, 1.00]

Each cell contains the average value, and the 10th and 90th percentiles in square brackets, across all census tracts within a state.

communities except for Mississippi, where the lowest congestion is in small urban areas. There are some differences across the population groups; however, they may be small to be statistically significant. Hypothesis testing or other inference needs to be considered further to make statistical statements on the differences.

Table 3.1 also provides ranges of the access measures (10th and 90th percentiles) of the state median access values across all census tracts within one state; these ranges are indications of the spread of the distribution of the access measures within each state. The 90th percentile of the travel distance is larger than 10 miles and it is larger than 0.90 (or 90%) for the congestion measure across all states. Those communities or census tracts with a travel distance larger than 25 miles are deemed without access or unserved, and not included in the calculation of the state level summaries in Table 3.1.

Disparity Measures   I illustrate here the use of the ID and the SRI as measures of disparity in the two spatial access dimensions, availability and accessibility. In both cases, higher values indicate greater disparity. In particular, the ID is an overall measure of the difference between the accessibility (or availability) computed across all the states for each population group (i.e. Medicaid/CHIP, non-Medicaid, and overall population). Based on the notion that, in a fair setting, each population group should utilize an amount of healthcare resources proportional to the size of the group, these indices measure the extent to which healthcare resources are disproportionately utilized across states. SRI is also considered because it is a reference-invariant index; it includes a disparity *aversion parameter* α, which incorporates the societal level of opposition to inequity. The SRI index for availability and accessibility computed for the seven states is shown in Figure 3.2, while the ID values are shown in Table 3.2. The SRI is computed for values of the aversion parameter α ranging from 0.5 to 20.

The difference between the non-Medicaid and Medicaid populations is striking. The SRI values for the non-Medicaid population vary from a minimum value of less than 5% to a maximum value between 20% and 25%. The SRI values for the Medicaid population vary from a minimum value of 0% to a maximum value of less than 5%. For all values of the aversion parameter α, the SRI for the non-Medicaid population is several times greater, indicating much greater disparity. As shown in Table 3.2, the ID values for the Medicaid population and the non-Medicaid population are equal to 17.58 and 83.25, respectively. These results agree with the conclusion indicated by

TABLE 3.2   ID Values Computed among the Seven States for Accessibility and Availability for the Three Population Groups, i.e. Medicaid/CHIP, Non-Medicaid, Overall Population

	Reference point: Median across all states		
	Medicaid/CHIP	Non-Medicaid	All population
Accessibility	17.58	83.25	24.17
Availability	9.28	15.46	11.87

Lower values are better.

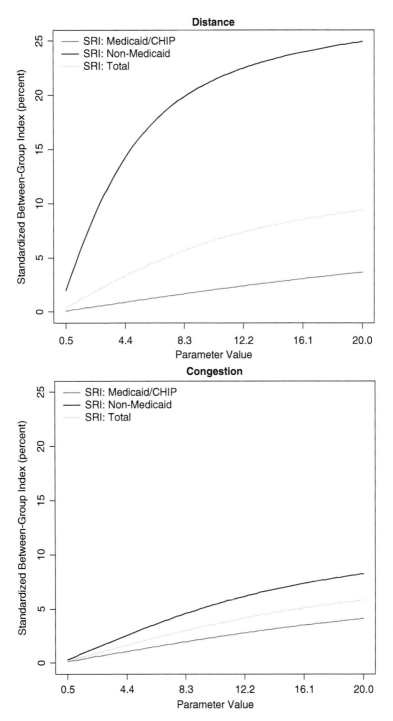

FIGURE 3.2 SRI computed among the seven states for accessibility and availability for the three population groups, i.e. Medicaid/CHIP, non-Medicaid, overall population vs disparity aversion parameter. (Lower values are better.)

the SRI values, i.e. that the non-Medicaid population experiences greater disparity across states than the Medicaid population.

The disparity measures only provide insights on whether there are disparities; they can be complemented with an analysis on *where* the disparities between Medicaid and non-Medicaid population are statistically significant as provided in the next section.

Significance Maps: Comparing Access for Medicaid vs Non-Medicaid Populations
Most existing research on quantifying and/or identifying disparities compares whether any differences between two or more population groups exist (i.e. the difference is $\delta = 0$). However, considering multiple levels of differences can help in gaining an understanding of how large differences are, if they exist. In the collaborative paper on access to pediatric primary care (Gentili et al. 2018), we considered the difference between the population groups taking three different levels in accessibility and availability:

- $\delta = 0$, $\delta = 1$ or $\delta = 2$ miles for the travel distance (accessibility measure).
- $\delta = 0.0$, $\delta = 0.1$ or $\delta = 0.2$ patient-to-provider caseload ratio or congestion (availability measure).

Figure 3.3 presents the significance maps for the different levels of disparity between the Medicaid-eligible children and non-Medicaid children for California where each point on the map corresponds to a census tract where the Medicaid-eligible children have a statistically significantly greater distance (lower accessibility) or greater congestion (lower availability) than the non-Medicaid children, at the 0.01 significance level. From these maps, we see the reduction in the number of communities experiencing disparities with the increase in the level of disparity considered. These maps can assist policy makers to target interventions to improve access to pediatric primary care since they pinpoint where improvements in access are most needed and at what level of enactment given limited resource.

In the collaborative research paper (Gentili et al. 2018), we also considered hypothesis testing procedures comparing the medians of the access measures for the two populations for all seven states. We found that while for all states we identified a statistically significant disparity at $\delta = 0$, only California showed a statistically significant disparity at $\delta = 1$ mile for the travel distance; thus all other states did not have statistically significant disparities at the higher comparison levels. This finding is important since it suggests that for California, incentivizing providers to accept public insurance could improve spatial access for Medicaid-eligible children.

Geographic Disparities Mapping the access measures to uncover geographic disparities is a widely used approach in the existing literature, commonly without further inferences on identifying communities for targeted interventions to improve access. The significance maps in the previous section only compare disparities between two population groups, but it is also important to make inferences on which communities to target for improving the access of the entire population, or for a sub-population.

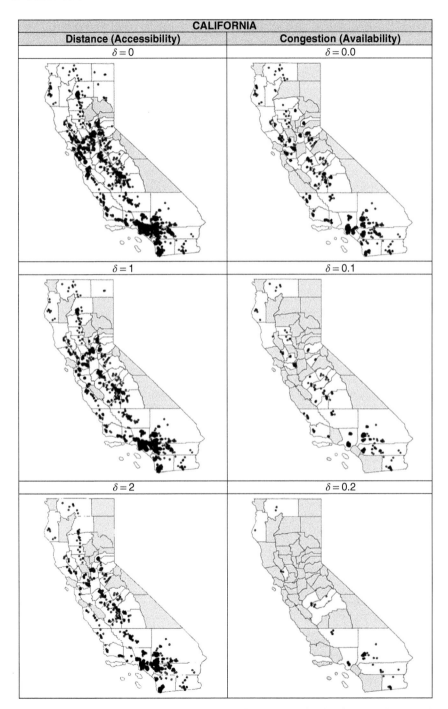

FIGURE 3.3 Accessibility and availability *significance maps* for the disparities between the Medicaid-eligible children and the non-Medicaid children. The gray-shaded regions on the maps correspond to counties where Medicaid-eligible children do not experience a significantly worse accessibility or availability.

In the previous section, I introduced the idea of threshold maps, which can identify the communities with a significantly lower or higher access than a given threshold or access standard. Figure 3.4 presents such threshold maps for California where the access standards (Kaiser Family Foundation n.d.) are as follows:

1. Ten miles for primary care, which is the Medicaid managed care organizations (MCOs) access standard for California for the Medicaid-eligible and the non-Medicaid sub-populations.
2. A 75% patient-to-provider caseload ratio or congestion for the Medicaid-eligible. The California access standard on wait time is at most 10 days but this is not easily mapped to a specific congestion level.

The maps in Figure 3.4 identify the communities where the access standards are not met. The top two maps compare the set of communities identified as having an average travel distance larger than 10 miles for the Medicaid (left) and non-Medicaid (right) sub-populations. From previous inferences, I pointed out that there is a statistically significant difference in the travel distance for the two populations. From these two plots, I also noted that both sub-populations have a large number of communities for which the access standard is not met; and there are generally more communities with higher distance than the 10 mile access standard for the Medicaid population than for the non-Medicaid population. Moreover, the middle left map shows the communities where there is a congestion level higher than 75% patient-to-provider caseload ratio for the Medicaid population, suggesting that many of these communities will not meet the access standard on wait time (less than 10 days to an appointment) since many providers that are within 25 miles will not take (new) Medicaid patients/appointments. These maps and findings can be useful for decision making in the state of California since they suggest that access is not met for a large number of communities according to the state access standards.

In our collaborative research, we defined *served* as a community with at least 80% of the population with a travel distance of less than 25 miles; *underserved* as a community with between 50% and 80% of the population with a travel distance of less than 25 miles; and *unserved* as a community with less than 50% of the population with a travel distance of less than 25 miles. Other criteria may be considered, depending on a state's standards or policies on access. Mapping the classification of communities into served, underserved, and unserved can be used as an intervention map for addressing systematic geographic disparities using targeted interventions.

The middle right map in Figure 3.4 shows the geographic distribution of the communities classified as served, underserved, and unserved for California. Table 3.3 provides the number of communities in need of interventions by classifying the census tracts as served, underserved, and unserved for all seven states. The California maps clearly pinpoint where interventions are most needed, with some large connected rural areas in most need of interventions. Since most of the unserved areas are in rural communities, telehealth, mobile health or other similar care approaches can be considered to address the reduced access to pediatric primary care. Among the seven states, there are some variations in terms of the percentage of communities that

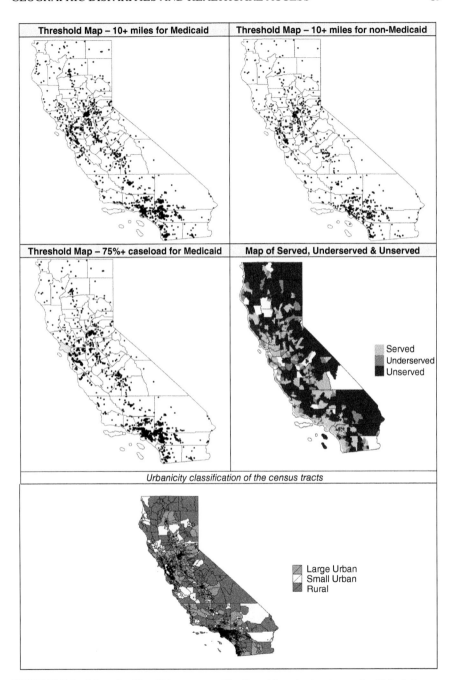

FIGURE 3.4 Maps for identifying geographic disparities: the top two and middle left maps are threshold maps based on three different access standards; and the middle right map is a map of the census tracts that are served, underserved, and unserved. The bottom map shows the urbanicity classifications of census tracts in the state according to the reclassification of their RUCA code.

TABLE 3.3   Percentage of Census Tracts in each State that are Served (at least 80% of the Population with a Travel Distance of less than 25 miles), Underserved (with between 50% and 80% of the Population with a Travel Distance of less than 25 miles), and Unserved (with less than 50% of the Population with a Travel Distance of less than 25 miles)

State	Served (%)	Underserved (%)	Unserved (%)
California	89	6	5
Georgia	82	11	7
Louisiana	85	9	6
Minnesota	84	9	7
Mississippi	84	12	4
North Carolina	84	11	5
Tennessee	82	12	7

are identified to be unserved however the percentage is small enough to be achievable with targeted interventions.

Case Study: Access to H1N1 Vaccine during the 2009 Vaccination Campaign

In this section, I will return to the following question: *Are the disparities in access due to variations in influencing factors?* I will illustrate the applicability of the methodology for the *geographically varying association map* to the analysis of the supply distribution in the context of an emergency response, the 2009 H1N1 influenza vaccination campaign in the United States. The implementation of the optimization model for estimating spatial access to vaccine during the vaccination campaign is introduced and described to a great extent in a collaborative journal article (Heir Stamm et al. 2017). The empirical results in this collaborative research can inform the development of more equitable and effective distribution plans for future public health emergency response efforts, including the identification of specific opportunities for better utilizing the existing healthcare service infrastructure and more accurately matching supply and demand.

Data Sources and Data Analytics   The focus of our study is vaccine accessibility and availability in nine states in the southeast region of the United States: Alabama, Arkansas, Florida, Georgia, Louisiana, Mississippi, North Carolina, South Carolina, and Tennessee. The collaborative study made use of three types of data from the nine southeast states, namely those that characterize vaccine supply, vaccine demand, and independent variables (geographic, socioeconomic, and healthcare service infrastructure) that may be associated with vaccine accessibility. The primary data source consisted of the vaccine shipment data from the Centers for Disease Control and Prevention, including the street addresses of facilities that received shipments and the quantities of vaccine shipped to each facility on or prior to 9 December 2009. In total, more than 13.3 million vaccines were received during this period at approximately 12 300 facilities across the nine states.

We obtained data for race/ethnicity at the census tract level from ESRI (2006). The percent of census tract population living below the federal poverty level is obtained from the Public Health Disparities Geocoding Project (2000). Using the area and population count of each census tract obtained from the US Census Bureau, we calculated its population density. Finally, we geocoded all influenza-relevant healthcare provider locations (not only those who received vaccine) using the 2009 NPPES database, including primary care providers, specialists associated with vaccination target groups, public health clinics, school-associated healthcare providers, pharmacies, and other locations associated with influenza prevention and/or treatment. Based on this, we estimated the density of providers relative to the population density to quantify the availability of possible service locations, and we explored this variable to determine the degree to which larger service infrastructure issues contribute to differences in accessibility of vaccine. For both the population and provider density estimates, we employ two-dimensional kernel density smoothing (Berman and Diggle 1989). Specifically, we assume that the population and provider network are point processes, and we estimate their spatially varying intensity functions.

Inference on the Geographically Varying Association Map   An optimization-based access model was used to measure vaccine accessibility across the nine-state region in the Southeast during the early stage of the vaccination campaign using a decentralized modeling approach presented in the collaborative research article (Heir Stamm et al. 2017).

We estimated and made inference on the association patterns between the H1N1 vaccine accessibility and multiple factors, including income, proportion of the population belonging to a minority racial/ethnic group, population density, and density of healthcare providers relative to the population. We used the spatially varying coefficient model along with inferences on the geographically varying association map described in the previous section. For the implementation of the model, we used R statistical software using the *mgcv* library (Wood 2006).

I will briefly describe the most relevant results here to illustrate how such methodology can be used to make inference on disparities in association with variations of factors influencing healthcare access. We found that population density and provider density have statistically significant spatial associations with spatial access to vaccine during the vaccination campaign, suggesting potential systematic disparities with respect to these two factors. We do not find significant associations between accessibility and the socioeconomic factors. Figure 3.5 presents the point map of the census tracts in which there is a statistically significant association between vaccine accessibility and provider density as an illustration. Some states exhibit positive association between population density and congestion in densely populated areas, while others exhibit negative association in such areas. The former indicates too few vaccines per person, or under-serving; the latter points to too many vaccines per person, or over-serving. The results indicate a tendency to over-serve areas with high population density, yet under-serving occurs in areas of both low and high population density in five of the states in this study.

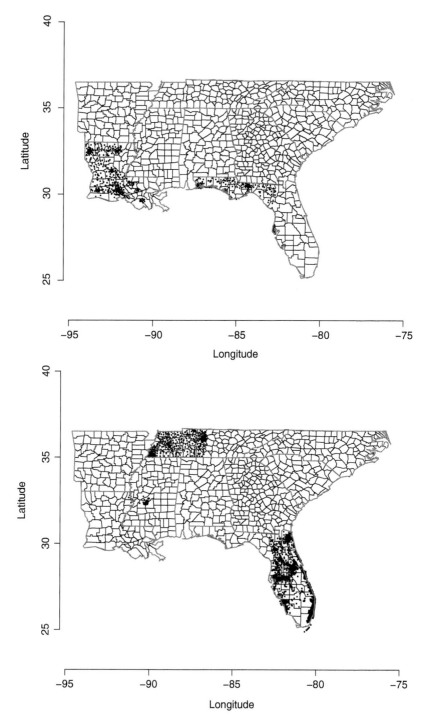

FIGURE 3.5 Significance maps for identifying locations where there is a statistically significant association of provider density to the availability of vaccine, where the association can be positive (top map) or negative (bottom map).

CONCLUSIONS

This chapter has reviewed the concept of health(care) disparities, particularly with applicability to healthcare access. With this chapter, I intended to not only review major disparity measures but to point out the need for more advanced statistical modeling to make inferences on systematic disparities for identifying inequities in access and other outcomes. I highlighted that reducing disparities in healthcare access involves important considerations as to what sub-populations and/or disparities are to be targeted. I also presented one specific example that is relevant to making inference on disparities for pediatric primary care access and how to use the modeling approaches to target interventions that could reduce disparities given a population group to be targeted (e.g. children with Medicaid insurance) or based on geographic variations alone. I also briefly presented a case study in which I illustrated how to make inference on the association between spatial access measures and factors known to influence access in the context of the 2009 H1N1 vaccination campaign.

ACKNOWLEDGMENTS

This chapter draws substantially upon the research of Stewart Curry, who has investigated the existing research on disparity measures, and of recently published research papers in the field; Stewart provided a good portion of the material introduced in the overview section of systematic disparity measures. The author is thankful to Stewart for also reviewing this chapter and for providing used suggestions on improving the presentation. I also gratefully acknowledge the contributions of Monica Gentili, Pravara Harati, Jessica Heir Stamm, Jean O'Connor and Julie Swann, who have been given their permission to illustrate the concepts and methodologies presented in this chapter using the studies from our collaborative research.

REFERENCES

Assuncao, R.M. (2003). Space varying coefficient models for small area data. *Environmetrics* **14**: 453–473.

Atkinson, A.B. (1970). On the measurement of inequality. *Journal of Economic Theory* **2**: 244–263.

Baicker, K., Chandra, A., and Skinner, J.S. (2005). Geographic variation in health care and the problem of measuring racial disparities. *Perspectives in Biology and Medicine* **48**(1): S42–S53.

Bayoumi, A.M. (2009). Equity and health services. *Journal of Public Health Policy* **30**(2): 176–182.

Berman, M. and Diggle, P.J. (1989). Estimating weighted integrals of the second-order intensity of spatial point patterns. *Journal of the Royal Statistical Society: Series B* **51**(1): 81–92.

Berman, S., Dolins, J., Tang, S.-F., and Yudkowsky, B. (2002). Factors that influence the willingness of private primary care pediatricians to accept more medicaid patients. *Pediatrics* **110**(2): 239–248.

Biewen, M. (2002). Bootstrap inference for inequality, mobility and poverty measurement. *Journal of Econometrics* **108**(2): 317–342.

Borrell, L.N. and Talih, M. (2011). A symmetrized Theil index measure of health disparities: an example using dental caries in U.S. children and adolescents. *Statistics in Medicine* **30**(3): 277–290.

Braveman, P. and Gruskin, S. (2003). Defining equity in health. *Journal of Epidemiology and Community Health* **57**(4): 254–258.

Brown, T.M., Parmar, G., Durant, R.W. et al. (2011). Health professional shortage areas, insurance status, and cardiovascular disease prevention in the reasons for geographic and racial differences in stroke (REGARDS) study. *Journal of Health Care for the Poor and Underserved* **22**(4): 1179–1189.

Browning, C.R., Cagney, K.A., and Wen, M. (2003). Explaining variation in health status across space and time: implications for racial and ethnic disparities in self-rated health. *Social Science and Medicine* **57**(7): 1221–1235.

Cao, S., Gentili, M., Griffin, P. et al. (2017). Disparities in preventive dental care among children in Georgia. *Preventing Chronic Disease* **14**: 170176.

Chandra, A. and Skinner, J. (2003). *Geography and Racial Health Disparities*. National Bureau of Economic Research.

Chen, J.T., Rehkopf, D.H., Waterman, P.D. et al. (2006). Mapping and measuring social disparities in premature mortality: the impact of census tract poverty within and across Boston neighborhoods, 1999–2001. *Journal of Urban Health: Bulletin of the New York Academy of Medicine* **83**(6): 1063–1084.

Cowell, F.A. and Mehta, F. (1982). The estimation and interpolation of inequality measures. *Review of Economic Studies* **49**(2): 273–290.

Cressie, N.A.C. (1993). *Statistics for Spatial Data*. New York, NY: Wiley.

Dai, D. (2010). Black residential segregation, disparities in spatial access to health care facilities, and late-stage breast cancer diagnosis in metropolitan Detroit. *Health and Place* **16**(5): 1038–1052.

Dubin, R.A. (1998). Spatial autocorrelation: a primer. *Journal of Housing Economics* **7**(4): 304–327.

ESRI (2006). *Community Sourcebook America with ArcReader*. Redlands, CA.

Fleurbaey, M. and Schokkaert, E. (2009). Unfair inequalities in health and health care. *Journal of Health Economics* **28**: 73–90.

Gelfand, A.E., Kim, H.-J., Sirmans, C.F., and Banerjee, S. (2003). Spatial modeling with spatially varying coefficient processes. *Journal of the American Statistical Association* **98**(462): 387–396.

Gentili, M., Isett, K., Serban, N., and Swann, J. (2015). Small-area estimation of spatial access to pediatric primary care and its implications for policy. *Journal of Urban Health* **92**(5): 864–909.

Gentili, M., Serban, N., Harati, P. et al. (2018). Quantifying disparities in accessibility and availability of pediatric primary care with implications for policy. *Health Services Research* **53**(3): 1458–1477.

Gordon-Larsen, P., Nelson, M.C., Page, P., and Popkin, B.M. (2006). Inequality in the built environment underlies key health disparities in physical activity and obesity. *Pediatrics* **117**(2): 417–424.

Gotway, C.A. and Young, L.J. (2002). Combining incompatible spatial data. *Journal of the American Statistical Association* **97**: 632–648.

Grady, S.C. (2006). Racial disparities in low birthweight and the contribution of residential segregation: a multilevel analysis. *Social Science and Medicine* **63**(12): 3013–3029.

Harper, S. and J. Lynch (2009). Measuring Health Disparitieshttps://open.umich.edu/find/open-educational-resources/public-health/measuring-health-disparities (accessed June 2019).

Harper, S. and Lynch, J. (2012). *Methods for Measuring Cancer Disparities: Using Data Relevant to Healthy People 2010 Cancer-Related Objectives*. National Cancer Institute.

Harper, S., Lynch, J., Meersman, S.C. et al. (2008). An overview of methods for monitoring social disparities in cancer with an example using trends in lung cancer incidence by area-socioeconomic position and race-ethnicity, 1992–2004. *American Journal of Epidemiology* **167**(8): 889–899.

Harper, S., King, N.B., Meersman, S.C. et al. (2010). Implicit value judgments in the measurement of health inequalities. *Milbank Quarterly* **88**(1): 4–29.

Haughton, J. and Khandker, S.R. (2009). *Handbook on Poverty and Inequality*. Washington, DC: The World Bank.

Hayward, P., Cramer, B., Nepaul, A. et al. (2008). *The Spatial Context of Health Disparities: A Literature Review*. Hartford, CT: Connecticut Department of Public Health.

Healthy People 2020. (2010). About healthy people. http://www.healthypeople.gov/2020/about/default.aspx (accessed July 2018).

Heir Stamm, J., Serban, N., Swann, J.L. et al. (2017). Quantifying and explaining accessibility with application to the 2009 H1N1 vaccination campaign. *Health Care Management Science* **20**(1): 76–93.

Kaiser Family Foundation.(n.d.) Medicaid MCO Access Standards: Primary Carehttps://www.kff.org/other/state-indicator/medicaid-mco-access-standards-primary-care/ (accessed January 2019).

Kramer, M.R., Cooper, H.L., Drews-Botsch, C.D. et al. (2010). Metropolitan isolation segregation and Black-White disparities in very preterm birth: a test of mediating pathways and variance explained. *Social Science and Medicine* **71**(12): 2108–2116.

Krieger, N., Chen, J.T., Waterman, P.D. et al. (2002). Geocoding and monitoring of US socioeconomic inequalities in mortality and cancer incidence: does the choice of area-based measure and geographic level matter? the public health disparities geocoding project. *American Journal of Epidemiology* **156**: 471–482.

Krivobokova, T., Kneib, T., and Claeskens, G. (2010). Simultaneous confidence bands for penalized spline estimators. *Journal of the American Statistical Association* **105**(490): 852–863.

Laporte, A. (2002). A note on the use of a single inequality index in testing the effect of income distribution on mortality. *Social Science and Medicine* **55**(9): 1561–1570.

Levy, J.I., Chemerynski, S.M., and Tuchmann, J.L. (2006). Incorporating concepts of inequality and inequity into health benefits analysis. *International Journal for Equity in Health* **5**(2) https://doi.org/10.1186/1475-9276-5-2.

Luo, W. and Qi, Y. (2009). An enhanced two-step floating catchment area (E2SFCA) method for measuring spatial accessibility to primary care physicians. *Health and Place* **15**(4): 1100–1107.

Mackenbach, J.P. and Kunst, A.E. (1997). Measuring the magnitude of socio-economic inequalities in health: an overview of available measures illustrated with two examples from Europe. *Social Science and Medicine* **44**(6): 757–771.

Maika, A., Mittinty, M.N., Brinkman, S. et al. (2013). Changes in socioeconomic inequality in Indonesian children's cognitive function from 2000 to 2007: a decomposition analysis. *PLoS One* **8**(10) https://doi.org/10.1371/journal.pone.0078809.

Morrill, R., Cromartie, J., and Hart, G. (1999). Metropolitan, urban, and rural commuting areas: toward a better depiction of the United States settlement system. *Urban Geography* **20**(8): 727–748.

Morrison, E.E. (2009). *Health Care Ethics: Critical Issues for the 21st Century*. Ontario, Canada: Jones & Bartlett Publishers.

Nobles, M., Serban, N., and Swann, J. (2014). Measurement and inference on pediatric healthcare accessibility. *Annals of Applied Statistics* **8**(4): 1922–1946.

O'Donnell, O., van Doorslaer, E., Wagstaff, A., and Lindelow, M. (2008). *Analyzing Health Equity Using Household Survey Data: A Guide to Techniques and Their Implementation*. Washington, DC: The World Bank.

Pearcy, J.N. and Keppel, K.G. (2002). A summary measure of health disparity. *Public Health Reports* **117**(3): 273–280.

Perloff, J.D., Kletke, P., and Fossett, J. (1995). Which physicians limit their medicaid participation, and why. *Health Services Research* **30**(1): 7–26.

Public Health Disparities Geocoding Project (2000). U.S. census tract poverty data 2000. Harvard School of Public Health.

Raghunathan, T.E. (2006). Combining information from multiple surveys for assessing health disparities. *Allgemeines Statistisches Archiv* **90**: 515–526.

Regidor, E., Calle, M.E., and Dominguez, V. (2003). Trends in the association between average income, poverty and income inequality and life expectancy in Spain. *Social Science and Medicine* **56**(5): 961–971.

Serban, N. (2011). A space–time varying coefficient model: the equity of service accessibility. *The Annals of Applied Statistics* **5**(3): 2024–2051.

Sergeant, J.C. and Firth, D. (2006). Relative index of inequality: definition, estimation, and inference. *Biostatistics* **7**(2): 213–224.

Singh, G.K. and Siahpush, M. (2006). Widening socioeconomic inequalities in US life expectancy, 1980–2000. *International Journal of Epidemiology* **35**(4): 969–979.

Skinner, J., Weinstein, J.N., Sporer, S.M., and Wennberg, J.E. (2003). Racial, ethnic, and geographic disparities in rates of knee arthroplasty among medicare patients. *New England Journal of Medicine* **349**(14): 1350–1359.

Talih, M. (2013). A reference-invariant health disparity index based on Renyi divergence. *Annals of Applied Statistics* **7**(2): 1217–1243.

Tassone, E.C., Waller, L.A., and Casper, M.L. (2009). Small-area racial disparity in stroke mortality an application of Bayesian spatial hierarchical modeling. *Epidemiology* **20**(2): 234–241.

Theil, H. (1967). *Economics and Information Theory*. Amsterdam: North Holland.

US Department of Health and Human Services (2003). *National Healthcare Disparities Report*. Rockville, MD: Agency for Healthcare Research and Quality.

US Department of Health and Human Services (2000). *Healthy People 2010: Understanding and Improving Health*. Washington, DC: US Government Printing Office.

Wagstaff, A. (2002). Inequality aversion, health inequalities and health achievement. *Journal of Health Economics* **21**(4): 627–641.

Wagstaff, A., Paci, P., and van Doorslaer, E. (1991). On the measurement of inequalities in health. *Social Science and Medicine* **33**(5): 545–557.

Waller, L.A., Louis, T.A., and Carlin, B.P. (1999). Environmental justice and statistical summaries of differences in exposure distributions. *Journal of Exposure Analysis and Environmental Epidemiology* **9**(1): 56–65.

Waller, L.A., Zhu, L., Gotway, C.A. et al. (2007). Quantifying geographic variations in associations between alcohol distribution and violence: a comparison of geographically weighted regression and spatially varying coefficient models. *Stochastic Environmental Research and Risk Assessment* **21**(5): 573–588.

Wood, S.N. (2006). *Generalized Additive Models, an Introduction with R*. Chapman & Hall.

4

LINKING ACCESS TO HEALTH OUTCOMES

The United States Institute of Medicine (IOM) defined access as the "timely use of personal health services to achieve the best possible outcome" (Institute of Medicine 1993). Access to healthcare does not guarantee good health and appropriate health outcomes. Nevertheless, access to healthcare is critical to ensuring that society enjoys optimal health, economic opportunities, productivity, and well-being. Facilitating access can be viewed as mediating appropriate utilization of healthcare resources to preserve or improve individual and population health. Appropriate access to healthcare can result in less disparate outcomes, reduced healthcare costs by preventing medical crises, and lower use of the emergency room (ER) to treat preventable conditions (Penchansky and Thomas 1981; Wyszewianski 2002).

The underlying premise of this chapter, thus of this book, is that healthcare access is an actionable approach for improving public health but it does not address health outcomes entirely. Healthcare access is necessary to utilize healthcare services toward achieving good outcomes, in interaction with other factors influencing outcomes.

In the first two chapters of this book, I differentiated between realized and potential access, where *realized access* refers to the direct utilization of healthcare services, and *potential access* refers to the opportunity to utilize services (Khan 1992; Guagliardo 2004; McGrail and Humphreys 2009). Under this conceptual framework, it is the realized access that directly impacts health(care) outcomes; however, appropriate healthcare utilization follows when potential access to healthcare services exists and it is tailored to the needs of a population of interest. When studying the link between healthcare access and outcomes, it is thus important to understand the relationship with respect to both potential access (indirect link) and realized access (direct link). *Does the potential access lead to increased utilization of appropriate healthcare services and to improved outcomes? Does the realized access result in reducing severe outcomes and in maintaining health and wellness? Does the realized access comply with recommended care? If not, is this because of lack of potential access or other factors?*

Healthcare System Access: Measurement, Inference, and Intervention, Nicoleta Serban.
© 2020 John Wiley & Sons, Inc. Published 2020 by John Wiley & Sons, Inc.

On one hand, to improve outcomes, healthcare access needs to be complemented by improvements in other factors, for example, community opportunities and norms, health education, health status and health history, expectations, belief system, among others. Some of the factors are also actionable, such as raising the level of health education, and they can impact directly on the health outcomes. Other factors are not actionable while they can influence outcomes to a great extent, thus simply acting as confounding variables as I will describe later in this chapter.

On the other hand, there are also factors that directly constrain healthcare access, including system constraints, for example, mobility or access to means of transportation; or information about preferences, for example, seeing a specialist versus a primary care provider. Such factors can be specified as constraints or preferences in the estimation of healthcare access as presented in Chapter 2 of this book. In analyzing the link between access and outcomes, it is important to distinguish between confounding factors and access constrains or preferences, particularly, in targeting interventions and policies.

In studying the relationship between access and outcomes, not the least important is establishing the primary objectives in targeting interventions. For this, the outcomes of interest need to be clearly delineated along with other factors influencing the link between access and outcomes. The outcomes can focus on one or more of the system levels, specifically, the people, processes, organizations, and society levels characterizing the healthcare system (Figure 2.2).

The health outcomes can be delineated following other multilevel representations of the healthcare system, for example, as a pyramid with the clinical level on the bottom, followed by the administrative level and then by the policy level (Statistics Canada and Canadian Institute for Health Information 2012). Under this representation, health outcomes would be derived at the clinical level to manage individual-level healthcare; further clinical outcomes can be aggregated into relevant indicators at the administrative and policy levels for decision making. Another representation is from the stakeholders' perspectives, with health outcomes differentiated by provider, patient, payer, regulatory, industry, academic, and society (Velentgas et al. 2013).

Such frameworks for characterizing health outcomes suggest that there are various types of outcomes of interest in the context of health(care) interventions and policy, particularly, those targeting healthcare access. I will expand on different types of outcomes in the next section.

OVERVIEW OF HEALTH OUTCOMES

The World Health Organization (WHO) defines an *outcome measure* as a "change in the health of an individual, group of people, or population that is attributable to an intervention or series of interventions." In this book, the central theme is healthcare access, which can influence outcomes related to many facets of the health and well-being of people as well as more generally of the healthcare system. In this section, I will describe several examples of outcomes, particularly those which can be improved with adequate healthcare access. The main categories of outcomes include:

- *Clinical outcomes*, referring to measurements of organs' functions, commonly tailored to a specific condition, for example, the forced expiratory volume in one second as a percentage of predicted volume (%FEV1) for lung function of patients with cystic fibrosis (CF) (Wang et al. 1993; Hankinson et al. 1999), or the fasting blood glucose for patients with diabetes. Such measures are meaningful for making decisions on diagnosis and treatment by health professionals but not directly observed by the patients, unless measured and shared by the health professionals with them.

- *Wellbeing outcomes*, referring to *health status measures*, e.g. body mass index (BMI), risk of developing chronic or acute conditions and number of oral cavities; *individual-reported measures*, e.g. how much pain a patient may be in, whether a patient can carry out usual activities; and *population health measures*, e.g. morbidity, mortality, prevalence of a condition. Such measures may not necessarily target a specific health condition. They generally reflect various aspects of wellbeing and health.

- *Healthcare outcomes*, referring to utilization of healthcare services, such as emergency department visits, physician office (PO) visits, medication adherence or treatment compliance with recommended care, as well as healthcare expenditure of the related utilization measures. Because clinical and wellbeing measures are not readily available in many studies, healthcare outcomes are used as proxies.

- *System outcomes*, referring to overall outcomes at the system or society level, measuring, for example, performance of the system, disparities in wellbeing or healthcare outcomes; or risk of chronic conditions by race, income; and referring to organizational and provider outcomes such as emergency department volume. System outcomes can be intended or unintended consequences of public health policies and legislation.

Other reports and studies have provided different frameworks for distinguishing among types of outcomes. Velentgas et al. (2013) overview two established frameworks, particularly in the context of comparative effectiveness research (CER), and provide their own classification of outcomes, differentiated into clinical, humanistic, and economic and utilization outcome measures. According to this classification, *clinical outcomes* involve a diagnosis or assessment by a health care provider; *humanistic outcomes* are health-related quality of life (HRQoL) outcomes and more generally patient-reported outcomes; and the *economic and utilization outcomes* include measures of health resource utilization, representing the payer and the societal perspective. Clinical outcomes by Velentgas et al. (2013) overlap with the definition of clinical outcomes in the framework I propose, where the primary focus is on a diagnosed condition, with outcomes derived from the assessment by a healthcare provider as well as from the individual's reported experience with the diagnosed condition. Moreover, the economic and utilization outcomes are healthcare outcomes in my definition; however, I contend that healthcare outcomes are more general since they can capture interaction with the healthcare system beyond utilization and expenditure. Because the measures by Velentgas et al. (2013)

focus on CER studies, system outcomes are not of interest and thus are not included in their classification.

Another classification by the Canadian Health Institute is into *patient-related* and *health system performance-related outcomes*, primarily defined in the context of interventions and decision making toward improving health and healthcare (Statistics Canada and Canadian Institute for Health Information 2008). Patient-related outcomes are further represented by health, health-related and non-health related outcomes. Health outcomes are those that lead to changes in health status in response to an intervention. Health-related outcomes are healthcare utilization measures that can be used as proxies of the health status (e.g. emergency department visits). The non-health related outcomes are those reported by the patients, for example, satisfaction with the healthcare provided. Health system performance-related outcomes can be indicators based on the patient-related outcomes and other factors influencing health.

Comparing this last framework with the classification of outcomes adopted in this book, patient-related outcomes can be those differentiated into clinical, well-being, and healthcare outcomes whereas the health system performance-related outcomes can be a subset of the system outcomes. The (patient-related) health outcomes defined by the Canadian Health Institute (Statistics Canada and Canadian Institute for Health Information 2008) are overall measures of the health status such as HRQoL (quality-adjusted life year [QALY]) or healthy year equivalents (HYEs), used for a global assessment of a health(care)intervention. These measures are not necessarily targeting improvement in one specific condition but in the overall health; thus, they are relevant in improving access in some dimensions but not others. For example, financial access can be linked to QALYs but distance to specialized care may be linked to more specific clinical and/or wellbeing outcomes. Health status measured by such global measures rely on information and data not widely available, thus health-related outcomes (e.g. healthcare measures) can be used as proxy measures for health status.

While these two other frameworks provide similar classifications, I prefer to use the classification introduced in this book since it provides a mapping to both frameworks, and it also has broader applicability in studies of the links between health outcomes and healthcare access.

I will conclude this section by highlighting that existing research has introduced a broad spectrum of outcomes that were studied within varying public health contexts. Without attempting to be comprehensive, I am providing below multiple examples of outcomes that I have encountered in my research inquiries over the years:

- *General wellbeing outcomes*: morbidity, mortality, disability-adjusted life years (DALYs), HRQoL, QALYs (Deswal et al. 2004; Beratarrechea et al. 2014; Gulliford et al. 2017).

- *Patient-reported outcomes*: behavioral or lifestyle changes; (patient-provider) satisfaction; ability to demonstrate taking medications appropriately; ability to interpret labels and health messages; self-reported health status; limitations in activities of daily living (ADLs); self-reported measures of adult health (fair/poor general health, functional impairment, time off work/school, depressive symptoms, and suicidal ideation); client-reported functioning; case manager clinical ratings to predict subsequent client functional status; self-reported medication underuse; the number of days in a month of poor physical and mental health (Hendryx et al. 1999; Berkman et al. 2011; Beratarrechea et al. 2014; Briesacher et al. 2015; Hargreaves et al. 2015; Venkataramani et al. 2016).

- *Healthcare outcomes*: costs incurred by the patient; compliance with recommended guidelines; hospitalization rates; use of emergency care; supply of secondary care resources; readmission rates after inpatient rehabilitation; nursing home resident hospitalizations (Giuffrida et al. 1999; Berkman et al. 2011; Beratarrechea et al. 2014; Oliver et al. 2014; Briesacher et al. 2015).

- *Women, maternal, and infant health*: mammography screening and uptake of influenza vaccine; birth spacing; antenatal care during pregnancy; birth and newborn care preparedness; emergency obstetrical care; initiation of breastfeeding; maternity care coordination; use of family planning services; number of obstetrical encounters; routine prenatal and illness-related services; excessive pregnancy weight gain; pre-pregnancy BMI; preterm birth; low birthweight; perinatal death; prevalence of gestational diabetes and hypertension; mortality rates for four leading causes of death for women in the United States (heart disease, stroke, lung cancer, and breast cancer); infant mortality (Wisdom et al. 2005; Gavin et al. 2006; Bhutta et al. 2010; Berkman et al. 2011; Cilenti et al. 2015; Haraldsdottir et al. 2015; Harris et al. 2015).

- *Mental and behavioral health*: co-morbidity; timely diagnosis; quality of life including level of stress or sense of belonging; BMI; rates of medication; compliance with recommended care; alcohol and/or drug consumption; rates of depression management by GPs; rates of mental health care claims; referrals; prescribing and counseling rates (Statistics Canada and Canadian Institute for Health Information 2008; Harrison et al. 2012; Moran et al. 2019).

- *Diabetes care*: average A1C level and uncontrolled A1C; blood cholesterol; blood pressure; compliance with recommended care for foot and eye examination; BMI; co-morbidity; mortality; frequencies of physician visits; health insurance coverage; screening for diabetes complications; treatment for hyperglycemia, hypertension, and dyslipidemia; medical history; self-reported medication underuse as a result of cost; symptom burden; and 12-Item Short-Form physical and mental functioning scores (Harris 2000, 2001; Piette et al. 2004; Statistics Canada and Canadian Institute for Health Information 2008; Prentice et al. 2013).

All the outcomes described above reflect some aspects of the health of a population with a focus on a specific type of healthcare and/or condition. Moreover, some health outcomes can be directly impacted by healthcare access but some only indirectly. It is important to establish the association model between outcomes and access, with the specification of the *outcome data type* (e.g. longitudinal, dichotomous, or numeric), *outcome classification* (e.g. clinical, system), *whether univariate or multivariate* (e.g. mortality versus both mortality and morbidity), or *whether a specific condition to be targeted* (e.g. diabetes) as well as the access dimension to be consider in the study. Further details are provided in the next section.

MODELING THE RELATIONSHIP BETWEEN ACCESS AND OUTCOMES

Health outcomes research is a methodology used to evaluate the link between treatments or interventions delivered and the actual outcomes achieved, to determine *what works and what doesn't* in healthcare. As I highlighted earlier in this chapter, the ways that health interventions generate health outcomes involve the complexities of human biology, individual preferences, environment, and system constraints, among others. Such complexities are also pertinent to the link between health outcomes and healthcare access.

Studies related to linking health outcomes to access measures have provided evidence of statistical significance of this linkage. These studies address various health outcomes and specialties, including breast cancer (Dasgupta et al. 2012), cardiac diseases (Graves 2010), colon cancer (Haas et al. 2011), neonatal mortality (Kazembe and Mpeketula 2010), diabetes care (Statistics Canada and Canadian Institute for Health Information 2008; Ahern et al. 2011; Prentice et al. 2013), and pediatric asthma (Teach et al. 2006), among many others. Many studies focus on the relationship between health outcomes and the financial dimension of access (Ayanian et al. 1993; Piette et al. 2004; Oswald et al. 2007; Currie et al. 2008). Primary care is also at the forefront of many studies of the link between outcomes and access (Laditka et al. 2003; Aakvik and Holmas 2006).

In many such related studies, a first simple approach to identify the potential dependence between outcomes and access is to simply contrast the maps of access measures and health outcomes. Although visual analytics could be useful in inferring general trends about the geography of the association between outcomes and access, more advanced statistical models are needed for informed evaluation of interventions.

Regression analysis is the most common tool in modeling the relationship between health outcomes and healthcare access. For dichotomous observed outcomes or discretely observed count outcomes, the most common modeling approach is the generalized linear model (Giuffrida et al. 1999; Johnson and Rimsza 2004; Mulvihill et al. 2007; Oswald et al. 2007; Grembowski et al. 2008; Fisher and Mascarenhas 2009; Long et al. 2013; Balcazar et al. 2015; Delphin-Rittmon et al. 2015; Han et al. 2015; Haraldsdottir et al. 2015; Hargreaves et al. 2015; Venkataramani et al. 2016). Other models include probabilistic Markov models for costs and outcomes of increasing access to bariatric surgery in obese adults (Gulliford et al. 2017); the proportional-hazards regression analysis to control for age, race, marital status, household income, coexisting diagnoses, and disease stage in modeling health insurance versus outcomes among women with breast cancer (Ayanian et al. 1993); and propensity score-adjusted multivariate regressions for linking outcomes to usual source of care (Witt et al. 2017), among many others. For the most part, these studies address two main questions: *Is there a statistically significant association between outcomes and access? Does this association systematically vary across population subgroups?* However, informing policy and making decisions requires going beyond these exploratory questions; multiple aspects of the relationship between outcomes and access need to be evaluated:

1. *What are the characteristics of the communities where this association is negative or positive? Are there inequities or positive deviances suggested by this association?*
2. *Are there common characteristics of significant positive or negative associations across multiple outcomes and/or across similar conditions?*
3. *Where are interventions needed to address reduced access and severe outcomes?*

Informing interventions by addressing these questions involves additional efforts to develop rigorous models for statistically assessing the significance of the association between outcome and access measures globally and locally. This is critical when many possible interventions could be competing for limited budgets. Drawing on the most effective decisions to intervene on improving health outcomes (and possibly in specific areas) cannot be realized without a large amount of information, principled analysis, and rigorous modeling of the link between access and outcomes. Toward supporting a principled outcome analysis, there are important aspects to be considered as outlined next.

Selection of the Outcome(s) of Interest

Generally when assessing health outcomes, it is not just one outcome of interest. There may be multiple outcomes that can be used in evaluating the enactment of an intervention or a policy. For example, for patients with diabetes, clinical outcomes of interest could include blood pressure, glycosylated hemoglobin, fasting blood glucose; wellbeing outcomes include whether the patient develops diabetic retinopathy, BMI; and healthcare outcomes include the rate of emergency department visits or hospitalizations. When seeking the link to healthcare access, one or all such outcomes may be considered depending on the end point of the intervention to be targeted. Velentgas et al. (2013) defined them as *composite endpoints*. They point out that the study power for a given sample size may be increased when such composite measures are used as compared with individual outcomes, since by grouping numerous types of events into a larger category, the composite endpoint will occur more frequently than any of the individual components.

While I attempted to group the health outcomes into the four categories, including clinical, wellbeing, healthcare, and system outcomes, I will admit that there is a fine line between the four categories. For example, a wellness outcome can also be a clinical outcome (e.g. BMI) and a system outcome can also be a healthcare outcome (e.g. expenditure). Moreover, health outcomes across all categories are also highly correlated with each other since one outcome can drive or impact other outcomes. Because of the strong dependence, studies on the link between outcomes and access commonly target one primary outcome. Modeling the relationship between outcomes and access requires advanced statistical modeling, thus analyzing multiple outcomes simultaneously will not only add to the complexity of the statistical modeling but also to the complexity of the interpretation of the relationship and its implication in decision making.

Moreover, clinical outcomes are only indirectly related to access while healthcare and system outcomes can be directly impacted as I also pointed out in the introduction to this chapter. In fact, addressing healthcare and system outcomes is a precursor of improving clinical and wellbeing outcomes. Thus many policies and interventions focus on healthcare and system outcomes. In the case studies of this chapter, I will illustrate the relationship between access and outcomes for both clinical (in a study for patients with CF) and healthcare outcomes (in a case study for children diagnosed with asthma).

Outcome Data Type

Similarly to the discussion in the previous section, outcomes can take various data types. Below I will cover most common types.

- *Binary* or *dichotomous* outcomes can take only two levels, i.e. they are categorical factors with only two categories. Examples of dichotomous outcomes include whether an individual is obese, whether he/she has a specific condition (e.g. diabetes), or whether he/she has a severe outcome (e.g. hospitalization). More generally, the qualitative outcomes are categorical factors with multiple categories. Examples of qualitative outcomes are the multiple stages of a condition (e.g. diabetes without diabetic retinopathy, with diabetic retinopathy or blindness), clinical health status (e.g. provided by clinical risk grouping such as the 3M™ Core Grouping Software), or rurality of provider practice location for providers accepting Medicaid.

- *Discrete count* outcomes are counts or number of occurrences of an event, condition or action. Examples of count outcomes include the number of emergency department visits with an asthma diagnosis, number of opiate prescriptions, and number of children at risk of caries among others.

- *Continuous numerical* outcomes are those that take values in a given interval of numbers, can be clinical measurements or lab results, or they can be represented by the average, median, or some other summary of the outcomes of the individuals in a population. Examples of numeric outcomes are the fasting blood glucose level of an individual, percentage of adults with diabetes, and the rate of hospitalizations among patients with acute conditions, among many others.

Another important aspect in establishing the outcome data type is the level of granularity of the observed outcome of interest, for example, outcomes can be observed at the individual level but also in aggregate for a sub-population. Commonly, dichotomous outcomes are observed at the individual level. Count and numerical outcomes can be observed both at the individual level (e.g. number of prescriptions filled within a year by a patient, BMI) but also aggregated over a population (e.g. number or prevalence of children with asthma).

Individual or aggregated outcomes can vary across communities within a geographic region, particularly when studying the link between outcomes and access. For geographically varying outcomes, it is important to note that they are not independent; they are spatially dependent. Outcomes of proximal communities will tend to be more similar than those of communities far away from each other. This is because of the similarities in the population and environment characteristics of neighboring communities.

Spatial dependence in geographically varying outcomes can be weak if the division of the geographic region is not highly granular, for example, the county division in some states of the United States like California. But if the division of the geographic region is highly granular, spatial dependence between the geographic units can be strong and thus rigorous modeling of the link between outcomes and access needs to account for the spatial dependence. Disregarding spatial dependence results in estimation of the variability in the data to be lower than it actually is, possibly resulting in misleading statistical significance of the link between outcomes and the explanatory variables of interest, for example, healthcare access.

Outcomes can also be observed longitudinally or varying over time. Below examples of such outcomes are provided:

Example 1: *Temporally varying numeric outcomes* – the outcome is observed at equally spaced time points, and it can be observed at the individual or (sub)population level. For example, the outcome can be the average, the count or the rate over a fixed period of time observed over multiple years. An example is the monthly number of psychological services received for a child diagnosed with attention deficit hyperactivity disorder (ADHD) over the course of the treatment of his/her condition. Another example is the daily volume of patients at an emergency department unit over the course of several years. A third example is the number of emergency department visits per Medicaid-insured child diagnosed with depression per year with comparisons across multiple states as shown in Figure 4.1.

Example 2: *Longitudinal observations of an individual-level numeric or count outcome* – an individual has multiple healthcare visits at a provider, with the same outcome recorded at each visit, over a period of time. An example of such outcome is provided in the first case study introduced in this chapter, where the outcome of interest is the %FEV1 for patients with CF as shown in Figure 4.2.

Example 3: *Longitudinal sequence of healthcare events* – an individual interacts with the healthcare system through a series of healthcare events including visits to the PO, emergency department encounters, hospitalizations, and medication. The events happen over a period of time, where the timing of the events and the order of the events is not known in advance, only known at the time of

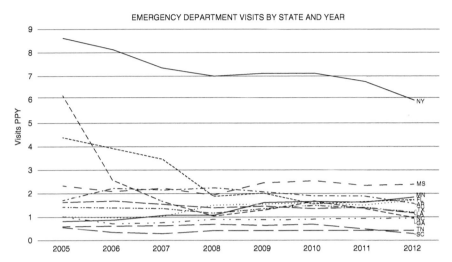

FIGURE 4.1 Emergency department utilization (number of visits per patient per year or PPPY) for Medicaid-insured adolescents diagnosed with depression, by state from 2005 to 2012. *Note:* PPPY is calculated as the aggregated count for emergency department events divided by the total number of enrollment months for all the adolescents with those services multiplied by 12.

the occurrence. An example of such outcome is provided in the third case study introduced in this chapter, where the outcome is a sequence of health-care utilization of individual children diagnosed with asthma. An illustration of utilization sequences is shown in Figure 4.3.

Example 4: Temporally varying binary outcomes – the outcome is observed at equally spaced time points, and it is commonly an individual dichotomous outcome. An example is whether the patient had an emergency department visit over the course of a year recorded for multiple years consecutively. Another example is whether the symptoms of a targeted condition have ameliorated, recorded monthly over the course of a year.

Why is it important to clearly delineate the data type of an outcome? The modeling approaches will be different depending on the data type, whether observed geographically, temporally, or longitudinally as shown in the next section.

Modeling Approaches

The common modeling framework for assessing the relationship between health outcomes and healthcare access is a regression in which the relationship can be estimated marginally (without accounting for other factors) or conditionally (accounting for other factors). Regression analysis is primarily applied in health services research in its simplest version, the classic multiple linear regression assuming linear relationships; or the classic logistic regression where the outcome variable is binary and the underlying relationship to the explanatory factors is

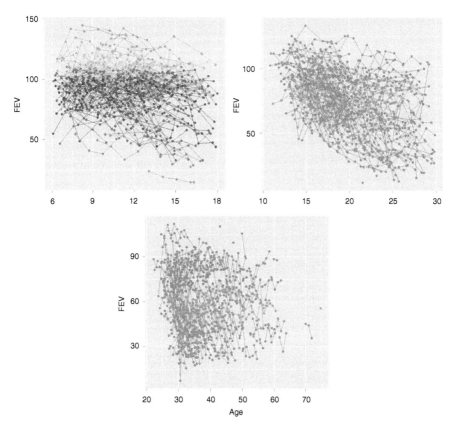

FIGURE 4.2   The %FEV1 versus age of patient of 200 randomly selected patients with cystic fibrosis categorized by age group: (a) children (less than 18 years old); (b) young adults (between 18 and 30); and (c) adults (more than 30 years old). Each connected line corresponds to the outcome versus age of one patient.

expressed linearly. These two approaches assume that the outcomes observed over multiple individuals or sub-populations are independent or uncorrelated, that the relationship does not change in time or geographically, and that there is only one outcome of interest or to be targeted for interventions. These are clearly important limitations in outcome studies.

Statistical modeling and machine learning are areas of research offering a broad spectrum of modeling approaches that address such limitations. I will provide a brief account of some modeling approaches that can be employed in health outcomes research, particularly when the outcome data present the challenges discussed above.

Useful models particularly for geographically varying outcomes are the spatial regression models, which can be applied in studies when the outcome of interest is observed over multiple communities within a geographic region, for example. In Chapter 3, I described the spatial-varying model, in which the relationship between

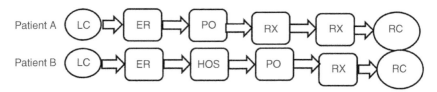

FIGURE 4.3 Two examples of utilization sequences. ER, an event at the emergency department; PO, a physician office visit; and RX, a prescription fill. The left censoring (LC) and right censoring (RC) events refer to the fact that the utilization sequence has been censored, that is, we do not observe the entire utilization sequence, but only over a period of time.

the response variable and the explanatory variable varies spatially or geographically (Gelfand et al. 2003; Waller et al. 2007). In contrast to the modeling setting in Chapter 3, where the response variable of interest was the healthcare access measure, in an outcome study, the response variable is instead a health outcome measure. Specifically, we seek to model the expectation of the response or outcome variable $Y(s)$ given a set of factors, $X_1(s), \ldots, X_r(s)$, where the primary factor of interest is a measure (or more) of healthcare access:

$$g(E\{Y(s) \mid X_1(s), \ldots, X_r(s)\}) = \alpha_1(s)X_1(s) + \cdots + \alpha_r(s)X_r(s)$$

where $E\{\ \}$ stands for expectation, $g()$ is a known link function, and $\alpha_1(s), \ldots, \alpha_r(s)$ are unknown (smooth) functions varying over the space domain $\mathcal{R}$, referred herein as *spatial association maps*. The link function is the identity function when the outcome $Y(s)$ is numeric; the link is the logit or probit function when the outcome is binary; or the link is the log function when the outcome is a count variable. Under this model, a statistically significant and spatially varying association coefficient between an access measure and the outcome response indicates a potential link between outcome and access, given confounding and other explanatory factors being included in the model.

The space-varying coefficient model is actually an extension of the time-varying coefficient model, in which we instead model the relationship between the outcome variable and the explanatory factors as varying in time smoothly (Assuncao 2003; Gelfand et al. 2003; Waller et al. 2007; Serban 2011). The time-varying coefficient model can be used for modeling outcomes that are observed over many time points, not necessarily equally spaced.

The space-varying or time-varying coefficient model is a particular case of a larger class of models in the field of non-parametric regression. The more general model is:

$$g(E\{Y \mid X_1, \ldots, X_r\}) = \alpha_1(X_1) + \cdots + \alpha_r(X_r)$$

where the $\alpha_1(), \ldots, \alpha_r()$ are non-parametric functions varying with the predicting variables. This model is called the generalized additive model (Hastie and Tibshirani 1990). However, I prefer the simpler version of this model, the space-varying or time-varying coefficient model, since it is easier to interpret, particularly in outcome studies.

Longitudinal outcomes are also common in many outcome studies. The classic approach for modeling *longitudinal (numeric) outcomes* is the linear mixed model (LMM), which is an extension of the standard regression model with a random effect introduced to model the variability in repeated measures or longitudinal outcomes (Diggle et al. 2002; Fitzmaurice et al. 2011). Generally, the LMM follows the formula:

$$Y_i = X_i\beta + Z_i b_i + \varepsilon_i$$

where Y_i is the vector of continuous outcomes, for example, corresponding to BMI measurements associated with one patient observed at each PO office visit over multiple such visits:

- $X_i = \begin{bmatrix} X_{11}^{[i]} & \cdots & X_{1p}^{[i]} \\ \vdots & \ddots & \vdots \\ X_{n_i 1}^{[i]} & \cdots & X_{n_i q}^{[i]} \end{bmatrix}$ is the design matrix consisting of the explanatory variables.

- $\beta = \begin{bmatrix} \beta_1 \\ \vdots \\ \beta_p \end{bmatrix}$ is the vector of the fixed effects/coefficients.

- n_i is the recorded measurements for the ith patients and p is the number of fixed effects.

- $Z_i = \begin{bmatrix} Z_{11}^{[i]} & \cdots & Z_{1q}^{[i]} \\ \vdots & \ddots & \vdots \\ Z_{n_i 1}^{[i]} & \cdots & Z_{n_i q}^{[i]} \end{bmatrix}$ contains the q covariates corresponding to the random effects associated with random effects coefficients $b_i = \begin{bmatrix} b_{i1} \\ \vdots \\ b_{iq} \end{bmatrix}$.

Moreover, $b_i \sim N_q(\mathbf{0}, \sigma^2 D)$ are the random effects and $\varepsilon_i \sim N(\mathbf{0}, \sigma^2 \mathbf{R}_i)$ are the residuals associated with the ith patient. Generally, it is assumed that σ^2 is an unknown scale parameter whereas D and $\mathbf{R}_i$ are unknown covariance matrices.

In LMMs applied to longitudinal outcomes, the random effects can be specified for the time covariate but also for other explanatory variables, for example, age of the individuals for which the outcomes are observed. The parameters in the vector β capture the population characteristics that are shared by all the patients, while b_i captures subject-specific variations. For instance, by including age as a random effect in the model, we not only capture how the mean response changes in the population as "age" increases, but also determine how individual longitudinal outcomes change as "age" increases.

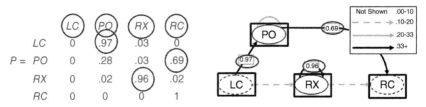

FIGURE 4.4   An example of a transition matrix (*P*) where only two events are represented (PO, physician visit; and RX, medication) along with the left censoring (LC) and right censoring (RC). On the left, the transition matrix is visualized as a network.

Individual-level utilization sequences are longitudinal realizations of patients' healthcare utilization in chronological order and with different interarrival times between events; modeling such individual-level sequences requires an approach that accounts for the order of events and the distribution of the interarrival times, an example of a modeling approach being the Markov renewal process (MRP) (Foufoula-Georgiou and Lettenmaier 1987). Under this model, for each pair of event types, e.g. an emergency department occurrence (ER) and a PO visit, a transition probability is estimated along with an inter-event time distribution. For example, the transition probability from ER to PO is the probability of a patient to have had an emergency department visit event followed by a physician visit, with the inter-event time between ER and PO being a random variable, assumed to have a parametric distribution. Although the Markov assumption (upon entry to an event, future events and future inter-event times depend only on the current event) is restrictive, the MRP model has advantages over more advanced statistical models; for example, the model output can be visualized using simple network graphs as illustrated in Figure 4.4. In this figure, the transition matrix is translated into a network, where the nodes are different healthcare events, including the left censoring (LC) and the right censoring (RC) events due to the fact that the utilization sequence has been censored, that is, we do not observe the entire utilization sequence, but only over a period of time. The links between the nodes have different strength and direction, depending on the probabilities of transition from one event to another. For example, there is no link between PO and medication (RX) in this network since the transition probabilities between the two events are 0.03 and 0.02 (provided in the accompanying transition matrix), which are very small probability values. In the same network, there is a link from LC to PO with probability 0.97, specifying that most patients represented by a utilization profile characterized by the transition matrix having PO as the first event observed.

However, the Markov model briefly introduced above is limited in many ways. The first limitation is that it does not account for missing data in utilization sequences. Utilization sequences derived from claims data are subject to data censoring, referring to missed events when a patient may not be eligible for health insurance or events occurring outside the study time period. The second limitation is an insufficient treatment of the effects of different event types on the prevalence of visits to a specific provider type. Each patient potentially visits multiple provider types repeatedly over the time period of interest. Thus, we have a competing-risks, repeated-events framework. A third limitation involves incorporating demographic and health-related covariates to explain variations in healthcare utilization.

To address the limitations presented above, another approach to modeling individual-level discrete sequences of events is the survival analysis, for example, an adaptation of the Cox model to counting process data (Borgan 1984). In particular, Cox's proportional hazards model allows for the inclusion of possibly censored survival times in the model and for covariates such as those incorporating knowledge about individual-level characteristics. Two other relevant methodology areas pertinent to modeling longitudinal utilization sequence are those of determining "long-term" survivors in a cohort (Farewell 1982; Kuk and Chen 1992; McLachlan and McGiffin 1993; Sy and Taylor 2000) and the use of the multivariate Weibull mixture model to capture heterogeneity in duration data (Nagode and Fajdiga 2000; Mosler and Seidel 2001; Mosler 2003; Bučar et al. 2004; Mosler and Scheicher 2008; Mair and Hudec 2009; Farcomeni and Nardi 2010). In recent research, my collaborators and I have introduced a parametric proportional hazards model to find the rate at which pediatric asthma patients visit different provider types given variables such as access to care, their current overall health condition, demographic variables, and history of healthcare utilization (Hilton et al. 2018).

Factors Influencing Health Outcomes

Earlier in this chapter, I highlighted that the relationship between outcomes and access is complex, being complemented or confounded by many factors, including community opportunities and norms, health education, individual or population health status and/or health history, expectations, or belief systems, among others. Thus when seeking to understand and explain variability in health outcomes, we need to clearly delineate the role of each factor, differentiated into:

- *Explanatory* factors referring here to healthcare access measures as they are of primary interest in an outcome study within the research framework of this book.
- *Confounding* factors being those that can affect the relationship between an explanatory variable (e.g. access measure) and the outcome variable so that the results do not reflect the actual relationship; this is because the confounding factors correlate with both the outcome and the explanatory variables. They are exogenous, that is, their relationship to the outcome variable is not of primary interest but their effects need to be *controlled* for when explaining the link between outcomes and access as the link may not be significant, or that a true effect is hidden by such factors.
- *Mediator* factors are those that explain the relationship between the dependent variable and the independent variable. They can be used in an outcome study when the explanatory variable of interest does not directly explain the outcome variable but it does so indirectly through a mediator variable.

I will note that the concept of "confounders" for independent variables in multi-variate regression analysis is more general than I defined here. The idea is that multivariate regression captures the so-called conditional relationship of an explanatory variable with the response or outcome variable conditional on other variables being in the model. The magnitude, the sign and the statistical significance of a conditional relationship depends on which other variables are in the model. But in the description provided here, I referred to confounding factors as only those that correct for the selection bias in observational studies.

While there are many confounding factors that could potentially affect outcomes, I will point out here those that have been previously linked to disparities in health-care for populations vulnerable to health inequities, like Medicaid-insured patients (Wang and Luo 2005; Hambidge et al. 2007). They can divide into *patient-level* factors including demographics (e.g. race, age, gender), disease specific (e.g. genotype class), and health status or clinical risk group (CRG); *socioeconomic factors* observed at the community level, including median household income, percentage of population below the poverty level, unemployment rate, and percentage of adults with a given level of education; and other *environment or community factors*, including area pollution, health provider density (Heier Stamm 2010), segregation (Nobles et al. 2014), and rurality (RUCA codes; United States Department of Agriculture 2016). The confounding variables can take various forms, they can stay the same (e.g. race) or vary geographically (e.g. community factors) or temporally (e.g. health status).

Interventions are often designed to change mediator variables that are causally related to the outcome variable of interest through interventional variables; thus, the relationship of the interventional variable to the outcome variable is mediated by mediator factors (Keele et al. 2015; Vander Weele 2016). For example, potential access to healthcare is an interventional factor toward improving outcomes because it can be altered through targeted interventions. However, potential access does not directly impact health outcomes. It is the realized access or healthcare utilization that directly impacts health(care) outcomes. Appropriate healthcare utilization follows when potential access to healthcare services exists and it is tailored to the needs of the population targeted. In this context, utilization of healthcare services can be viewed as mediating the relationship between potential access and health outcomes. Thus, establishing mediator variables is key to evaluating the impact of interventions on health outcomes.

In the next section, I will overview three case studies with different settings in terms of the data type for the health outcome of interest and different modeling procedures to illustrate the extent of outcome research studies in the context of the main theme of this book – healthcare access.

CASE STUDIES

Does Travel Distance to CF Centers Impact Clinical Outcomes?

Cystic fibrosis, a life-threatening disorder, is a second respiratory disease that shows great disparities in outcomes for patients (Schechter 2003). The disease is chronic, life-long, and debilitating to patients. Recent research has shown that a significant proportion of the variation in outcomes can be attributed to socioeconomic factors, but financial barriers appear to be of limited consequence, and therefore, unexplained disparities remain (Halfon and Newacheck 1993; Schechter et al. 2001, 2009; Wolfenden and Schechter 2009; Barr et al. 2011; Kovell et al. 2011; Taylor-Robinson and Schechter 2011). The analysis in this case study is based on a cross-sectional study and comparison of outcomes among different population groups (Wolfenden and Schechter 2009).

While there has been significant interest in the relationship between CF disease management and outcomes (Schechter and Margolis 1998; Schechter et al. 2001), there is little research that addresses the association with geographic distance to care and how the relationship varies across different age groups. Since CF is a rare condition, accessibility or geographic access to care is likely to be limited, with only approximately 120 accredited care centers across the United States. In one of my recent studies, my collaborators and I considered the impact of geographic distance from CF centers on lung function in children, young adults, and adults with CF (Johnson et al. 2018).

The study population consisted of patients with CF who received care at Cystic Fibrosis Foundation (CFF)-accredited centers and who were listed in the registry of the CFF during the years 1986–2011. According to the CFF, the registry currently captures data on 81–84% of all persons with CF in the United States (Knapp et al. 2016), thus our study population covered most of the patients with CF in the United States. However, we did not include the entire population in the CF registry; this is because of incomplete data for some patients as provided in the associated collaborative publication (Johnson 2018). After removing missing data relevant for this study, the population was reduced from 44 541 to 20 400 patients.

The health outcome of interest in this study was the %FEV1 (Wang et al. 1993; Hankinson et al. 1999). As defined earlier in this chapter, this is a clinical outcome. The outcome was considered longitudinally, that is, the outcomes of all recorded visits of one patient in the CFF registry were modeled as a sequence of time-dependent responses. This is called a longitudinal study in the statistical modeling literature.

The objective was to model the relation of geographic access to this clinical outcome, where the geographic access was measured as the travel distance between the zip codes of each patient's home location and the location of the center where the patient received care. Each patient's geographic access was determined as the road distance in miles. Because the association between health outcomes and geographic distance was nonlinear, we transformed travel distances into a discrete variable with three categories – high distance for distances greater than 75 miles; medium distance for distances between 25 miles and 75 miles; and low distance for distances less than 25 miles. The 25 mile limit for low distance was suggested by the US Department of Health and Human Services defining underserved areas for primary care, thus setting the limits of the expected travel for routine care.

As highlighted earlier in the chapter, when analyzing the link between access and outcomes, it is critical to identify confounding factors that can explain the bias selection in the study population. In this study, patient-level confounding factors included the patient's gender, age at the time of FEV measurement, insurance status, and geno-type, all of which have been shown in the literature to be predictors of %FEV1 in patients with CF (Schechter et al. 2001).

We employed mixed-effects modeling to assess the statistical significance of the association between geographic proximity to CF centers and the clinical outcome, %FEV1. The model included random effects to capture the within-individual and age-specific variability. Importantly, we considered that the relationship between out-come and access could be different by age group, differentiated into: children con-sisting of patients less than 18 years old; young adults consisting of patients between 18 and 30: and adults consisting of patients more than 30 years old. This is because the outcome variable has a multimodal distribution that depends on age as shown in Figure 4.5. Importantly, the variations in the outcome variable by age are confounded with the relationship between the outcome and access. For example, children depend on their parents availability and willingness to travel; the middle age group tend to move more since the geographic access variability will be due to age; last, the older group tend to consist of those who have a less severe CF and thus better outcomes.

Figure 4.6 is a visual approach to evaluate the relationship between access and the clinical outcome, presenting the variations in travel distance by four levels of %FEV1, for each age group and for patients who did and did not move. For children, the median distance from a care center is higher than that for adults with the exception of the heathiest adults. As patients aged, the heathiest patients tended to be the farthest away from their CF care centers. For children who moved over the study period, the difference in the mean travel distance between the groups differentiated by %FEV1 was not significant. For young adults, the difference was also not significant.

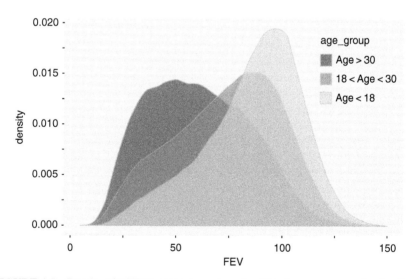

FIGURE 4.5   Density of %FEV1 across age categories. This figure compares the density of the distribution of the %FEV1 outcome variable across children, young adults, and adults. This figure shows the shift in the %FEV1 outcome variables with age.

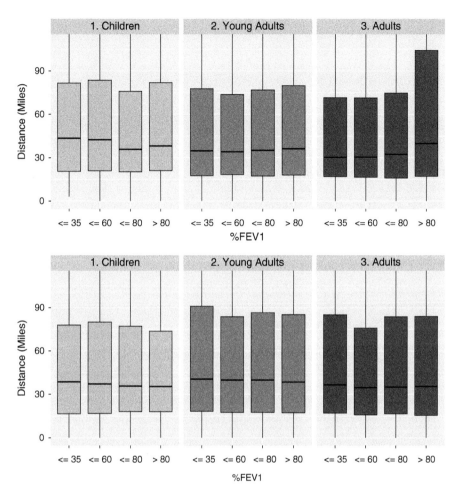

FIGURE 4.6 Travel distance (access measure) versus %FEV1 (outcome measure) by age group differentiated by patients who did move (a) and those who did not move (b). Each age category is represented (children, young adults, and adults). The boxplots present the distribution of the distance by four different levels of %FEV1.

For children who did not move, those in the high %FEV1 group lived on average 1.43 miles farther from a care center while adults who did not change distance categories and were in the high %FEV1 category lived on average of 2.94 miles farther. These insights underline the variation in the relationship between access and outcome by age group as I previously described. They also point to different relationships between outcomes and access in terms of significance and direction for the CF patients who moved and those who did not move further away from a CF center.

To differentiate by age group, there are two possible modeling approaches. One approach is to consider three different models, separated by age group. Alternatively, one could include the age group variable as a predictor or controlling factor and add

TABLE 4.1   Model Results from Applying the Mixed Effects Model using Interaction terms between Age Groups and Distance Categories

	Point estimate	Lower 95% CI	Upper 95% CI	p-value
Intercept	114.42	113.46	115.38	<0.001
Age	−1.49	−1.52	−1.46	<0.001
Male (ref. female)	1.02	0.45	1.59	<0.001
Severe mutation	−2.36	−3.00	−1.72	<0.001
Medium distance (ref. low distance)	−0.15	−0.61	0.30	0.51
High distance (ref. low distance)	0.21	−0.23	0.64	0.35
Young adults	−0.44	−1.16	0.28	0.23
Adults	−4.87	−5.76	−3.97	<0.001
Young adults: medium distance	−0.15	−0.67	0.36	0.56
Young adults: large distance	−0.98	−1.47	−0.49	<0.001
Adults: medium distance	−0.08	−0.61	0.44	0.75
Adults: large distance	0.77	0.27	1.26	0.00
Urban	−0.63	−0.90	−0.36	<0.001
Medicaid insurance	−6.79	−7.40	−6.18	<0.001
Median income	−5.08	−5.56	−4.61	<0.001
Year 2001–2005	−0.97	−1.06	−0.88	<0.001
Year 1996–2000	−1.48	−1.65	−1.32	<0.001
Year 1991–1995	−2.37	−2.61	−2.13	<0.001
Year 1986–1990	−2.09	−2.44	−1.73	<0.001

interaction terms of the age-group variable with the access measure and possibly other confounding factors. The results of the model with the interaction terms are shown in Table 4.1 and the results for the models considering the two sub-populations separately are provided in the associated research paper (Johnson et al. 2018).

On the one hand, this study found no strong evidence of an effect of geographic distance from care centers on %FEV1 in patients who did not change distance categories during the study period. On the other hand, for patients who did change geographic distance categories, the average %FEV1 was slightly higher for older adults who moved further from their CF center and marginally worse for young adults who moved farther from a CF care. As distance increased, the outcomes were better for older adults and worse for young adults.

The study did not find significant effects on lung function based on interactions between the geographic distance and socioeconomic status or urban/rural characteristics. However, it found significant relationships between median income, geographic distance to a CF center, and urban/rural designations. CF centers were located in urban areas, many of which were also in zip codes with a higher median income. Thus, patients with the smallest distances to care were also more likely to have high median incomes and urban environments.

As first suggested by Figure 4.6 as well as by the statistical modeling, an important challenge in characterizing the association between the clinical outcomes and distance to care was the high level of mobility in adults. When patient mobility exists, it is difficult to determine the impact of mobility versus the impact of distance, given that a mobile population is inherently different.

In conclusion, we found that geographic distance to CF centers has no significant association with lung health in patients who did not move too far or too close from a CF center during the course of the study period. Among those who did, the association that we found between better lung function and geographic distance in older adults is more likely from relocation following lung function rather than distance affecting lung function. Overall, we found that socioeconomic and genetic factors appear to impact clinical outcomes to a greater extent than access to the care centers.

Is Geographic Access Associated with Severe Healthcare Outcomes for Pediatric Asthma?

In Chapter 2 a modeling approach focusing on measuring access and making inference on disparities between Medicaid and non-Medicaid sub-populations for pediatric asthma was presented. I will return to pediatric asthma in the case study in this section. In Chapter 2, I underlined the burden of the asthma condition among children diagnosed with this condition. But asthma not only impairs quality of life, it also results in severe outcomes, particularly in ER visits and hospitalizations, which in many cases could be preventable. Asthma is the second most common reason for pediatric ER visits that lead to hospitalizations (Agency for Healthcare Research and Quality 2008).

In this second case study, based on one of my collaborative research papers (Garcia et al. 2015), I will evaluate the relationship between geographic access and health outcomes for pediatric asthma, with a focus on how differences in geographic access potentially impact severe health outcomes, including emergency department visits and hospitalizations for asthma-diagnosed children. It is not uncommon to consider utilization of emergency department care and/or hospitalizations as health outcome measures in chronic disease management (Li et al. 2003; Lee et al. 2007; Ludwick et al. 2009), particularly for pediatric asthma (Ford et al. 2001; Beck et al. 2012).

Similar to the case study in Chapter 2, the population under consideration consists of children ages 5–17 estimated to have a current diagnosis of asthma in two states Georgia (GA) and North Carolina (NC). In this study, a severe outcome is defined as an emergency department visit or hospitalization that was caused by the child's asthma condition. The response variable of interest in the statistical model is the outcome rate calculated as the ratio of emergency department visits or hospitalizations to the estimated number of children with asthma at the county level for each age group. For Georgia, emergency department visits and hospitalizations were obtained from the Online Analytical Statistical Information System (OASIS) database. For North Carolina, the emergency department visits and hospitalizations were obtained from the Healthcare Cost and Utilization Project (HCUP) state databases, which contain de-identified individual records from all hospitals.

The relationship between severe health outcomes and access was considered for multiple access measures, including access to asthma specialized care and primary care separately. (In Chapter 2, I provided an access measure that accounted for both types of care into one measure.) The approach to obtaining the two access measures was somewhat simpler than the one presented in Chapter 2, by not including the smoothing penalty to correct for geographic similarity in the access measure. The estimation access procedures for the specialized asthma care and for primary care were detailed in two of my collaborative publications (Garcia et al. 2015; Gentili et al. 2018).

Figure 4.7 presents the travel distance to primary care and specialized care for the two states. In these maps we capture only the population with access, that is, when the travel distance is lower than 25 miles for primary care, and lower than 30 and 45 miles for specialized care for urban and rural communities, respectively. The largest difference between the two states is in the level of access for specialized asthma care – North Carolina has significantly better access than Georgia. A question of interest is whether severe health outcomes would reduce significantly if access in Georgia was similar to that of North Carolina. This question can be investigated using a statistical model with the response variable being the health outcome of interest and the primary explanatory variable being the access measure of interest as provided next.

We quantified the impact of geographic access on severe outcomes using logistic regression with replications, and we fitted separate models for hospitalizations and emergency department visits at the county level in each state. Because the access measures were derived at the census tract level, we included both the average and the variance summaries of the access measures within each county as explanatory factors.

Most importantly, we included a series of controlling factors, as main effects and in interaction with the access measures. Since the severe outcomes are derived as utilization of hospital care, to control for access to hospital care only the number of hospitals in each county is included as a factor in the model. (The data on hospital location are available from the Directory of US Hospitals at www.the-ihi.com.) Socioeconomic variables extracted from the American Community Survey were restricted to data on households that have at least one child under the age of 18 (20). They included a variable specifying whether the response variable is for children in one of three age ranges (5–9, 10–14, 15–17). For income and education, we selected among potential variables by investigating the strength of the association of these variables with the response variable. The variables selected were the median family income and the percent of adults with less than a high school diploma.

A simple visual display pointing to potential relationships with the outcome and among the covariates included in the regression model is a correlation plot where the outcome is transformed using the logit link function used in logistic regression. The correlation plots for Georgia and North Carolina are shown in Figure 4.8. The plots on the left show the Person correlation, a measure of linear relationship between two variables, and the plots on the right show the Kendall tau correlation, a measure of the nonlinear relationship between two variables. From these two plots, the correlation between transformed emergency department visit rate and the predictors included in the model is weak, with the strongest correlation for the county-average distances to specialist and primary care. The correlation between covariates is also weak.

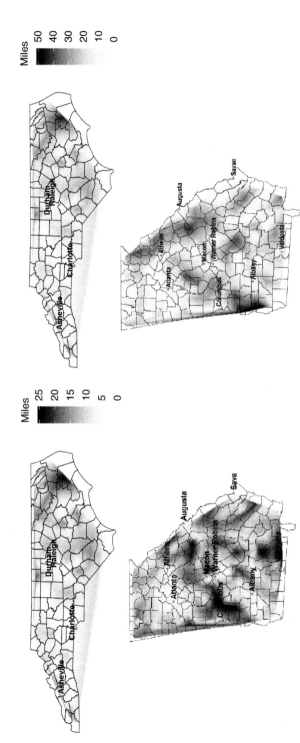

FIGURE 4.7 Travel distance (access measure) to primary care (a) and to asthma specialized care (b) for North Carolina (top) and for Georgia (bottom).

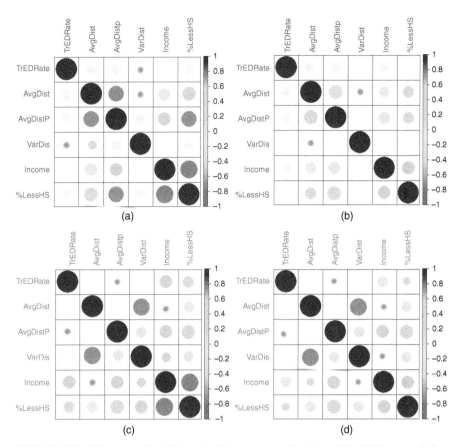

FIGURE 4.8 The correlation displays for Person correlation (a) and Kendall tau correlation (b) for Georgia (top) and North Carolina (bottom). The size and the shade are indications of how strong or weak the correlation is between any two variables.

Applying the logistic regression with model selection, the models applied to each of the two outcomes show different significant relationships, although somewhat consistent across the two states. The detailed results of the models are provided in the collaborative paper (Garcia et al. 2015). I will summarize here some of the important findings only.

For example, in Georgia none of the access variables are significantly associated with the occurrence of emergency department visits as main effects (i.e. not in interaction with other factors) but access to primary care is significantly associated with the occurrence of hospitalizations. Therefore, we would expect that improving access to primary care would have a greater impact on the hospitalization rate than the emergency department visit rate. Moreover, a different set of access variables are associated with severe outcome rates when comparing Georgia with North Carolina. For example, unlike in Georgia, the main effects of all the access variables are significant in the corresponding model for North Carolina. Contrasting the models for hospitalizations, there are more significant interaction terms involving the access variables in North Carolina than in Georgia. This is an important finding because it points to a state-by-state analysis. Different states will show significance for different forms of access measures, suggesting different interventions in improving access, and ultimately outcomes.

We also used the regression model to predict the reduction of emergency department visits occurring with improvements in access, more specifically, with reductions in distance to access asthma providers. This prediction approach can be used to understand the direct impact of access onto reduction of severe outcomes. Specifically, we allow travel distance to decrease to 15 miles for primary care, to 5 or 15 miles for specialist care, or both, then project the rate of ER visits. I will warrant that such an analysis of predicting outcomes when changing the level of access needs to be interpreted with caution since we do not capture a causal relationship between outcomes and access.

Figure 4.9 shows the geographic distribution of locations with a positive improvement in outcome for one of the interventions and the number of county/age pairs in each state with a predicted reduction in the number of emergency department visits for each of the four interventions. Reducing travel distance to both specialized and primary care versus to only primary care to 15 miles or less shows a reduction in the number of emergency department visits in one new county in Georgia only. Thus, the maps for the intervention with less than 15 miles for both specialized and primary care look identical to those in Figure 4.6. In contrast, further reducing specialist care to 5 miles versus 15 miles adds 10 additional counties to those showing improvement, although the improvement in emergency department visits is small. Moreover, there is a significant spatial trend in the emergency department visits reduction with a more significant reduction in urban areas when the distance is reduced to 5 miles. This suggests that if geographic access is improved only at the level of 15 miles, primarily rural areas should be targeted for intervention.

Moreover, the decrease in distance from 15 to 5 miles generally improves outcomes only marginally, while the joint improvement of access to primary and specialist care does not lead to a noticeably greater impact on the reduction of emergency department visits than improving specialist distances alone. This suggests that access to specialist care plays an important role in reduction of severe outcomes, while a level of access similar to the comparative state of North Carolina will suffice.

Are the Healthcare Outcomes for Pediatric Asthma Aligned with the Recommended Care Guidelines?

In the third case study in this chapter, I will present a study on *healthcare outcomes* for pediatric asthma, with a focus on assessing them against the recommended guidelines for pediatric asthma (National Heart Blood and Lung Institute 2007). Healthcare outcomes of interest are the occurrence of emergency department encounters, hospitalizations, PO visits and medication, all in all referring to variations in realized access or healthcare utilization. If realized access does not conform to the recommended

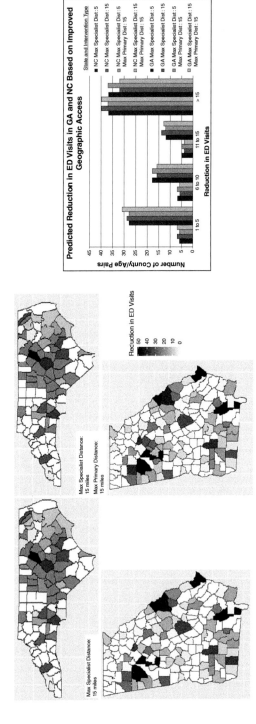

FIGURE 4.9 Geographic distribution of the reduction in the number of emergency department visits when access to primary and specialist care is improved for North Carolina (top maps) and Georgia (bottom maps).

guidelines for pediatric asthma, then interventions and efforts to improve access may be considered.

Because asthma is a chronic condition, it requires healthcare management over the course of the condition's progression, commonly spanning multiple years. In order to capture appropriate utilization, the patient-level longitudinal utilization needs to be observed over a period of several years, accounting for multiple types of healthcare events. This leads to a *utilization sequence,* which is a longitudinal realization of a patient's healthcare utilization in chronological order and with different interarrival times between healthcare events. An illustration of a utilization sequence is shown in Figure 4.3.

Detailed utilizations at the event level along with the time stamps of the events are only available in electronic health records or administrative claims data. For this particular study, the main data source is the 2005–2012 Medicaid Analytic Extract (MAX) medical claims data acquired from the Centers for Medicare & Medicaid Services (CMS), consisting of identifiable individual-level claims data for all Medicaid-enrolled beneficiaries. Such data allow tracking of patients' utilization sequences over a period of many years for a large population.

The study population is similar to previous case studies on pediatric asthma in this book, except that the focus is now on the Medicaid-enrolled children only. It also focuses only on those children with persistent asthma (National Committee for Quality Assurance 2011). This case study is based on one of my collaborative research papers (Hilton et al. 2017), which presents new methodology on modeling healthcare utilization sequences toward making inferences on patient-level utilization profiles. The methodology is general; it can apply to other conditions or healthcare settings, for example, ADHD treatment for young children (Moran et al. 2019).

In this study, the set of possible events includes *ER visits, hospitalizations (HOS), physician's office visits and clinic visits (PO), asthma short-term medication (ASM) and asthma controller medication (ACM).* An example of a utilization sequence given this set of events is as follows: Consider a patient who visited the ER for an asthma attack on 1 January 2010, who subsequently received a prescription for an inhaler that was filled about one month later, along with a referral to a primary care physician, who the patient visited two months later. The patient then visited the same physician within three months of the other visit, and then refilled another asthma prescription three months later. The resulting utilization sequence is (ER, ACM, PO, PO, ACM) with time stamps scaled to a one-year interval: (0.0, 0.08, 0.25, 0.50, 0.75).

Given the utilization sequences for more than 1.5 million children, one approach to profile patient-level utilization is using a discrete sequence clustering analysis, assuming that an utilization sequence follows a MRP (Foufoula-Georgiou and Lettenmaier 1987) briefly introduced in this chapter. The proposed MRP modeling is further integrated within a machine learning algorithm (Hilton et al. 2017) that captures heterogeneity of children's utilization behaviors, inspired by existing research on modeling longitudinal, categorical data (Schach and Schach 1972; Smyth 1997; Ramoni et al. 2002; Pamminger and Frühwirth-Schnatter 2010). The unsupervised classification algorithm groups children with similar longitudinal utilization patterns, for example, children who regularly receive medication and children who visit a PO regularly. The model output consists of utilization profiles, which can be used to assess utilization behaviors longitudinally relative to recommended care guidelines. The utilization profiles can be visualized as networks, where the nodes are the type of care and the vertices provide information about the probability of transitioning from one type of care to another accompanied by the estimated average time of transition.

While we considered 10 states in the collaborative research paper (Hilton et al. 2017), here I am presenting the utilization profiles for Georgia and North Carolina to be consistent with the previous case study. Figure 4.10 presents the utilization profiles for the two states.

Both states have a utilization profile characterized by a high probability of controller and short-term medication with a high probability link of following up with controller medication (ACM) after short-term medication (ASM), corresponding to Profile 1 in the utilization networks. This profile also presents some level of PO utilization, with a strong link (high probability) of medication prescription after a PO visit. Only Georgia has some severe outcomes (hospitalizations) but those are followed by medication without a return to hospitalizations. Thus, children in this profile have their asthma controlled by medication with no severe outcome after taking the medication. This profile consists of most of the children in the study population of each state, 72.2% and 89.7% in Georgia and North Carolina, respectively.

Two other profiles in Georgia do not present severe outcomes also (Profiles 2 and 3); they are characterized by visits to the PO with a high probability of follow-up but with only short-term medication (Profile 2) or no medication (Profile 3). Only Profile 4 in Georgia includes nodes corresponding to severe outcomes (ER visits and hospitalization); this same profile does not include a node corresponding to controlled asthma medication. This profile includes 12% of the children with asthma in Georgia; these children are those who need to be targeted for interventions to improve the health outcomes related to their asthma condition since based on the presence or absence of specific utilization nodes, this utilization profile will primarily include children with uncontrolled asthma.

North Carolina has only three profiles, with Profiles 2 and 3 including severe outcomes without a node for the asthma controller medication. These two profiles, a total of 10% of children, consist of those children with uncontrolled asthma, thus a priority for targeted interventions.

Based on these utilization networks, I will point out several take home points:

- The majority of children have their asthma condition controlled, with high utilization of controller medication, but they achieve this with limited utilization of POs. This is in contrast to the national guidelines recommending 2–12 visits annually for asthma care when asthma is controlled, and more frequently for those whose asthma is not well-controlled (National Heart Blood and Lung Institute 2007).

- A relatively small proportion of children have severe outcomes, and their asthma is uncontrolled. Particularly for these children, ER visits or hospitalizations are not followed up by visits to the PO as recommended by care practices.

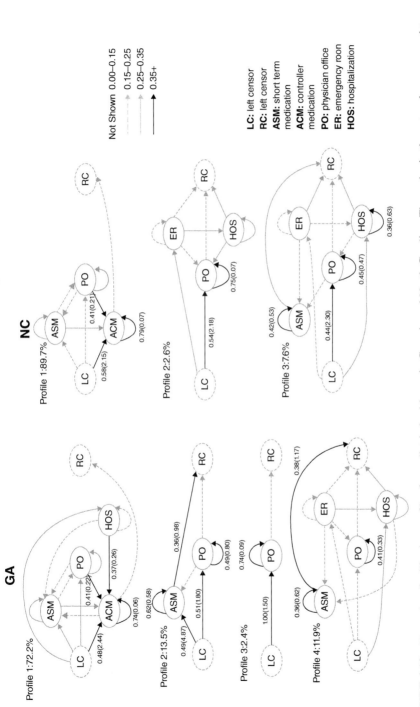

FIGURE 4.10 Networks of utilization profiles for pediatric healthcare in Georgia and North Carolina. The nodes in the networks correspond to healthcare events and the links correspond to the probability of transitioning from one event to another. The numbers accompanying the links correspond to the transition probabilities, with the average time between events in parentheses. ACM, asthma controller medication; ASM, asthma short-term medication; ER, emergency room; HOS, hospitalization; LC, left censoring; PO, physician office; RC, right censoring.

- Both states present a similar proportion of children with severe healthcare outcomes; however, previous studies provided in this book showed that North Carolina has much better access to specialized asthma care than Georgia, while they both have similar access to primary care. An explanation for this discordance in the results is that the study on utilization profiles includes Medicaid-enrolled children only, who generally tend to have much lower access to specialized asthma care as shown in the case study in Chapter 2. Thus, the higher access to specialized asthma care in North Carolina as estimated in the previous section does not necessarily translate to better access for the Medicaid population.

The methodology applied to study utilization of care with respect to recommended care guidelines does not control for factors influencing utilization, for example, the health status or the clinical risk of a patient, among others. In another research paper (Hilton et al. 2018), my collaborators and I introduced a survival analysis approach to study longitudinal utilization of care while including controlling and explanatory factors. In particular, we studied how access to primary care, measured as the travel distance, impacts utilization of asthma care. However, the model is challenging to interpret. An alternative simpler approach to including controlling and explanatory factors in the overall analysis is to consider the clustering membership as a response outcome variable; for this model, because the response variable is a qualitative variable with multiple levels, a multinomial regression model can be applied, where the baseline is the utilization profile that most closely follows recommended care (Moran et al. 2019).

CONCLUSIONS

The study of health(care) outcomes is the precursor of decision making in healthcare delivery, specifically, in advancing healthcare access. Important ingredients in studying health(care) outcomes are identifying most appropriate outcomes within the specific context of the study, deriving the outcomes or approximates of the outcomes of interest given the data availability, and developing rigorous methodologies for understanding the link between outcomes and various aspects of healthcare delivery. This chapter provides the fundamentals for the ingredients in studying health(care) outcomes with a focus on analyzing the link between outcomes and access.

Two case studies illustrate the modeling of the relationship between outcomes and access, highlighting that the relationship can be complex, depending on the age, location, or other characteristics of the study population. The first case study focuses on the relationship between access and clinical outcomes while the second study focuses on the relationship between access and healthcare outcomes. Importantly, the hypothesis that there is a significant link between outcomes and access given other confounding factors does not necessarily hold for some healthcare settings. A third case study focuses on the study of healthcare outcomes, with a focus on assessing them against the recommended guidelines for pediatric asthma. This study can be used to identify the sub-population with severe outcomes who have not accessed the healthcare system following the recommended care, more specifically, the sub-population for which the realized access is not sufficiently tailored to the needs of those seeking care. All three studies are illustrations of how health outcomes can inform decision making on healthcare access. It is thus paramount to develop rigorous statistical models to understand the significance, direction and magnitude of the link between outcomes and access.

ACKNOWLEDGMENTS

This chapter draws substantially upon the recent research presented in three journal articles. In this regard, the author gratefully acknowledges the contributions of Ben Johnson, Michael Schechter, Erin Garcia, Anne Fitzpatrick, Ross Hilton, and Richard Zheng who have given their permission to illustrate the concepts and methodologies presented in this chapter using the studies from our collaboration. The author is also thankful to Julie Swann for providing useful suggestions on improving the presentation of this chapter.

REFERENCES

Aakvik, A. and Holmas, T.H. (2006). Access to primary health care and health outcomes: the relationships between GP characteristics and mortality rates. *Journal of Health Economics* **25**(6): 1139–1153.

Agency for Healthcare Research and Quality (2008). Statistical Brief #52. Healthcare Cost and Utilization Project (HCUP). Rockville, MD.

Ahern, M., Brown, C., and Dukas, S. (2011). A national study of the association between food environments and county-level health outcomes. *The Journal of Rural Health* **27**(4): 367–379.

Assuncao, R.M. (2003). Space varying coeffcient models for small area data. *Environmetrics* **14**: 453–473.

Ayanian, J.Z., Kohler, B.A., Abe, T., and Epstein, A.M. (1993). The relation between health-insurance coverage and clinical outcomes among women with breast-cancer. *New England Journal of Medicine* **329**(5): 326–331.

Balcazar, A.J., Grineski, S.E., and Collins, T.W. (2015). The Hispanic health paradox across generations: the relationship of child generational status and citizenship with health outcomes. *Public Health* **129**(6): 691–697.

Barr, H.L., Britton, J., Smyth, A.R., and Fogarty, A.W. (2011). Association between socioeconomic status, sex, and age at death from cystic fibrosis in England and Wales (1959 to 2008): cross sectional study. *BMJ* **343**: d4662.

Beck, A., Simmons, J.M., Huang, B., and Kahn, R.S. (2012). Geomedicine: area-based socioeconomic measures for assessing risk of hospital reutilization among children admitted for asthma. *American Journal of Public Health* **102**(12): 2308–2314.

Beratarrechea, A., Lee, A.G., Willner, J.M. et al. (2014). The impact of mobile health interventions on chronic disease outcomes in developing countries: a systematic review. *Telemedicine and E-Health* **20**(1): 75–82.

Berkman, N.D., Sheridan, S.L., Donahue, K.E. et al. (2011). Low health literacy and health outcomes: an updated systematic review. *Annals of Internal Medicine* **155**(2): 97–107.

Bhutta, Z.A., Lassi, Z.S., Blanc, A., and Donnay, F. (2010). Linkages among reproductive health, maternal health, and perinatal outcomes. *Seminars in Perinatology* **34**(6): 434–445.

Borgan, Ø. (1984). Maximum likelihood estimation in parametric counting process models, with applications to censored failure time data. *Scandinavian Journal of Statistics* **11**(1): 1–16.

Briesacher, B.A., Madden, J.M., Zhang, F. et al. (2015). Did Medicare Part D affect national trends in health outcomes or hospitalizations? A time-series analysis. *Annals of Internal Medicine* **162**(12): 825.

Bučar, T., Nagode, M., and Fajdiga, M. (2004). Reliability approximation using finite Weibull mixture distributions. *Reliability Engineering & System Safety* **84**(3): 241–251.

Cilenti, D., Kum, H.-C., Wells, R. et al. (2015). Changes in North Carolina maternal health service use and outcomes among medicaid-enrolled pregnant women during state budget cuts. *Journal of Public Health Management and Practice* **21**(2): 208–213.

Currie, J., Decker, S., and Lin, W. (2008). Has public health insurance for older children reduced disparities in access to care and health outcomes? *Journal of Health Economics* **27**(6): 1567–1581.

Dasgupta, P., Baade, P.D., Aitken, J.F., and Turrell, G. (2012). Multilevel determinants of breast cancer survival: association with geographic remoteness and area-level socioeconomic disadvantage. *Breast Cancer Research and Treatment* **132**(2): 701–710.

Delphin-Rittmon, M.E., Flanagan, E.H., Andres-Hyman, R. et al. (2015). Racial-ethnic differences in access, diagnosis, and outcomes in public-sector inpatient mental health treatment. *Psychological Services* **12**(2): 158–166.

Deswal, A., Petersen, N.J., Ashton, C.M., and Wray, N.P. (2004). Impact of race on health care utilization and outcomes in veterans with congestive heart failure. *Journal of the American College of Cardiology* **43**(5): 778–784.

Diggle, P., Heagerty, P., Liang, K.L., and Zeger, S. (2002). *Analysis of Longitudinal Data*. Oxford University Press.

Farcomeni, A. and Nardi, A. (2010). A two-component Weibull mixture to model early and late mortality in a Bayesian framework. *Computational Statistics & Data Analysis* **54**(2): 416–428.

Farewell, V.T. (1982). The use of mixture models for the analysis of survival data with long-term survivors. *Biometrics*: 1041–1046.

Fisher, M.A. and Mascarenhas, A.K. (2009). A comparison of medical and dental outcomes for medicaid-insured and uninsured medicaid-eligible children: a US population-based study. *Journal of the American Dental Association* **140**(11): 1403–1412.

Fitzmaurice, G.M., Laird, N.M., and Ware, J.H. (2011). *Applied Longitudinal Analysis*, 2e. Hoboken, NJ: Wiley.

Ford, J.G., Meyer, I.H., Sternfels, P. et al. (2001). Patterns and predictors of asthma-related emergency department use in Harlem. *Chest* **120**(4): 1129–1135.

Foufoula-Georgiou, E. and Lettenmaier, D.P. (1987). A Markov renewal model for rainfall occurrences. *Water Resources Research* **23**(5): 875–884.

Garcia, E., Serban, N., Swann, J., and Fitzpatrick, A. (2015). The effect of geographic access on severe health outcomes for pediatric asthma. *Journal of Allergy and Clinical Immunology* **136**(3): 610–618.

Gavin, N.I., Benedict, M.B., and Adams, E.K. (2006). Health service use and outcomes among disabled medicaid pregnant women. *Womens Health Issues* **16**(6): 313–322.

Gelfand, A.E., Kim, H.-J., Sirmans, C.F., and Banerjee, S. (2003). Spatial modeling with spatially varying coefficient processes. *Journal of the American Statistical Association* **98**(462): 387–396.

Gentili, M., Serban, N., Harati, P. et al. (2018). Quantifying disparities in accessibility and availability of pediatric primary care with implications for policy. *Health Services Research* **53**(3): 1458–1477.

Giuffrida, A., Gravelle, H., and Roland, M. (1999). Measuring quality of care with routine data: avoiding confusion between performance indicators and health outcomes. *British Medical Journal* **319**(7202): 94–98.

Graves, B.A. (2010). Access to cardiac interventional services in Alabama and Mississippi: a geographical information system analysis. *Perspectives in Health Information Management* **7**(Spring): 1b.

Grembowski, D., Spiekerman, C., and Milgrom, P. (2008). Linking mother and child access to dental care. *Pediatrics* **122**(4): E805–E814.

Guagliardo, M.F. (2004). Spatial accessibility of primary care: concepts, methods and challenges. *International Journal of Health Geographics* **3**(3): 1–13.

Gulliford, M.C., Charlton, J., Prevost, T. et al. (2017). Costs and outcomes of increasing access to bariatric surgery: cohort study and cost-effectiveness analysis using electronic health records. *Value in Health* **20**(1): 85–92.

Haas, J.S., Brawarsky, P., Iyer, A. et al. (2011). Association of area sociodemographic characteristics and capacity for treatment with disparities in colorectal cancer care and mortality. *Cancer* **117**(18): 4267–4276.

Halfon, N. and Newacheck, P.W. (1993). Childhood asthma and poverty: differential impacts and utilization of health services. *Pediatrics* **91**: 56–61.

Hambidge, S.J., Emsermann, C.B., Federico, S., and Steiner, J.F. (2007). Disparities in pediatric preventive care in the United States, 1993–2002. *Archives of Pediatrics and Adolescent Medicine* **161**(1): 30–36.

Han, X.S., Nguyen, B.T., Drope, J., and Jemal, A. (2015). Health-related outcomes among the poor: medicaid expansion vs. non-expansion states. *PLoS One* **10**(12): e0144429.

Hankinson, J.L., Odencrantz, J.R., and Fedan, K.B. (1999). Spirometric reference values from a sample of the general US population. *American Journal of Respiratory and Critical Care Medicine* **159**(1): 179–187.

Haraldsdottir, S., Gudmundsson, S., Bjarnadottir, R.I. et al. (2015). Maternal geographic residence, local health service supply and birth outcomes. *Acta Obstetricia et Gynecologica Scandinavica* **94**(2): 156–164.

Hargreaves, D.S., Elliott, M.N., Viner, R.M. et al. (2015). Unmet health care need in US adolescents and adult health outcomes. *Pediatrics* **136**(3): 513–520.

Harris, M.I. (2000). Health care and health status and outcomes for patients with type 2 diabetes. *Diabetes Care* **23**(6): 754–758.

Harris, M.I. (2001). Racial and ethnic differences in health care access and health outcomes for adults with type 1 diabetes. *Diabetes Care* **24**(3): 454–459.

Harris, D.E., Aboueissa, A.M., Baugh, N., and Sarton, C. (2015). Impact of rurality on maternal and infant health indicators and outcomes in Maine. *Rural and Remote Health* **15**(3): 3278.

Harrison, C.M., Britt, H.C., and Charles, J. (2012). Better outcomes or better access – which was better for mental health care? *Medical Journal of Australia* **197**(3): 170–172.

Hastie, T. and Tibshirani, R. (1990). *Generalized Additive Models*. Chapman & Hall/CRC.

Heier Stamm, J. (2010). Design and analysis of humanitarian and public health logistics systems. PhD thesis. Georgia Institute of Technology, Atlanta.

Hendryx, M.S., Dyck, D.G., and Srebnik, D. (1999). Risk-adjusted outcome models for public mental health outpatient programs. *Health Services Research* **34**(1): 171–195.

Hilton, R., Zheng, Y., Serban, N. et al. (2017). Patient-level longitudinal utilization for pediatric asthma healthcare: drawing inferences from millions of claims. *Medical Decision Making* **38**(1): 107–119.

Hilton, R., Zheng, Y., and Serban, N. (2018). Modeling heterogeneity in healthcare utilization using massive medical claims data. *Journal of the American Statistical Association* **113**(521): 111–121.

Institute of Medicine (1993). *Access to Health Care in America*. Washington, DC: National Academy Press.

Johnson, W.G. and Rimsza, M.E. (2004). The effects of access to pediatric care and insurance coverage on emergency department utilization. *Pediatrics* **113**(3 Pt 1): 483–487.

Johnson, B., Ngueyep, R., Schecheter, M. et al. (2018). A study of the impact of geographic access on health outcomes for cystic fibrosis. *Pediatric Pulmonology* **53**(3): 284–292.

Kazembe, L.N. and Mpeketula, P.M.G. (2010). Quantifying spatial disparities in neonatal mortality using a structured additive regression model. *PLoS One* **5**(6): e11180.

Keele, L., Tingley, D., and Yamamoto, T. (2015). Identifying mechanisms behind policy interventions via causal mediation analysis. *Journal of Policy Analysis and Management* **34**(4): 937–963.

Khan, A.A. (1992). An integrated approach to measuring potential spatial access to health care services. *Socio-Economic Planning Sciences* **26**(4): 275–287.

Knapp, E.A., Fink, A.K., and Goss, C.H. (2016). The Cystic Fibrosis Foundation Patient Registry: design and methods of a national observational disease registry. *Annals of the American Thoracic Society* **13**(7): 1173–1179.

Kovell, L.C., Wang, J., Ishman, S.L. et al. (2011). Cystic fibrosis and sinusitis in children: outcomes and socioeconomic status. *Otolaryngology-Head and Neck Surgery* **145**(1): 146–153.

Kuk, A.Y. and Chen, C.-H. (1992). A mixture model combining logistic regression with proportional hazards regression. *Biometrika* **79**(3): 531–541.

Laditka, J.N., Laditka, S.B., and Mastanduno, M. (2003). Hospital utilization for ambulatory care sensitive conditions: health outcome disparities associated with race and ethnicity. *Social Science and Medicine* **57**(8): 1429–1441.

Lee, J.E., Sung, J.H., Ward, W.B. et al. (2007). Utilization of the emergency room: impact of geographic distance. *Geospatial Health* **1**(2): 243–253.

Li, G.H., Grabowski, J.G., McCarthy, M.L., and Kelen, G.D. (2003). Neighborhood characteristics and emergency department utilization. *Academic Emergency Medicine* **10**(8): 853–859.

Long, W.E., Cabral, H.J., Garg, A. et al. (2013). Are components of the medical home differentially associated with child health care utilization, health, and health promoting behavior outcomes? *Clinical Pediatrics* **52**(5): 423–432.

Ludwick, A., Fu, R., Warden, C., and Lowe, R.A. (2009). Distances to emergency department and to primary care provider's office affect emergency department use in children. *Academic Emergency Medicine* **16**(5): 411–417.

Mair, P. and Hudec, M. (2009). Multivariate Weibull mixtures with proportional hazard restrictions for dwell-time-based session clustering with incomplete data. *Journal of the Royal Statistical Society: Series C (Applied Statistics)* **58**(5): 619–639.

McGrail, M. and Humphreys, J. (2009). Measuring spatial accessibility to primary care in rural areas: improving the effectiveness of the two-step floating catchment area method. *Applied Geography* **29**(4): 533–541.

McLachlan, G. and McGiffin, D. (1993). On the role of finite mixture models in survival analysis. *Statistical Methods in Medical Research* **3**(3): 211–226.

Moran, A., Serban, N., Danielson, M.L. et al. (2019). Assessing adherence to evidence-based care practices for preschool children diagnosed with ADHD in the medicaid system. *Psychiatric Services* **70**(1) https://doi.org/10.1176/appi.ps.201800204.

Mosler, K. (2003). Mixture models in econometric duration analysis. *Applied Stochastic Models in Business and Industry* **19**(2): 91–104.

Mosler, K. and Scheicher, C. (2008). Homogeneity testing in a Weibull mixture model. *Statistical Papers* **49**(2): 315–332.

Mosler, K. and Seidel, W. (2001). Theory & methods: testing for homogeneity in an exponential mixture model. *Australian & New Zealand Journal of Statistics* **43**(2): 231–247.

Mulvihill, B.A., Altarac, M., Swaminathan, S. et al. (2007). Does access to a medical home differ according to child and family characteristics, including special-health-care-needs status, among children in Alabama? *Pediatrics* **119**(Suppl 1): S107–S113.

Nagode, M. and Fajdiga, M. (2000). An improved algorithm for parameter estimation suitable for mixed Weibull distributions. *International Journal of Fatigue* **22**(1): 75–80.

National Committee for Quality Assurance (2011). Improving Outcomes in Asthma: Advancing Quality Using NCQA HEDIS Measures.

National Heart Blood and Lung Institute (2007). Expert Panel Report 3: Guidelines for the Diagnosis and Management of Asthma. Technical report.

Nobles, M., Serban, N., and Swann, J. (2014). Measurement and inference on pediatric healthcare accessibility. *The Annals of Applied Statistics* **8**(4): 1922–1946.

Oliver, G.M., Pennington, L., Revelle, S., and Rantz, M. (2014). Impact of nurse practitioners on health outcomes of medicare and medicaid patients. *Nursing Outlook* **62**(6): 440–447.

Oswald, D.P., Bodurtha, J.N., Willis, J.H., and Moore, M.B. (2007). Underinsurance and key health outcomes for children with special health care needs. *Pediatrics* **119**(2): E341–E347.

Pamminger, C. and Frühwirth-Schnatter, S. (2010). Model-based clustering of categorical time series. *Bayesian Analysis* **5**(2): 345–368.

Penchansky, R. and Thomas, J.W. (1981). The concept of access: definition and relationship to consumer satisfaction. *Medical Care* **19**(2): 127–140.

Piette, J.D., Wagner, T.H., Potter, M.B., and Schillinger, D. (2004). Health insurance status, cost-related medication underuse, and outcomes among diabetes patients in three systems of care. *Medical Care* **42**(2): 102–109.

Prentice, J.C., Dy, S., Davies, M.L., and Pizer, S.D. (2013). Using health outcomes to validate access quality measures. *American Journal of Managed Care* **19**(11): E367–E377.

Ramoni, M., Sebastiani, P., and Cohen, P. (2002). Bayesian clustering by dynamics. *Machine Learning* **47**(1): 91–121.

Schach, E. and Schach, S. (1972). A continuous time stochastic model for the utilization of health services. *Socio-Economic Planning Sciences* **6**(3): 263–272.

Schechter, M.S. (2003). Non-genetic influences on cystic fibrosis lung disease: the role of sociodemographic characteristics, environmental exposures, and healthcare interventions. *Seminars in Respiratory and Critical Care Medicine* **24**(6): 639–652.

Schechter, M.S. and Margolis, P.A. (1998). Relationship between socioeconomic status and disease severity in cystic fibrosis. *The Journal of Pediatrics* **132**(2): 260–264.

Schechter, M.S., Shelton, B.J., Margolis, P.A., and Fitzsimmons, S.C. (2001). The association of socioeconomic status with outcomes in cystic fibrosis patients in the United States. *American Journal of Respiratory and Critical Care Medicine* **163**(6): 1331–1337.

Schechter, M.S., McColley, S.A., Silva, S. et al. (2009). Association of socioeconomic status with the use of chronic therapies and healthcare utilization in children with cystic fibrosis. *Journal of Pediatrics* **155**(5): 634–U667.

Serban, N. (2011). A space–time varying coefficient model: the equity of service accessibility. *The Annals of Applied Statistics* **5**(3): 2024–2051.

Smyth, P. (1997). Clustering sequences with hidden Markov models. In: *Advances in Neural Information Processing Systems*, 648–654. MIT Press.

Statistics Canada and Canadian Institute for Health Information (2008). A Framework for Health Outcomes Analysis. Ottawa, ON.

Statistics Canada and Canadian Institute for Health Information (2012). Health Outcomes of Care: An Idea Whose Time Has Come. Ottawa, ON.

Sy, J.P. and Taylor, J.M.G. (2000). Estimation in a cox proportional hazards cure model. *Biometrics* **56**(1): 227–236.

Taylor-Robinson, D. and Schechter, M.S. (2011). Health inequalities and cystic fibrosis. *BMJ* **343**: d4818.

Teach, S.J., Guagliardo, M.F., Crain, E.F. et al. (2006). Spatial accessibility of primary care pediatric services in an urban environment: association with asthma management and outcome. *Pediatrics* **117**(4 Pt 2): S78–S85.

United States Department of Agriculture (2016). Rural-Urban Commuting Area Codes. https://www.ers.usda.gov/data-products/rural-urban-commuting-area-codes.aspx (accessed March 2019).

Vander Weele, T.J. (2016). Mediation analysis: a practitioner's guide. *Annual Review of Public Health* **37**: 17–32.

Velentgas, P., Dreyer, N.A., Nourjah, P. et al. (eds.) (2013). *Developing a Protocol for Observational Comparative Effectiveness Research: A User's Guide*. Rockville, MD: Agency for Healthcare Research and Quality.

Venkataramani, A.S., Brigell, R., O'Brien, R. et al. (2016). Economic opportunity, health behaviours, and health outcomes in the USA: a population-based cross-sectional study. *The Lancet Public Health* **1**(1): E18–E25.

Waller, L.A., Zhu, L., Gotway, C.A. et al. (2007). Quantifying geographic variations in associations between alcohol distribution and violence: a comparison of geographically weighted regression and spatially varying coefficient models. *Stochastic Environmental Research and Risk Assessment* **21**(5): 573–588.

Wang, F. and Luo, W. (2005). Assessing spatial and nonspatial factors for healthcare access: towards an integrated approach to defining health professional shortage areas. *Health & Place* **11**(2): 131–146.

Wang, X., Dockery, D.W., Wypij, D. et al. (1993). Pulmonary function between 6 and 18 years of age. *Pediatric Pulmonology* **15**(2): 75–88.

Wisdom, J.P., Berlin, M., and Lapidus, J.A. (2005). Relating health policy to women's health outcomes. *Social Science and Medicine* **61**(8): 1776–1784.

Witt, W.P., Fullerton, C.A., Chow, C. et al. (2017). Effect of having a usual source of care on health care outcomes among children with serious emotional disturbance. *Academic Pediatrics* **17**(1): 45–52.

Wolfenden, L.L. and Schechter, M.S. (2009). Genetic and non-genetic determinants of outcomes in cystic fibrosis. *Paediatric Respiratory Reviews* **10**(1): 32–36.

Wyszewianski, L. (2002). Access to care: remembering old lessons. *Health Services Research* **73**(6): 1441–1443.

5

HEALTHCARE INTERVENTIONS FOR IMPROVING ACCESS

Health interventions typically aim to prevent, treat or cure health problems at the patient level while *healthcare interventions* aim to improve the healthcare system and the population health. Since healthcare access is a system outcome, the focus of this chapter is on healthcare interventions, differentiated into multiple modalities, including health policy, e-healthcare, community-based, and network interventions. The *health policies* of interest are addressing improvements in healthcare for the public health. *E-healthcare and community-based interventions* refer to alternative modalities for healthcare delivery. *Network interventions* refer to location or reallocation of healthcare resources as presented in more detail in this chapter.

This chapter primarily focuses on "*What works best and for whom*" with the goal of improving healthcare access and ultimately health outcomes. It builds upon the understanding of measurement and inference on healthcare access and the link to health outcomes discussed in the previous chapters. But it goes beyond quantifying the impact of healthcare interventions on healthcare access and health outcomes to address a broad spectrum of questions such as:

- How will the system respond if a particular intervention is to be implemented? At what level would the interventions need to be enacted to close the gaps in healthcare access disparities?
- What communities and sub-populations are most in need of intervention? What intervention should be considered and for which sub-population or community?
- What are the benefits of an intervention? Is it cost-saving or cost-effective? Does it reduce severe outcomes? Does it reduce disparities in health outcomes? Does the intervention have unintended consequences?
- What is the impact of advocacy in promoting health policy? How important is informed decision making?

Healthcare System Access: Measurement, Inference, and Intervention, Nicoleta Serban.
© 2020 John Wiley & Sons, Inc. Published 2020 by John Wiley & Sons, Inc.

Addressing questions such as these requires extensive population health data to link changes in outcomes to intervention strategies. It also involves knowledge across many domains, including health systems, health economics, statistical modeling, optimization, and simulation. Generally, such questions are addressed within specific contexts, for example, the improvement in access for the Medicaid population with the increase in the Medicaid acceptance rates among providers (Nobles et al. 2014; Cao et al. 2017b); the cost-effectiveness of telehealth programs (Kirkizlar et al. 2013; Bergmo 2015); the cost-effectiveness of preventive care (Philips and Holtgrave 1997); or the cost reduction of dental care from the utilization of Silver Diamine Fluoride (SDF) for arresting carries (Johnson et al. 2019).

Different approaches can be used to improve access for different types of care. Increasing Medicaid acceptance rates is a highly cited intervention for improving access for the Medicaid population. Telemedicine and mobile health are emerging healthcare service interventions, advanced to address access barriers to healthcare across many services, particularly for the population in rural communities and/or for specialized care. Expanding the independence or scope of practice of licensed healthcare professionals (e.g. nurse practitioners (Kaiser Family Foundation 2012), dental hygienists) and allowing provision of specific healthcare services to be delivered by a larger network of providers (e.g. pharmacists being allowed to prescribe contraception medication) have recently been at the forefront of many debates in health policy making. Specific services have the potential to avoid high healthcare costs while reducing the need of care, for example, preventive care services.

As highlighted in this chapter, there is not one "magic bullet" type of healthcare intervention that addresses all needs related to healthcare access. In fact, together all such interventions can best tackle the conundrum of the trade-off between Equity, Effectiveness, and Efficiency in healthcare access.

A TAXONOMY OF HEALTHCARE INTERVENTIONS

An *intervention* may be defined as an interceding act that has the intention of modifying an outcome (MedicineNet n.d.). *Healthcare interventions* typically aim to intercede with healthcare system outcomes, in a way that monitor, promote, alter, tailor or transform the healthcare system. The focus in this book and hence in this chapter, is on interventions that target improvements in healthcare access. As highlighted in the introduction to this chapter, there are many such interventions with different objectives toward improving access. The multiple types of healthcare interventions discussed in this chapter are as follows:

- *Health Policy*
- *Network Intervention*
- *Community-based Healthcare*
- *E-Healthcare*

Health Policy

> Health policy refers to decisions, plans, and actions that are undertaken to achieve specific healthcare goals within a society. An explicit health policy can achieve several things: it defines a vision for the future, which in turn helps to establish targets and points of reference for the short and medium term. It outlines priorities and the expected roles of different groups; and it builds consensus and informs people.
>
> (World Health Organization n.d.)

In other words, health policies are the actions, decisions, regulations or laws enacted at the healthcare (eco)system and organization levels, while impacting the people, processes, and organization levels, following the multilevel framework of the healthcare system described in Chapter 2 (Figure 2.2). Health policies can impact one or more of the dimensions of healthcare access, and generally they focus on specific healthcare services. Health policies can exist at the organizational, local, or national levels. Some well-accepted broad categories of health policies are found in the framework by Penchansky and Thomas (1981).

Affordability Most developed countries have opted for a universal healthcare system. However, in the United States, financial access is not universal; it has been one of the most debated aspects of the national health policy agenda. Because healthcare is so expensive in the United States, affordability is generally thought of as the affordability of health insurance rather than the services themselves. In the United States, health insurance is fragmented into:

- *Medicare*, the national federal healthcare insurance program for people over 65 years old.
- *Medicaid*, a public insurance program for populations with low income, disability and/or in foster care or otherwise in state custody.
- *Children's Health Insurance Program (CHIP)*, also a public insurance program but only for children of families with an income level that does not qualify for Medicaid.
- *Exchange healthcare programs*, available for those who need to seek healthcare benefits outside all the other types of programs.
- *Private employer-sponsored health insurance* available to those who work, or their dependents, and may be either self-funded by the employer or a group health plan purchased by the employer from the commercial health insurance market.
- *Uninsured*, those who may not qualify for federal or state programs, do not have employer-sponsored healthcare benefits, and do not acquire healthcare insurance through the exchange programs.

While some people without insurance may have access to some programs for services such as mental and behavioral health services or cancer screening, most do not.

This fragmentation of the financial access in the United States is the result of a patchwork of state and federal laws. One of the most important federal laws that dramatically shifted the health policy landscape, including the affordability of health insurance, was the 2010 Patient Protection and Affordable Care Act (PPACA). The PPACA has been revisited, debated, and amended for the last decade. To provide greater financial access to individuals most likely those uninsured, it allows states to apply to expand Medicaid or deliver Medicaid services using new care models with an enhanced federal financial match to help offset those costs; requires employer-sponsored health plans to allow dependent children to remain on those plans until age 26; and regulates to provide certain tax incentives to encourage the purchase of insurance by individuals. However, despite the broad reach of the PPACA, because of the way that the United States Constitution is written, much of the legal authority to regulate and promote the affordability of health services and private health plans is reserved to the states. This often results in substantive differences across the states and regions of the country.

While affordability is a necessary condition of accessing the healthcare system, a precursor of the realized utilization of the healthcare system, it is not a sufficient condition. As I highlighted in the earlier chapters of this book, other access dimensions are equally important. Most importantly, affordability is closely related to other dimensions of access. For example, limited affordability implies limited availability of providers accepting patients without the ability to pay for healthcare services. Federal Qualified Health Centers (FQHCs) and alike as well as emergency departments are mandated to accept any patient regardless of the ability to pay, however, the healthcare services provided in such organizations are limited.

Moreover, while approximately 40% of the United States population was enrolled in insurance programs such as Medicare and Medicaid in 2018, hence deemed to have financial access, their access to healthcare services is limited because of reduced access in other dimensions. Thus, it is paramount to consider policies and interventions that address access beyond affordability or financial access.

Availability and Accessibility   As I underlined above, the healthcare system in the United States is fragmented, with various types of healthcare insurance programs, each program being served by a different network of providers, depending on varying reimbursement rates and how streamlined the administrative process is. This may result in a larger or smaller network of providers available to a healthcare insurance program, which can impact the level of availability of some or all healthcare services. Lack or reduced availability of the providers results in large travel distances to reach a provider within the network of available providers, thus reducing accessibility. The two access dimensions, accessibility and availability, are closely interrelated; as I highlighted earlier in the book, they are commonly studied together under the so called concept of spatial access.

Systematic disparities exist in the provider networks across various types of healthcare insurance programs, particularly, when contrasting public versus commercial programs (Berman et al. 2002; Centers for Medicare & Medicaid Services 2016; Cao et al. 2017b; Wishner and Marks 2017). Moreover, regardless of the insurance status, for some sub-populations, particularly those in rural communities, access to healthcare services is also reduced, particularly for specialized healthcare. Such systematic disparities can result in inequities in healthcare delivery, and ultimately, inequities in health outcomes.

There are several approaches to expanding the network of providers available for specific healthcare services and/or for sub-populations in need of healthcare, where some approaches involve adding providers to the network while others involve using the existing providers in the network under less restrictive practice specifications for licensed professionals. The former type of approaches include the classic approach of allocation or re-allocation of resources using network interventions and more novel approaches such as mobile healthcare or telemedicine described later in this section. Health policies generally focus on the latter type of approaches since they only require changes in some of the existing laws and regulations.

Recent debates in many healthcare policy areas, contraception, preventive dental care, vaccination, among others, have focused on giving prescription authority to licensed professionals in many healthcare domains; expanding the scope of practice; relaxing supervision (so called independent practice); and reimbursement for the services provided by public insurance programs. *Giving prescriptive authority* means that a healthcare provider has legal ability to prescribe prescription medication. *Expanding the scope of practice* means allowing more procedures, actions, and processes that a healthcare provider is legally permitted to do. *Relaxing independent practice* means that "any individual permitted by law provides care and services, without direction or supervision, within the scope of the individual's license and consistent with individually granted clinical privileges." (Joint Commission on Accreditation of Healthcare Organizations 2016) *Reimbursement of services* refers to direct payment by the insurance programs to the provider that has delivered the services. Health policies related to these four areas addressing access barriers are generally state governed, with wide variations across states. Below are some examples of such policies.

> *Giving prescriptive authority to pharmacists*: Pharmacists have long been an underutilized resource in the healthcare system. An illustration of utilizing this resource aiming to increase access to a specific type of service is the expansion of prescription authority of pharmacists to prescribe short-acting contraception to women, without a doctor's visit or authorization. Such policy has been enacted in a handful of states as of 2018, including California, Oregon, Maryland, Hawaii, Colorado, New Jersey, New Mexico, and Washington, with New Hampshire passing a bill to study the impact of such health policy as a first step (American Pharmacists Association 2016; Rodriguez et al. 2016; National Alliance of State Pharmacy Associations 2018).
>
> *Scope of practice and independent practice for pharmacists*: Expansion of scope of practice and supervision of pharmacists in administering vaccination has been enacted in all 50 states, the District of Columbia, and Puerto Rico but with some variations in terms of the extent of pharmacists' authority across states. Such variations are in three areas: types of vaccines that can be administered;

the age of the patient to whom a pharmacist can administer a vaccine; and the pharmacist's scope of practice to screen, recommend, prescribe, and administer immunization. These policy differences across states can significantly reduce access to vaccination for populations that are most vulnerable to conditions that can be prevented by immunization (American Pharmacists Association 2015; Goad 2015).

Scope of practice and independent practice for NPs: Preventive healthcare and wellness have been one of the primary areas of advancement of recent health policy, specifically, the PPACA. Many studies forecast that the resulting increase in the demand of care due to the PPACA provisions may not be adequately supported by the supply of healthcare services (Colwill et al. 2008; Hofer et al. 2011; Petterson et al. 2012; Anderson 2014; HRSA 2013). Health policies toward addressing this shortage include expanding scope of practice and independent practice of the NPs as the current supply of NPs could bear the additional demand for primary care (Arifkhanova 2017). About half of the states permit NPs to practice and/or prescribe drugs without physician supervision or collaboration; in about 21 states, NPs have full practice authority and in the rest of the states, they require some level of physician supervision (Arifkhanova 2017; Rudner and Kung 2017). Figure 5.1 displays the variations on the scope of practice for NPs across states.

Scope of practice and independent practice for dental hygienists: Preventive dental care is also an important area of intervention, particularly for children. Oral disease is cited as the greatest unmet health need among United States children (Newacheck et al. 2000), and significant disparities exist (US Department of Health and Human Services 2000). Recent health policies have promoted relaxation of supervision requirements for dental hygienists in public health and safety net settings, allowing hygienists to perform specific preventive services without the physical presence of a dentist (Naughton 2014). Currently, three states do not allow general supervision, and four states allow general supervision only for some services and/or under specific settings. General supervision can facilitate improved access to dental care for sub-populations vulnerable to healthcare inequities because dental hygienists do not need to be directly supervised by dentists at the time of service provision (Greenberg et al. 2008; Naughton 2014).

Medicaid reimbursement for NPs and dental hygienists: Supervision constraints may also apply in the direct reimbursement for the services delivered by NPs through the public insurance programs, again with wide variations in the services provided and the type of supervision required (2012). Thus even when supervision of NPs is relaxed, if the NPs are not directly reimbursed, their ability to practice independently in schools, nursing homes, and other similar settings is limited. Similarly, direct Medicaid reimbursement of the services provided by dental hygienists is mandated only in 18 states, with variations in the age of the patient, the healthcare setting, and the registration requirements (American Dental Hygienists' Association n.d.-b). Direct

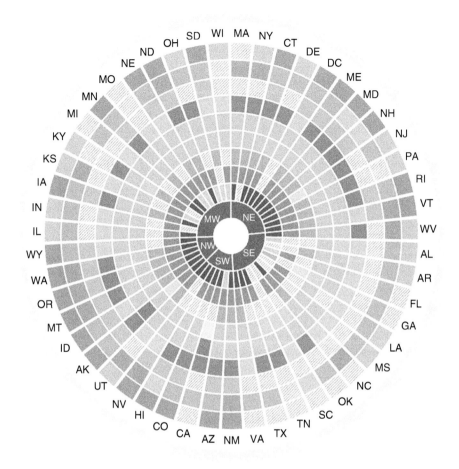

Color Key:

Full

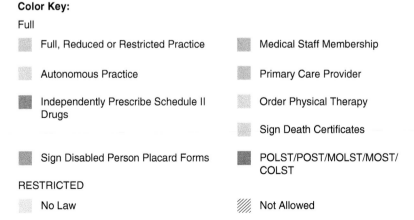

Full, Reduced or Restricted Practice	Medical Staff Membership
Autonomous Practice	Primary Care Provider
Independently Prescribe Schedule II Drugs	Order Physical Therapy
	Sign Death Certificates
Sign Disabled Person Placard Forms	POLST/POST/MOLST/MOST/COLST

RESTRICTED

No Law	Not Allowed

FIGURE 5.1 NPs scope of practice by state. *Source:* American Association of Nurse Practitioners and Barton Associates (https://www.bartonassociates.com/locum-tenens-resources/nurse-practitioner-scope-of-practice-laws).

reimbursement could provide dental hygienists the opportunity to reach out to areas and sub-populations with reduced access to dental care, particularly rural communities, schools, and nursing homes. If direct reimbursement is restricted, dental hygienists need to be affiliated to dentists who accept Medicaid to be reimbursed for their services; however, for most states, a relatively small percentage of dentists accept Medicaid thus restricting dental hygienists' ability to serve dental shortage areas even if supervision is not required for basic preventive dental services.

Acceptability   Closely related to affordability and availability of healthcare services is acceptability of insurance programs by healthcare providers. In the United States, most commercial or private insurance programs are differentiated into Health Maintenance Organization (HMO) and Preferred Provider Organization (PPO) insurance plans. HMO plans cover services provided only within that HMO's network with some opportunities to see a non-network provider. PPO plans differentiate providers into in-network and out-of-network providers, with a higher co-payment or cost to the patient when services are delivered by out-of-network providers. In comparison, public insurance programs such as Medicaid and CHIP cover services provided only by the participating healthcare providers. Generally, the network of providers participating in public insurance programs is limited to only a percentage of available providers for a particular healthcare service, with a substantively reduced network for specialized healthcare. Last, Medicare is an insurance program that is private-public insurance, where the decision making and the coverage is made by different entities, some private, and some governmental-based. Moreover, approximately 33% of those qualifying for Medicare are enrolled in Medicare Advantage plans, which are fully private (Kaiser Family Foundation 2017).

Health policy has been primarily focused on approaches to increase the participation of healthcare providers in the public insurance programs since it greatly limits availability and accessibility of healthcare services. Policies or interventions that target improving healthcare access for the population with public insurance (referred to as *Medicaid* herein) target the healthcare provider participation in Medicaid programs, which can be of two types: interventions that target increased caseload of those providers already participating in Medicaid: or increased number of providers participating in Medicaid. While it is difficult to design a policy that would exclusively result in changes in one of the two types of improvements, considering the types of changes separately is useful for analyzing the sources of limited accessibility for Medicaid populations, and for evaluating the likely success of interventions. These types of structural changes may be achieved through policies that increase Medicaid payment levels or promote Medicaid managed care contracts that allow healthcare providers greater flexibility.

Accommodation   Healthcare consumerism and healthcare costs are pushing more care to more convenient locations (Landers 2010). For example, some basic healthcare services are being provided in new on-site clinics at chain retail stores, at home, in schools or in the form of telehealth or telemedicine. Below I will provide a brief account for three of the emerging approaches to overcome access barriers, including in-home healthcare, in-school healthcare, and telehealth; with this I will highlight important considerations on the healthcare delivery and the health policy, underlying the implementation of these approaches.

Network Interventions

Network interventions for improving healthcare access include opening new facilities or expanding the caseload at some of the existing facilities given an expanded budget. For the healthcare system, facilities can be clinics, provider groups, individual practices, public health department centers, and school centers, among many others. Selecting telemedicine sites or where to integrate practices could also be viewed as network interventions. Thus all modalities of care discussed above can be integrated in a network intervention, where the decision making is on *where* and *how* to intervene.

Given the multiple possible settings for network interventions, the decision making can be quite complex, depending on the needs for healthcare of various sub-populations, available resources, policies in place and integration within the larger healthcare network. The set of decisions to be made in a network intervention can be complex also because the main objectives to be achieved cannot all be optimized. Such decisions could lead to specific geographic areas to have inadequate access to healthcare or the intervention cost may be too high to be a feasible solution. In this complex decision environment, when designing and implementing network interventions, several considerations need to be taken into account.

Are there healthcare needs to be met? Is there a population group or a geographic area with higher needs to be prioritized? Identifying the need for an intervention is at the core of all 3 E's: efficiency, effectiveness, and equity. Measurement and inference of the outcome of interest, as presented earlier in the chapter, are the basis for addressing such questions.

What type of intervention will be implemented? Will the intervention be selected from multiple modalities or settings, e.g. school-centers, telemedicine? Generally, when network interventions are considered, one specific setting for the intervention is considered because the decision making is commonly initiated by an organization with a specific intervention focus.

What are the implementation and setting constraints? There are many possible constraints to the implementation of network interventions but the most substantive ones are: (i) the primary target for the implementation, e.g. serving a high demand area, reducing disparities in access, meeting access standards; (ii) implementation and operating costs; (iii) health policies restricting or facilitating provision of care, reimbursement of specific services within different settings or for scope of practice and supervision of licensed healthcare providers; (iv) availability of appropriate providers and staff at the sites considered for interventions and for the type of care provided; and (v) the set of healthcare services to be delivered as part of the intervention and the participation in various health insurance programs.

In an ideal world, network interventions would consider all possible settings of care within the set of implementation constraints; this can be viewed as an optimization approach of a centralized planner, for example, Veterans Administration or the Military Health System, which have the flexibility to consider multiple modalities, specifically, to choose between telemedicine, open a new clinic or contracting a provider or organization for provision of care for the planner's patient population. Such an "ideal world" approach, while in most case is not realistic, can inform the decision making on what and where is needed given the trade-off between the 3 E's.

It is however more realistic to begin with one very specific setting of care, thus "how" to intervene is established a priori, then consider an optimal decision on "where" to intervene for the highest impact to the system outcomes. When selecting "where" to locate healthcare sites, there are four primary categories of decision making: (i) finding a set of optimal sites; (ii) locating optimal sites in a new area; (iii) measuring the effectiveness of past location decisions; and (iv) improving existing location patterns (Rahman and Smith 2000). Examples of such network interventions are many, with a few examples presented below. Amir et al. (2017) expanded on many such examples within a survey of facility location problems or network interventions in healthcare.

- *Community Health Centers* (CHCs) can increase access across all dimensions for medically underserved communities. Due to limited resources to invest and operate CHCs, it is important to identify the best location and number of new CHCs in a geographical network, as well as what services each CHC should offer at which caseload level (Griffin et al. 2008). Such a network intervention can improve access by as much as 20% across multiple outcomes (Griffin et al. 2008). This is a classic example of a network intervention, applying to other types of healthcare facilities not only CHCs.

- *Service integration* is particularly critical in healthcare delivery (Suter et al. 2009; Czako and Poreisz 2013), where medical services are usually provided by small, autonomous groups of providers who specialize in specific pathologies. Patients often get treatment for individual health conditions rather than receiving coordinated care for their overall health. For example, a typical Medicare patient is seen by two primary care physicians and five specialists per year; patients who have a few chronic conditions can visit as many as 16 physicians in a year (Pham et al. 2007; Bodenheimer 2008). Integration/coordination of services in the healthcare system thus involves the deliberate integration of patient care activities between two or more participants involved in a patient's care; the objective is to facilitate appropriate and timely delivery of healthcare services (McDonald et al. 2007). Integration of healthcare services requires targeted network interventions where the decisions involve matching providers practicing at different locations and/or within different healthcare delivery modalities (e.g. office vs telemedicine). Such interventions have been widely considered in the existing research and practice, including for telehealth (Soares et al. 2013; Mehrotra 2014), co-location of specialist providers in primary care offices (Sullivan et al. 2006; Briggs et al. 2007; Rumball-Smith et al. 2014), and training of primary care providers in specialized care (Baker et al. 2009; Blount and Miller 2009).

- *Loan repayment* is commonly used to encourage providers to choose areas of practice with higher need, such as rural areas (Geletko et al. 2014; Nicholson et al. 2015). For most programs, providers applying for a loan repayment program choose their area of service, while guaranteeing to dedicate a proportion of their caseload to public insurance for a period of a few years, for example. Studies have shown loan repayments to be one of the most successful ways to encourage generalist physicians to locate in underserved areas (Pathman et al. 2004); however, there is less success in maintaining the practices in these areas in the long term (Sempowski 2004). A network intervention targeting areas for locating providers participating in such programs can have a higher impact in terms of improving access and reducing costs (Johnson et al. 2017).

- *Telemedicine* provides patients with access to locally unavailable medical services and substitutes face-to-face contact with telecommunication with physicians. Telemedicine is a network intervention because it relies on the current network of providers to provide tele-healthcare while adding locations to the network from which telemedicine can be practiced. It is one approach of integrated health services, where integration refers to the process of combining and coordinating services in such a way that both service users and providers benefit. Many implementations have been adopted to date, with wide applicability in Canada (Praxia Information Intelligence and Gartner Inc. 2011). Within the framework of network interventions, designing telemedicine health networks is a complex decision making process, with constraints on intervention costs; on the available provider network; on health policy such as reimbursement, targeted population; and on varying healthcare needs among, many others. Implementation of telemedicine while accounting for all such constraints to obtain optimal locations of telemedicine sites is an "ideal" allocation of existing resources; however, such an ideal allocation can be used in designing telemedicine interventions since they rely on the current network of providers.

- *Home healthcare* is the provision of patient care delivered in the home. While home healthcare does not involve setting up sites for healthcare delivery, it can be viewed as a network intervention or location problem since it falls under the area of improving existing location patterns. The logistics of decisions related to the human resource (HR) planning in home healthcare is very complex, involving decisions on which care workers deliver care services and to which patients, as well as on scheduling patient visits assigned to each care worker (Cissé et al. 2017). Figure 5.2 is an illustration of the layout of the decision making in HR management in home healthcare. The network intervention of home healthcare management aims to determine optimal service deployment in terms of location and routing. When strategically implemented, home healthcare has many benefits for both those receiving care and those providing

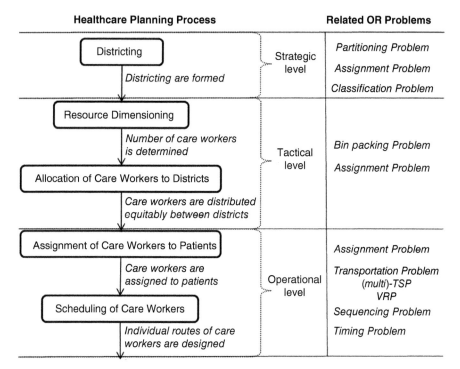

FIGURE 5.2   Human resources planning in home healthcare. *Source:* Courtesy of Cissé et al. (2017).

care with respect to all dimensions of healthcare access. However, the planning effort required to manage home-based services is highly complex because it involves questions at different levels of decision, such as districting, staff management, routing, and scheduling. Thus, considering home healthcare as a network intervention with all its implications in terms of strategic and optimal deployment is paramount to improve the experience and to reap the benefits in the provision of home-based care. I will expand on this modality of healthcare below.

Community-Based Healthcare

In-Home Healthcare   Home healthcare is defined by the National Clinical Home-care Association as "the provision of medical supplies and/or clinical services directly to patients in the community" (World Health Organization 2015). The largest population targeted for home healthcare is the elderly population, with the majority (70%) of patients being 65 years of age and older (Mitzner et al. 2009). Around the world, home healthcare potentially has a large market. Only in the United States, the number of people over 65 is expected to exceed 70 million by 2030 (Landers 2010). Many countries have made substantive investments in home healthcare delivery. Denmark allocated about 1.6% of its GNP (Gross National Product) in 2005 (about $4 billions) for the care of 200 000 patients. In European countries, around 1–5% of the public health budgets are spent on home healthcare services (Emilianoa et al. 2017).

Home healthcare can reduce pressure on family members, balancing fulltime employment, parenting, and caregiving (World Health Organization 2015). According to the National Association for Home Care & Hospice, "Home care reinforces and supplements care provided by family members and friends and maintains the recipient's dignity and independence, qualities that can be lost even in the best institutions. Home care also allows patients to take an active role in their care." It has also been shown to be a cost-effective way to increase access to primary healthcare services for the populations vulnerable to inequities in health and healthcare such as children and the elderly (The National Association for Home Care & Hospice 2010; Romagnoli et al. 2013).

Home healthcare consists of a wide range of healthcare services, the most popular being medical/skilled nursing services (75%), followed by personal care (44%), and therapeutic services (37%) (Mitzner et al. 2009). More specific services include exercising, checking vital signs such as blood pressure, psychological or social assessment, wound care, medication education, pain management, disease education and management, physical therapy, speech therapy, medication reminders, administering medications, and occupational therapy (Mitzner et al. 2009; World Health Organization 2015; Cissé et al. 2017). Home care can also be an integral component of the post-hospitalization recovery process (transitional care), especially during the initial weeks after discharge when the patient still requires some level of regular physical assistance (World Health Organization 2015).

While home healthcare directly addresses accommodation as the primary access dimension, it relies on the availability of providers to provide such care. Several challenges may arise in this context (Cissé et al. 2017). Most often, home healthcare requires continuity of care, ensuring that each patient is assigned to a restricted set of care workers. Not all services can be provided in the same time or in an order convenient to a healthcare provider; for example, one service should be planned three days after another service. Healthcare delivery requires to also account for the expertise and qualifications of the care workers. Patients may also have preferences for a care worker, gender, or language.

Home healthcare can be provided by community health workers/volunteers, nurses, social workers, general practitioners/family doctors, nutritionists, physiotherapists, geriatricians, and specialized physicians such as psychiatrists and cardiologists (World Health Organization 2015). However, the constraints in the delivery of home care reduce the availability of providers, thus health policies for improving availability and accessibility of healthcare as discussed in the previous section are highly relevant in this context also.

Medicare and Medicaid programs in the United States can lead the way in health policy to advance and facilitate home healthcare as they are the largest payers of home healthcare services (The National Association for Home Care & Hospice 2010). In 2009, Medicare spending accounted for approximately 41% of home health expenditures and Medicaid has seen nearly a decade of double-digit growth associated with shifting preferences away from institutional care toward home and community-based settings (The National Association for Home Care & Hospice 2010).

In-School Healthcare   School absenteeism due to illness and/or doctor visits can be a substantive determinant of overall being and education level. Chronic conditions can interfere with a child's ability to succeed in school. Specifically, an increase in missed school time caused by chronic illnesses can lead to a decline in school performance. Challenges faced by parents to take their children to receive healthcare services, such as long travel distances, and missing work, can be significant enough to delay or preclude care all together for their children, potentially resulting in severe outcomes that can then require emergency services, hospitalizations, and long-term poor health in some cases. Healthcare approaches to healthcare delivery that can accommodate parents and their children in seeking care when needed include not only home-based care discussed above but also school-based healthcare. School-based healthcare can come in two forms: school-based health centers (SBHCs); or school programs.

SBHCs are generally located on or inside school groups, and the delivery of services often is provided by a NP or physician assistant while being integrated with the mission and activities of the school community (Brindis 2016). SBHCs provide services to students in pre-kindergarten through grade 12 but they can also open the door to the entire community. By 2013, the School Based Health Alliance estimated that there were 2300 SBHCs, approximately 1.8% of the public and private schools in the United States (Knopf et al. 2016).

The Community Preventive Services Task Force recommended the implementation and maintenance of SBHCs in low-income communities, based on sufficient evidence of effectiveness in improving educational and health outcomes (Community Preventive Services Task Force 2016). The American Academy of Pediatrics recommends SBHCs as "one model of a system of healthcare delivery that provides a healthcare 'safety net' for children and adolescents who are uninsured or underinsured or represent special populations who do not regularly access healthcare" (Community Preventive Services Task Force 2016).

SBHCs have the role of addressing access to appropriate healthcare for children in all its dimensions. Moreover, being integrated in the education system, they have a dual impact; they not only improve access to healthcare, but they can also promote better educational outcomes, and decrease risk-taking behaviors that often lead or contribute to negative health outcomes (Brindis 2016). SBHCs can meet students' physical health and mental health needs, which may not be addressed by a complex and fragmented healthcare system. SBHCs provide students easier access to health services; this reduces time missed at school and helps parents to avoid losing work time and spending extra time to transport their children to and from healthcare facilities (Knopf et al. 2016; Ran et al. 2016).

SBHCs can impact the uptake and utilization of many healthcare services. Services provided by SBHCs in the United States include comprehensive physical and mental health assessments (97%); vision, hearing, and other screening and prevention services (93%); and immunizations (85%) (Kwong et al. 2010; Knopf et al. 2016; Ran et al. 2016). In addition, a majority of SBHCs provide pregnancy testing (81%), contraceptive counseling (70%), and follow-up services for contraceptive users (59%) (Ran et al. 2016). They can address management of chronic conditions such as asthma, mental and behavioral health, and oral health, among others. Services can also be provided to school staff, student family members, and others within the surrounding community (Knopf et al. 2016).

In-school healthcare can be delivered by public health programs, for example, the Oral Health Initiative and other organizations have encouraged targeted oral health interventions such as school-based sealant programs (Griffin et al. 2016a). Generally, management of chronic conditions and preventions are candidates of school programs, however such programs need to reach a large enough population to be effective. Thus health conditions that are more common among children, such as dental cavities or asthma, are the best candidates to be targeted in the implementation of school-based programs. Moreover, school-based programs commonly target schools with a high percentage (>50%) of free and reduced lunch students thus targeting communities and child populations known to have many barriers in accessing healthcare.

Research on school dental sealant programs has shown their effectiveness in improving outcomes, specifically, in preventing caries and in reducing cost across a wide range of program settings (Griffin et al. 2016a,b). In one of my collaborative research papers, we showed that school-based programs can lead to net savings to Medicaid when the sealant program is staffed by dental hygienists and at a penetration level higher than 25%, i.e. the difference between total savings to Medicaid and the Medicaid spending on school-based services was positive under these settings (Johnson et al. 2017).

Noteworthy challenges in delivering care in schools are billing and financing for implementation and sustainability of school-based healthcare as well as the uptake of the services by students for whom those services are made available (Community Preventive Services Task Force 2016). Similar challenges as in other settings discussed above apply to the delivery of care in school programs, specifically, independent practice, and Medicaid reimbursement. For example, if dental hygienists are not reimbursed by the public insurance programs directly for their services, they only can provide preventive dental care under public health programs, which are financed by states, thus generally with low levels of penetration of the population targeted for such programs due to limited resources.

Moreover, there are wide variations in the specifications of school health policies across states. For example, policies on counseling and mental health services vary from no requirements to provide services (e.g. Alabama, Colorado, Iowa, Kansas, Rhode Island, Vermont, and other states) to allowing school districts to make their own guidance policies (e.g. California, Delaware, and other states) to requirements to provide psychological services in the form of consultation and counseling to parents, students, and school personnel (e.g. Arkansas, Montana, and other states) (National Association of State Boards of Education n.d.). Such policies can facilitate or hamper provision of care in schools and increase the disparities in health among children within and between states.

On one hand, because school-based healthcare can overcome educational obstacles and increase access to needed healthcare services, they can reduce severe health outcomes, some can be cost saving, and they can advance health equity (Knopf et al. 2016). On the other hand, they can also increase health inequities if national and/or state policies are not consistently implemented within and between states and locally.

E-Healthcare: Telemedicine and Mobile Healthcare

E-healthcare has emerged as another modality for delivering care to mitigate access barriers. It can play the role of the intermediary between a system's technology and patients' healthcare. E-healthcare is a new way of approaching healthcare, a network approach in which patients take a more central role in their own healthcare management. Two important implementations of e-healthcare that address the accessibility and accommodation dimensions of healthcare access are telehealth or telemedicine, and mobile healthcare.

Telehealth and/or *telemedicine* defines the exchange of information – data, images, and video – by electronic and telecommunication means to aid in healthcare delivery, and nonclinical practices such as continuing medical education and nursing call centers. The World Health Organization (2009) refers to both telehealth and telemedicine in one concept: "The delivery of healthcare services, where distance is a critical factor, by all healthcare professionals using information and communication technologies for the exchange of valid information for diagnosis, treatment and prevention of disease and injuries, research and evaluation, and for the continuing education of healthcare providers, all in the interests of advancing the health of individuals and their communities." Examples of telemedicine include two providers discussing a case over the phone, video consultation, and image transmission over fixed or mobile networks.

Telemedicine provides patients with access to locally unavailable medical services and often substitutes face-to-face contact with physicians. It closes the geographic gap between the licensed caregivers and/or the care receiver, with the primary objective of providing medical diagnosis and treatment. Its purpose is not only to increase access to healthcare but also to promote the efficiency, effectiveness, and quality of mainstream medicine. It is also at the frontier of the pursuit of a healthy lifestyle, patient empowerment, as well as preparedness and response to natural and man-made threats (Bashshur and Shannon 2009).

Examples of implementation of telehealth or telemedicine are widespread. A recent study on telemedicine worldwide by the World Health Organization (2009) found that teleradiology (use of image acquisition, storage, display, processing, and transport) has the highest rate of established programs. Other examples include telepathology, teledermatology, and telepsychiatry, which were featured as primary applications by the World Health Organization (2009). Initiatives in various specialties included cardiology/electrocardiography (a widely adopted application), consultation, dentistry, hematology, home care, immunology, mammography (yet another widely adopted application), patient monitoring, neurology, oncology, ophthalmology, rehabilitation, rheumatology, stroke treatment, ultrasonography, and urology. Several other more detailed examples are provided by Rouse and Serban (2015).

Mobile healthcare is the use of mobile networks and devices in healthcare delivery. It emphasizes leveraging health-focused applications on portable devices such as smartphones, sensors, and other mobile devices to drive health participation by consumers and clinicians (Federal Communications Commission 2010). Mobile technologies cannot physically carry drugs, doctors, and equipment between locations, but they can carry and process information in many forms (Qiang et al. 2011). Its primary objectives are remote monitoring and patient-centered care.

The field of mobile healthcare encompasses applications, devices, and communications networks that allow clinicians and patients to give and receive care anywhere at any time. Physicians download diagnostic data, lab results, images, and drug information to handheld devices like PDAs and smartphones. Emergency medical responders use field laptops to keep track of patient information and records. Patients use health monitoring devices and sensors that accompany them everywhere. Mobile healthcare promotes information symmetry between patients, providers, health organizations, and the healthcare system. Mobile healthcare offers convenience critical to improving consumer engagement and clinician responsiveness. It presents opportunities to enhance disease prevention and management by extending health interventions beyond the reach of traditional care (Estrin and Sim 2010).

At the heart of mobile healthcare applications for both prevention and chronic disease management is healthcare access. The oldest and most established use of mobile healthcare is access to an emergency department via the emergency phone call for ambulance services. Recently, because of the availability of various mobile provider apps, consumers can also receive information on locations of health facilities and resources even without accessing the Internet or the broadband network (Topol 2010). Applications for social networking are forging connections between patients and between healthcare providers to share knowledge and experiences, and they are now made available through mobile devices. In emergency responses, mobile healthcare applications have been used to collect medical information, report on areas in greatest need, and to direct emergency medical treatment (Qiang et al. 2011).

Therefore, mobile healthcare could in principle impact all five healthcare access dimensions (availability, accessibility, affordability, acceptability, and accommodation). Its potential for equitable healthcare delivery is greatest among all healthcare technologies primarily because of the extent of communication via mobile technology. Regardless of income, race, and ethnicity, mobile communication connects more than 75% of people worldwide.

MODELING APPROACHES

The 3 E's framework for decision making in health policy and interventions underlines the trade-off between overall input (efficiency), overall output (effectiveness), or differentially weighted output (equity). While there is some level of incompatibility among the three objectives, one could derive mathematical models for balancing the trade-offs between the 3 E's in the healthcare system (Mandell 1991; Balcik et al. 2010). However, making optimal decisions under this trade-off is a theoretical framework. For a practical implementation, there are steps to consider in making appropriate and informed decisions given many constraints and considerations. Important questions to address are:

- *Are interventions needed?*
- *Where are the interventions needed and for what population groups?*
- *What interventions are needed?*
- *How to evaluate interventions?*

At the core of these questions lies extensive data analytics and modeling as presented in all the chapters of this book. A broad spectrum of analytical methodologies come into play including system engineering, analytics, operations research, and risk management, among others, to design and evaluate healthcare interventions as presented in this chapter. In the next section, I will review several analytical methodologies commonly employed in the evaluation and design of healthcare interventions then focus the presentation on methodological approaches to address the above questions.

Overview of Modeling Approaches

The analytical approaches for modeling healthcare interventions can be structured into retrospective and prospective methodologies. *Retrospective methods* primarily can address questions about the status quo of healthcare access and its relationship to outcomes and the system as a whole. *Prospective methods* can be used to predict the impact of healthcare interventions on outcomes as well as to create "what-if" scenarios under which multiple interventions can be compared and evaluated.

Retrospective models are primarily derived from the areas of engineering, machine learning, and (bio)statistics fields. Among common tools are:

- *Association analysis*: regression, correlation and/or covariance estimation.
- *Multivariate analysis*: clustering, classification.
- *Statistical inference*: hypothesis testing, confidence intervals, confidence sets.

One of the most (and perhaps *the* most) used retrospective model is regression modeling. It seeks estimation of the association of explanatory variables (predictors or covariates) to a response variable of interest. However, because both the response and the explanatory variables come in many forms and with various dependency structures, regression methods span many modeling areas including time series analysis (Brockwell and Davis 1991; Box et al. 1994), spatial statistics (Anselin 1988; Cressie 1993; Waller and Gotway 2004), and functional data analysis (Ramsay and Silverman 2010), among others. Regression analysis has been the topic of many textbooks; it is taught in most undergraduate and graduate analytics programs. In previous chapters, I illustrated the applicability of regression modeling in the context of identifying disparities in healthcare access with respect to health(care) determinants and in the context of linking outcomes to healthcare access.

Regression models are also often used in predictive modeling by establishing relationships between sets of variables; if the statistical significance of these relationships is high, a predictive model can be constructed to predict the consequence of various actions. For example, such predictive models can be used to identify whether healthcare access impacts outcomes as illustrated in a case study in Chapter 4, suggesting where interventions may be needed for the highest impact (Garcia et al. 2015). They can also be used in assessing how outcomes will change with changes in some input variables that are controlled by a given intervention. In this chapter, I will briefly present the applicability of a simple regression model to evaluate the potential impact on access with the increase in the reimbursement rates for dental care within the Medicaid system (Johnson et al. 2017).

Many data mining and machine learning techniques fall under the area of multivariate data analysis. Clustering and classification methodologies often assume that data follow a multivariate distribution with multiple modes, one mode corresponding to a class or cluster (Hartigan 1975). Dimensionality reduction methods also assume that correlated observations lie in a multidimensional space that could be projected into a space of much lower dimensionality (Hastie et al. 2009). In dimensionality reduction, the multidimensional observations are transformed into lower-dimensionality vectors that are uncorrelated. Classic examples of such methods are principal component analysis or independent component analysis. Network and causal models range from simple lattice and random mixing network, to small-world graphs or incredibly detailed social networks where nodes represent people, and edges represent relationships and interactions. Many (potential) applications related to healthcare access are in emergency responses (Larson and Nigmatulina 2010). Illustrations of such methodologies are the study of healthcare outcomes for children diagnosed with asthma in Chapter 4 and the economic evaluation for preventive dental care for young children in this chapter.

Statistical inference complements any statistical modeling to further understand how uncertainty in the data informing the model propagates into the estimated output parameters and model summaries. Most common statistical inference in health services research and health policy is hypothesis testing, with a focus on the statistical significance of the relationships between health(care) outcomes, health determinants, system-related factors, among others. Statistical significance is commonly measured by *p-values*; however, many journals are recommending not to measure significance using p-values alone due to their misinterpretation, instead suggesting to complement statistical significance with confidence intervals (Wassertein and Lazar 2016).

Several challenges arise in statistical inference when multiple outcomes and/or population groups are compared jointly, and when there is dependence in the outcome measures to be studied simultaneously. Under multiple inferential comparisons, the significance or confidence levels need to be adjusted for multiple comparison; this is a challenging problem since the adjustment depends on the multiplicity level, e.g.

number of multiple joint hypothesis tests, and on the level of dependence between the joint comparisons. Some common approaches to correct for multiplicity are using the classic Bonferroni correction, the Holm–Bonferroni correction (Holm 1979), the Tukey correction for pairwise comparison (Tukey 1949), and the false discovery rate correction (Benjamini and Hochberg 1995), among many others.

Estimation of confidence bands for functions varying in time or space smoothly can be pointwise or simultaneous (Wasserman 2004). Pointwise confidence bands are most common in statistical inferences of spatially varying outcomes in healthcare access studies; however, they do not account for the dependence in the outcome measures across geography. Instead, joint inferences in the form of simultaneous confidence bands incorporate information about the dependence in the outcome measures, providing more reliable statistical inferences. In this book, I illustrated the applicability of simultaneous confidence bands for identifying communities with statistically significant disparities in healthcare access when comparing the Medicaid versus non-Medicaid insured populations (Chapter 3), and for identifying communities where the relationship between access and outcome is statistically significant (Chapter 4).

Prospective models assume specific structures, functionalities, and/or dynamics of the system rather than being fully informed by observed data. They also primarily provide prospective inferences with a focus on decision making under limited resources, trade-offs in the system (e.g. cost and quality-adjusted life years, QALYs), and/or uncertainty in the system. This area of methodological research has been the topic of handbooks, book chapters, and other publications (Pierskalla and Brailer 1994; Pierskalla 2009).

Prospective (structural) models are primarily derived from the areas of engineering, optimization, management, simulation, and stochastic modeling fields. Among common prospective methodologies useful in designing and evaluating healthcare interventions are:

- *Simulation*
- *System dynamics (SD)*
- *Optimization*

Examples of simulation models used in healthcare delivery are discrete-event simulations, agent-based models, or model-based simulations. They are commonly used in guiding the decision making and evaluate "what-if" scenarios. In simulation models for healthcare interventions, the variables of interest are "actors" or "agents" in the system (Tracy et al. 2018); for example, they can be represented by patients, caregivers, administrators, providers, and others. Commonly, the rules governing the interaction between the agents and the paths they follow are dictated by a structural model, often using prior understanding of the system's structure, flow, and functionality. The relationships specified by the model are evaluated using probability theory and statistics, to describe the variability of events. Specific examples in healthcare access interventions are for food access in low-income communities (Widener et al. 2018); for cost-effectiveness of telemedicine or mobile health, with many relevant references in a recent review (De la Torre-Díez et al. 2015); obstetrics services (Koike et al. 2016); or a multidisciplinary sleep center (Pendharkar et al. 2015).

SD models use a set of differential and algebraic equations representing dynamics found in real-life situations. SD models use the power of computer simulation to replicate the dynamics in a system. Using experimental or measured data to obtain coefficients and model parameters, SD models typically require tuning and validation to ensure they represent the real-life systems they are intended to replicate. Because SD methods capture complicated dynamics in large systems, interactions between different points in the system are often unknown. SD modeling is commonly complemented by sensitivity analysis, which could reveal unexpected behaviors when changing the values of the model parameters or when adding/removing components to/from the system. Specific examples are for modeling supply and demand for dental care (Brailsford and DeSilva 2015) or for ambulatory healthcare demands (Diaz et al. 2015).

Optimization tools are at the core of decision making, an essential aspect of operations research. They compute best values for a set of decision variables of a decision process by optimizing measure outcomes using mathematical representations. The components of an optimization model can be divided into four categories:

1. *Decision variables* representing the range of choices available.
2. *Parameters* or the inputs to the decision-making process.
3. *The objective function*, the goal or the function to be optimized.
4. *The constraints*, the rules that govern the operation of the system.

The mathematical representation of an optimization model depends on whether it represents centralized or decentralized systems. A centralized approach assumes that a centralized planner makes all the decisions in the system. Although not realistic in sociotechnical systems such as healthcare, centralized decision models may be useful for coordinating the operations of segments at the higher level of the system controlled by a single decision-making body (e.g. government). Decentralized models are more realistic, but designing such models to render effective operation of the overall system is the main challenge for both healthcare delivery and industrial supply chains (Uzsoy 2005).

This book includes many illustrations of optimization modeling for measuring and making inference on healthcare access. This chapter also illustrates how to use such models in evaluating and designing interventions. For the rest of the section, I will focus on a series of questions addressing the practical implementation of targeted healthcare interventions.

Question Addressing Practical Implementation: Are Interventions Needed?

The methodologies presented in previous chapters lay the foundation for addressing this very basic question: *Are healthcare interventions needed?* While it may be that some communities have limited resources allocated to healthcare delivery, it is possible that this is a systemic problem across all communities, not only for those communities known to be vulnerable to health(care) inequities. Not all healthcare delivery challenges and needs can be addressed by healthcare interventions.

Moreover, it is possible that prior hypotheses and/or beliefs on the need for intervening to improve healthcare delivery do not hold. An example is the study of the relationship between geographic access and health outcomes for patients with cystic fibrosis – my collaborators and I found the relationship not to be significant, with other factors such as the genetic make-up to be more important in explaining differences in outcomes (Johnson et al. 2018). Another example is the hypothesis that improving geographic access to specialized asthma care for children will reduce the rate of emergency department visits and hospitalizations due to asthma significantly. In my collaborative research, this hypothesis did not hold for all communities with high levels of severe asthma outcomes although for some communities we did see a reduction (Garcia et al. 2015). These examples do not necessarily suggest that no intervention is needed, but that those which were a priori assumed to have been improving the outcomes of interest will not address the unmet needs to the extent needed.

The modeling techniques introduced in previous chapters, specifically, in the analysis of disparities in healthcare access (Chapter 3) and the analysis of the relationship between outcomes and access (Chapter 4), have applicability in addressing this fundamental question. They span many of the retrospective models discussed above, including (spatially varying coefficient) regression and statistical inference on the relationships between access, outcomes, and other confounding or controlling factors. Previous chapters and the accompanying references provide extensive details on such modeling approaches.

Question Addressing Practical Implementation: Where Are the Interventions Needed and for Which Sub-Populations?

In Chapter 3, I presented various modeling approaches for identifying whether systematic disparities in healthcare access and other outcomes exist, more specifically, whether the disparities are localized in specific regions within a geographic space and/or characteristic to specific population groups that are most in need of improving access to care. In Chapter 4, I also presented approaches to identify communities where severe health outcomes can be reduced with the improvement in healthcare access, for example. Thus, interventions to improve health(care) outcomes and access can be targeted to the areas with the greatest potential for improvement and tailored to each community's needs.

Similar modeling techniques apply here, however the statistical inference on the outcomes of interest are assessing *not whether* there is statistical significance *but where* there is statistical significance. Statistical inferential approaches discussed in previous chapters include the so called *significance maps*, *threshold maps,* or *geographically varying slope map*s. These maps are point maps of locations where there is a statistically significant need for addressing improvement in healthcare access and/or health outcomes.

The discussion in the next section addressing the question on the type of interventions needed expands on modeling approaches on how to design and evaluate targeted interventions. The optimization approaches discussed in the next section can be informed by statistical inference methods used to identify where to target interventions. This will not only reduce cost of intervention and of healthcare delivery but also reduce disparities, aligning with the aim to balance the trade-off in the 3 E's framework.

Question Addressing Practical Implementation: What Interventions Are Needed?

The scope of interventions in improving healthcare access is very broad. In previous sections of this chapter, I have discussed several types of interventions that have been considered in improving healthcare access, including health policies focused on inde-pendent practice, scope of practice, reimbursement, in-home or in-school healthcare, and telemedicine or mobile healthcare, along with network interventions focused on identifying the best locations to make changes in the provider network. Such interventions may be designed to impact the overall system or be targeted to improve access locally.

One of the advantages of the optimization access models described in Chapter 2 is that they can be used to evaluate and design interventions given constraints on resources. In this section, I will provide an overview of modeling techniques that can be used to design and implement policy and network interventions.

Implementation of policy interventions will entail fixed and variable costs, for example, a one-time cost (e.g. changes in claims process), a cost per provider (e.g. working with a particular provider to encourage an increased caseload), or ongoing costs (e.g. changes in reimbursement rates), and can be targeted by area or overall. Considerations of the intervention cost and healthcare expenditure along with the benefits of the interventions are substantive in value-based decision making.

To analyze policy interventions, the access optimization models can be used to match patients with providers, then varying the parameters in the model constraints related to providers, where these parameters can be viewed as *system levelers*, for example, the maximum caseload or percent of providers accepting Medicaid in each county. More specifically, the enactment of the policy interventions can be quantified throughout the entire network, or selectively, in areas of greatest need for healthcare.

Particularly, to target interventions to a subset of areas, an additional layer to the access optimization model can be added by specifying a decision variable that models whether or not to enact an intervention at location k using binary values of 0 and 1 ($x_k \in 0,1\ \forall k$), and a decision variable that models the level of enactment at location k up to a maximum value ($y_k \in [0,Max]\ \forall k$). In addition to the specification of these decision variables, other constraints may be considered: (i) to stay below a total budget, with costs incurred for each location where an intervention is enacted; and (ii) to ensure the level of an intervention at location k is 0 unless choosing to enact that intervention there.

The locations of interventions can be identified using modeling approaches; or they can be specified depending on the intervention area of interest, for example, when funding is available only for a region or district. An illustration of this approach is provided in the case study presented in this chapter.

The decision variables can also be selected optimally. To this end, the objective, defined by an access outcome as described in Chapter 2, is optimized across different settings specified by x_k and y_k for the locations k at which the intervention is considered. This approach can be used to determine the interventions under the setting that would have the greatest impact.

This particular model falls in an optimization class broadly called "facility location" problems (Daskin 1995; Owen and Daskin 1998; Daskin and Dean 2004; Griffin et al. 2008); it allows one to charge a fixed cost for enacting an intervention at each location and a variable cost if applicable. The existing literature on facility location provides many approaches to solving such problems. Daskin and Dean (2004) review location models for healthcare facilities. One application in this area of research is optimizing availability of ambulances such that the emergency response is within some standard limits. However, facility allocation can have a broader application beyond optimal ambulance responses. Other relevant example are optimization for optimal location of CHCs (Griffin et al. 2008), location models to improve accessibility to rural health services (Murawski and Church 2009), and locating preventive healthcare facilities (Verter and Lappiere 2002), among many others.

To design and analyze network interventions, the optimization access models can be applied again but with two major additions. First, similar to the policy intervention model, additional decision variables need to be considered for whether to add a provider to each location k, for the caseload of that provider ($z_k \in [0, MaxCap]$ $\forall k$), and an associated budget constraint limiting the total fixed cost plus variable cost. Secondly, in contrast to the policy intervention model, designing network interventions needs to also allow patients to choose from the locations available to them based on the characteristics of the locations to be considered (e.g. distance, staffing type, and expected congestion). This latter layer is needed to study network interventions because new locations are added to the model from which the patients will choose.

For the policy and network interventions introduced above, one can examine the impact across population groups and across the network to ensure the intervention's changes "do no harm," or at least the disutility to others is not significant. The intervention's impact can be estimated at the state level by determining how the population-based weighted average access changes as the intervention is implemented, while simultaneously measuring variation in access experienced across areas or population groups (Nobles et al. 2014). This can be done after solving the optimization models above or by adding a term to the objective function to penalize for systematic disparities in access.

Furthermore, an intervention's effect can be quantified locally by mapping the differences between the status quo and a full enactment of it. The map identifies communities that drive changes in access and can be used to visualize the level of disparities in access before and after implementation. This approach can be complemented with rigorous statistical inference, to clearly delineate whether the changes are statistically significant for specific groups or overall.

Another large area of applicability of decision making in designing interventions to improve access to care is in addressing HR planning in home-based healthcare and identifying optimal collaboration among healthcare providers in integrated care services. Decisions related to the HR planning in home-based care using operations research include deciding about which care workers deliver care services and to which patients as well as scheduling patient visits assigned to each care worker (Cissé et al. 2017). Logistics transportation approaches that have been used for dispatching vehicles to deliver products to customer locations can be applied to this healthcare setting (Bennett 2010).

The optimization approaches for HR planning are different from the optimization access models presented in previous chapters; specifically, begin with a set of locations where the homes are: $\mathcal{G} = s \in 1, \ldots, S$ where S is the number of homes or communities to be reached by providers. These locations are assumed fixed, similarly to the optimization access problem. However, the assumptions on the providers delivering care are that the providers assigned to the homes do not have fixed locations and that the schedule or routing is for each provider separately. The optimization problem is to optimize the routing between patients, i.e. $(s_i, s_j) \in \mathcal{A}$ where $\mathcal{A}$ is the set of possible routes. A complete set of undirected arcs $(s_i, s_j) \in \mathcal{A}$ in the routing network connects all customer locations. The travel time d_{ij} on each arc is known.

According to the optimal route, each patient is assigned an allowed time from an allowable menu of equally spaced times, given constraints of the possible times of the provider and patient preferences. There are different objectives that could be considered, for example: (i) minimize the duration of a route which serves all patients; (ii) maximize the number of patients served by one provider route; or (iii) a weighted objective of both. Because the optimization problems are quite different from those presented in the context of the optimization access models, I will not expand on these modeling approaches but I refer to the existing research for further developments (Bennett 2010; Gutiérrez and Vidal 2013; Cissé et al. 2017).

Another area where optimization modeling can be used in designing and evaluating interventions is the integration of care services, in which professionals from different organizations work as a team, sharing resources and using a coordinated process to meet all of a patient's care requirements. The models described above have applicability in this area however the decision making and the computation efforts to perform such analysis are substantive. This area of research holds many promises particularly for the application of operations research modeling approaches.

Question Addressing Practical Implementation: How to Evaluate Interventions from an Economic Perspective?

A value-based model for designing interventions requires assessment of how access varies in response to potential changes in the system. Specifically, it requires analysis of the impact that optimal policy changes and network interventions would have on access and outcomes of the overall system, specific population subgroups, and areas of greatest shortage. Importantly, a value-based healthcare delivery needs to provide high value if the health benefits justify its costs. Value is measured in terms of the patient benefits achieved per cost spent. Measuring, valuing, and comparing costs and benefits are defined within the economic evaluation framework. Economic evaluations thus analyze the benefits of interventions given the costs, including not only financial costs but also number of years of life saved or quality of life. The importance of economic evaluations lies in the long-term impact of the care provided by the interventions facilitating healthcare access and improving outcomes. It consists of the synthesis of outcomes and costs of an intervention.

Several different types of economic evaluations have been considered in healthcare delivery, including cost-savings or cost reduction, cost–benefit, cost-effectiveness and cost–utility analyses. There is a great confusion across these types of economic evaluations while there is also some overlap between them (Jefferson et al. 2002; Zilberberg and Shorr 2010; Barrios et al. 2012). Two main aspects distinguish between the economic evaluations: what benefits are considered; and how they are quantified.

To begin with the simplest economic evaluation, *cost-savings analysis* is the net difference between the direct benefits versus the expenditure for the delivery of healthcare both measured in monetary terms, e.g. dollars. Generally, it is challenging to demonstrate cost-savings of interventions since the considered benefits from the interventions are limited to direct savings. Illustrations of cost-savings analysis are the economic evaluation of preventive dental care (Lee et al. 2018) and of immunization of young children (Goodell et al. 2009), counseling adults on the use of low dosage aspirin (Goodell et al. 2009), or for H1N1 vaccination (Khazeni et al. 2009).

A cost–benefit analysis (CBA) is more complex than a cost-saving evaluation; it compares costs and benefits of an intervention, where the benefits include direct (e.g. expenditure saved) and indirect benefits (e.g. productivity gains) as well as intangible benefits (e.g. satisfaction) (Centers for Disease Control and Prevention 2009a). CBA standardizes all costs and benefits in monetary terms, e.g. dollars where the costs of the intervention occur in the immediate future and benefits occur in the distant future. Common measures are the net benefit, that is, subtract costs from benefits, or the ratio benefit, dividing the program's net benefits by its net costs. When using the ratio benefit, the result is a summary measure that states, "for every dollar spent on a specific program, X dollars are saved." A CBA considers all cost and benefit components determining the potential return on investment of an intervention, including any costs that go into developing, implementing and executing the intervention. The decision rule is that if the net present value of the benefits outweighs the costs, the intervention has the potential to increase social welfare according to the Kaldor–Hicks criterion (Mishan 1982).

CBA is used when in the economic evaluation of an intervention, there is a monetary value that can be placed on the benefits or consequences of the intervention. In healthcare, CBA is thus less common since placing a monetary value on health can be highly debatable. Nonetheless, it has been applied in many studies related to depression, *in vitro* fertilization, and prevention of cardiovascular diseases, among others (Zarnke et al. 1997).

Unlike a CBA, a cost-effectiveness analysis (CEA) expresses benefits in natural health units instead of converting outcomes to dollars (Jefferson et al. 2002; Zilberberg and Shorr 2010; Barrios et al. 2012). A common CEA measure is the ratio of net intervention costs divided by net program effects, where the intervention costs are program costs minus the cost of illness averted by the program (Centers for Disease Control and Prevention 2009b). A CEA is used when a CBA is not a viable analysis option because the outcome of interest cannot be expressed in monetary value, e.g. quality of life.

The most complex economic evaluation is the cost–utility analysis (CUA) since it extends CEA to deal with the problem of multiple health outcomes. Often CEA and CUA are used interchangeably. CUA combines all health outcomes associated with an intervention in terms of increases in length of life and quality of life using a health index. Length of life adjusted by quality of life is known as a QALY, sometimes referred to as a disability-adjusted life year. In a CUA, one could compare interventions that affect different health outcomes by using a QALY – for example, when comparing interventions that affect obesity, nutritional outcomes, and cardiovascular disease. The summary measure in a CUA is cost per QALY or cost per disability-adjusted life year (Centers for Disease Control and Prevention 2009b). CUA uses one generic measure of health improvement allowing direct comparison on the same scale of different types of health effects.

CEA along with its extension CUA has been the topic of many review papers (Jefferson et al. 2002; Zilberberg and Shorr 2010; Barrios et al. 2012) and of many recommended guidelines. The Panel on Cost-effectiveness in Health and Medicine developed recommendations for the conduct of CEA in the mid-1990s (Weinstein et al. 1996). The *New England Journal of Medicine* published guidelines in 1994 and the *British Medical Journal* (*BMJ*) published guidelines in 1996 for economic submissions to the journals (Homik and Suarez-Almazor 2004). The major components of these guidelines are the design of the model, the source of outcomes and cost data, and analysis/interpretation of the results. CEA has also been applied to many health(care) settings, including in infectious diseases, epidemic responses (Zilberberg and Shorr 2010), in prevention (Philips and Holtgrave 1997; Goodell et al. 2009), in palliative care (Wichmann et al. 2017), in breastfeeding uptake and preventing or treating postnatal depression (Mallender et al. 2018), and more generally, in allocation of public funds for multiple services in Sweden (Svensson and Hultkrantz 2017).

Modeling economic evaluations involves multiple steps:

1. Establishing the perspective from which the evaluation is made.
2. Identifying and estimating the costs involved in the evaluation.
3. Identifying and estimating the benefits involved in the evaluation.
4. Establishing the decision modeling, including possible implementation settings, assumptions, and mathematical relationship.
5. Performing sensitivity analysis with respect to uncertain aspects in the decision making.

Perspective of the economic evaluation refers to the point of view one takes when conducting the evaluation (Zilberberg and Shorr 2010). Specifically, it determines which costs, benefits, and outcomes are likely to matter more than others. For example, economic costs are evaluated in terms of costs to the healthcare sector, costs to patients (out-of-pocket expenses) and costs to society; thus the value of care will be different depending on the perspective (Homik and Suarez-Almazor 2004). While a societal perspective counts in all costs, regardless of who incurs them, system/patient perspective will only consider costs specific to the system/patient. Generally, it is more challenging to take a societal perspective because externalities should be considered in economic evaluations; externalities are costs and benefit accruing to others than those directly involved in the delivery of care. Thus the perspective from which costs are being estimated should be stated clearly and justified (Husereau et al. 2013).

The other critical modeling component in an economic analysis is establishing the *costs* involved in the evaluation. There are three specific types of costs that can be considered: *direct* costs (both medical and non-medical), *indirect* costs (e.g. loss of wages for the patient and loss in production for society, or costs to social services, family and friends), and *intangible* costs (e.g. pain and suffering resulting from the disease and/or intervention). The costs are also differentiated depending on the perspective of the economic evaluation. For example, the costs to the patient involve direct medical costs (e.g. intervention), direct non-medical costs (e.g. transportation), and indirect costs (e.g. lost wages) whereas the costs to society include all costs.

Estimation of costs is carried out by first establishing the evaluation perspective and then investigating various components of the costs, including direct, indirect and intangible costs, depending on the type of economic evaluation. This latter step involves identification of the health resources involved in the delivery, and the consumption and the maintenance of the healthcare services. The valuation of the health resources is measured using appropriate physical units, for example, the amount of time spent on different activities or number of readmissions and emergencies. The resources are further measured using appropriate unit costs. These can be based on hospital staff salaries, marked prices, or price weights based on national tariffs or charges. Last, in estimating costs, one must elect to use either average costs or marginal costs, and *discounting* (time preference) must also be taken into account. An important recommendation of the Panel on Cost-effectiveness in Health and Medicine is to adjust costs for inflation and to discount both future costs and effectiveness estimates (Husereau et al. 2013).

In most economic evaluations, the primary focus is on direct costs since they are better understood by public health decision makers. For direct costs such as medication prescription and physician visits, market prices or administrative data can be used. When estimating such direct costs, an important distinction between charges and costs is warranted. Charges reflect the submitted reimbursement for the service delivered by a healthcare provider. In contrast, costs are meant to represent the actual consumption of resources (Zilberberg and Shorr 2010). Direct costs can also be estimated for non-medical items, for example, volunteer work, capital expenditures, including depreciation and opportunity costs, and shared overhead (Homik and Suarez-Almazor 2004).

A third aspect in economic analyses in healthcare delivery is establishing the outcomes and benefits of interest to be contrasted to the cost of care. Health outcomes can, for example, be cases of illness avoided, symptom-free days, successful treatments, lives saved, and life years gained. These benefits of such outcomes generally describe symptom relief, disease progression, or treatment effectiveness. The benefits in economic evaluations should include the value placed on the particular health state as a function of the outcome. One measure that puts value on the health outcome is the QALY. The QALY includes quantity and quality of life and incorporates the valuation patients place on each health state. The QALY is used by many economists and reimbursement agencies, and is primarily used in cost-effectiveness or CUA while in cost-reduction, cost-savings or CBA, the value needs to be converted into monetary units.

An economic analysis usually involves a decision analysis model that takes individual patients in a study population through a series of health states that may occur within a specific order and with fixed probabilities. One approach to the decision modeling is using patient-level healthcare trajectories observed from electronic health records (EHRs) or administrative claims data, for example, following a cohort of patients over multiple years of treatment for a targeted condition. The healthcare trajectories or pathways can be modeled using models for discrete sequences of events, including Markov models (Hilton et al. 2017; Lee et al. 2018; Moran et al. 2019) or survival analysis (Hilton et al. 2018). Such models are used to estimate the probability of a specific care trajectory within the study population and of the outcomes given specific treatment pathways. Claims data can also provide information about the direct expenditure of each trajectory; however, this would only reflect the cost from the system's perspective and not the cost from a patient or societal perspective. The economic evaluation can be performed directly for the population for which the care trajectories have been observed, or for a hypothetical population that could have benefited from the intervention of interest. Depending on the type of the economic analysis, varying data about the benefits given the outcomes need to be considered beyond those observed directly from EHRs or claims data.

When data on observed health(care) trajectories are not available and/or not feasible to acquire, the alternative approach is to consider a simulation decision model, in which a hypothetical cohort of patients is considered to evaluate the economic benefits of the intervention, assuming a series of health states with predetermined probabilities. Using a simulation model, the health(care) trajectories each (hypothetical) patient has incurred can be simulated based on a decision tree along with the associated costs and experienced outcomes. An illustration of a decision tree is shown in Figure 5.3; in this decision tree, there are three different treatment groups, one following the standard of care, another following the intervention treatment only, and a third will enter the intervention treatment after being exposed to the standard care treatment. The decision tree reflects all possible scenarios, each scenario occurring with a specified probability; those scenarios not reflected in the decision tree have

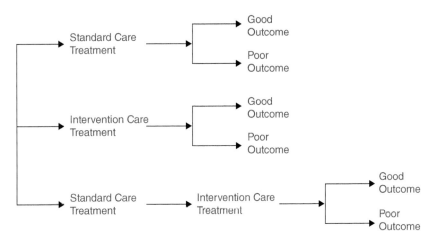

FIGURE 5.3 An illustrative decision tree with three different treatment arms and two outcomes per arm.

probability 0. For each arm in this example, a specified percentage of patients will have a good outcome and a certain percentage will have a poor outcome. Moreover, each arm of the tree will have an associated cost, which can be fixed or it can vary with a specified distribution. While this illustrative decision tree has only two different outcomes per arm, more outcomes can be considered. Most commonly, decision trees are modeled and simulated as Markov decision processes (Feinberg and Shwartz 2002).

A well-designed decision model is a tool that can simulate or mimic expected health(care) pathways and individual behaviors in relation to the intervention of interest. Decision models can simulate different "what-if" scenarios by making explicit assumptions about the probability of occurrence, prognosis of an outcome, duration, benefits, health-related quality of life, and costs. It is intended to evaluate how costs and benefits might change if the values of key parameters in the model change – this being explored through simulations.

It is important to keep in mind the reliance on high quality data upon which the economic analysis is based as it has an impact on the resulting quality of the analysis itself. An economic analysis requires the input of many types of data, and where data are not available, assumptions are made (Homik and Suarez-Almazor 2004). Decision models involve many assumptions and parameter estimates about the underlying targeted condition and mathematical relationship between probabilities, generally obtained from the literature. Thus the results derived from such models include a degree of uncertainty. *Sensitivity analyses* are designed to estimate how this uncertainty in the assumptions and parameter estimates may impact the results of an economic analysis, and it has been recommended to accompany economic evaluations (Husereau et al. 2013).

The most common sensitivity analysis is the assessment of how the variation in one assumption or parameter impacts the economic evaluation; that is, one parameter at a time, for example, the effectiveness of an intervention is varied while all others are assumed fixed. However, it is more realistic to consider a global sensitivity analysis, in which the *joint* variation in multiple assumptions or parameters impacts the economic evaluation; that is, multiple parameters are varied simultaneously. Global sensitivity analysis generally requires more computational effort since a larger parameter space is explored. Nonetheless, such analyses can provide necessary insights on when there are cost benefits of an intervention and what scenarios need to be targeted for the highest return on investment.

To place the economic evaluation within the framework of this book, economic analysis deals with the evaluation of resource allocation in health, whether this refers to managing health services, financing healthcare, or dealing with supply and demand in the healthcare field (Homik and Suarez-Almazor 2004). Two tenants of health economics, in particular, economic analysis, are equity and scarcity. Thus an overarching objective is to balance the benefit of resource allocation to a particular area against the benefits lost or harm that would occur in the other area not receiving the resources (Homik and Suarez-Almazor 2004). This makes economic analysis a necessary decision tool in public health, particularly in decision making for improving healthcare access.

CASE STUDIES: INTERVENTIONS TO IMPROVE DENTAL CARE ACCESS

Oral health was cited as the greatest unmet health need among United States children (Newacheck et al. 2000), a silent epidemic affecting the nation's poorest children (US Department of Health and Human Services 2000). Even with public-insurance coverage, low income and minority children receive preventive services at a lower level than their counterparts (Seale and Casamassimo 2003; Hughes et al. 2005; Flores and Tomany-Korman 2008), with only 46% publicly insured children receiving preventive dental care in 2013 (US Department of Health and Human Services 2014).

Public insurance programs such as Medicaid and CHIP remove most barriers related to financial access for dental care receipt for children (Liao et al. 2008; Decker 2011), hence other forms of access impact the utilization of dental care services to a greater extent (Fisher and Mascarenhas 2007). The Centers for Medicare & Medicaid Services (CMS) identified several key barriers to dental care, including limited availability of dental providers and low reimbursement rates (Centers for Medicare & Medicaid Services 2011). According to a 2009 survey, identifying a dentist accepting Medicaid remained the most frequently reported barrier to children seeking dental services (Government Accountability Office 2010). These barriers reflect multiple access dimensions, accessibility, availability, and acceptability.

In the case studies of this chapter, I will illustrate how healthcare interventions are to be implemented toward improving access to dental care, with a focus on addressing a series of questions: *Why important in policy making? Where to intervene? What communities and sub-populations to target? How much to intervene?*

Do the interventions have an impact on outcomes and cost? Which intervention is most effective and/or efficient?

Access Estimation for Medicaid-Enrolled Children: Why Important in Policy Making?

Existing research on dental care access has been limited to evaluations of the dental workforce at the state level (Georgia Health Policy Center 2012) or nationally (Health Policy Institute 2015), dentist-per-population ratio (Allison and Manski 2007; Beazoglou et al. 2010; Munson and Vujicic 2018) or minimum distance (Horner and Mascarenhas 2007), with the recent estimates provided by the Health Policy Institute (HPI) of the American Dental Association (ADA) being the first to account for both the supply and demand of dental care for children on public insurance nationwide (Health Policy Institute 2017). The HPI-ADA study used the two-step floating catchment area (2SFCA) to measure spatial access, capturing the interaction between two dimensions of access: availability and accessibility (Guagliardo 2004; Nasseh et al. 2017). Based on this study, the highlighted finding is that "... nationwide, the majority of publicly insured children live within 15 minutes of a Medicaid dentist and in some states it's as high as 99 percent" (Health Policy Institute 2017). Reports on spatial access are available for each state in the United States, with access estimates provided for varying levels of patient-to-provider ratios (Health Policy Institute 2017).

In one recent collaborative research paper, I have presented a series of limitations to the HPI-ADA approach, which can result in significant *overestimation of access* (Serban and Tomar 2018). Two primary limitations included: (i) the specification of the dentists' participation in the Medicaid program along with their dedicated caseload for the Medicaid-enrolled children; and (ii) the methodology used to obtain the access estimates. The specification of the caseload dedicated to children enrolled on Medicaid varies significantly across provider types (e.g. pediatric dentist, general dentist, or specialist), whether the provider's practice is in a rural or urban area, and across states (Serban et al. 2019). Figure 5.4 presents the distribution of the number of Medicaid-insured children seen a year by dentists across all dentists reimbursed by Medicaid programs across 48 states. This figure shows that over all providers, the median provider-level caseload is lower than the assumed minimum caseload in the HPI-ADA study of 500 patients; it also shows that the caseload varies with the urbanicity level of the dentist's practice location.

In addition, the approach used to derive the ADA-HPI estimates was the basic 2SFCA method dating from as early as 1997 (Peng 1997). I briefly discussed the 2SFCA approach and its extensions along with important limitations in spatial access estimation in Chapter 2. Importantly, I highlighted that the gravity models, particularly those derived based on catchment areas, generally overestimate access.

This potential overestimation of spatial access to dental care for Medicaid-enrolled children is more than just an academic concern. Potential interventions designed to improve access for dental care will not target those most in need of interventions to improve access if such estimates are to be used toward this end (Gentili et al. 2015; Cao et al. 2017b). The HPI-ADA estimates may also influence the decisions

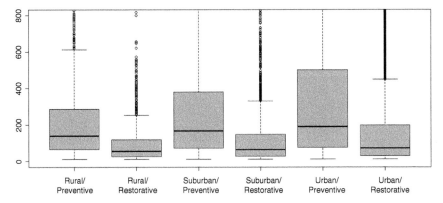

FIGURE 5.4   Provider-level caseload measured as the number of Medicaid-insured children seen per year by level of urbanicity of the practice address of the dentists and differentiated into preventive and restorative care. The provider-caseload was derived from the 2012 MAX claims data.

of state legislation, which have control over Medicaid policy and regulation of health professions. This example underlines the importance of using rigorous and principled approaches to model access for making informed interventions and policies. It also highlights the need for relying on relevant data in making informed decisions, as I will further expand on in Chapter 6.

Access Inference: *Where* to Intervene? *What* Communities and Sub-Populations to Target?

In a recent study, my collaborators and I developed access estimates for one state in the United States, Georgia (Cao et al. 2017b). The model was similar to the access measurement model introduced in Chapter 2. The approach was a mathematical model for matching need/demand and supply for particular healthcare services (e.g. preventive dental care) under a series of realistic constraints (e.g. Medicaid acceptance, Medicaid provider caseload, lack of access to a car) and preferences (e.g. preference of the closest provider if not excessively busy).

Similar to other case studies presented in this book, we used the National Plan and Provider Enumeration System (NPPES) data for all dental care providers, complemented by the Board of Dentistry data to identify providers that are active. We also used the InsureKidsNow.gov database to identify those providers reporting as participating in Medicaid. Important considerations in the estimation of the dental care supply were: (i) the specification of the supply, differentiated into supply for preventive and restorative care, for children and adults, and for Medicaid and non-Medicaid children; and (ii) specification of provider-level caseload by the type of provider. Not all dentists provide preventive care, such as orthodontics or maxillofacial surgery specialists. Pediatric dentists devote most of their caseload to preventive care for children while general dentists share their caseload between adults and children (Serban et al. 2019).

Need is not the same across all children. Need is driven by age and by risk of dental caries. For example, sealants are typically applied in children within specific age groups. Moreover, a higher risk of caries requires more frequent visits to the dentist. To estimate the need for dental care for children, we complemented the demographics data available from the American Community Survey with a model used to estimate the prevalence of risk of caries based on National Health and Nutrition Examination Survey (NHANES) data (Cao et al. 2017a). Thus, the need estimation model also accounted for financial access to dental care, differentiated into no financial access, public insurance, and other forms of affordability.

The optimization model took a system perspective in which children access the same set of providers with competitive access between children with varying financial access; while there is a preference for the shortest distance, not all children within one community visit the closest provider. Instead, the model accounted for other constraints and preferences such as wait time for an appointment or whether a provider accepts new patients through what we call congestion experienced at a provider, an availability access barrier. Most importantly, the model can be used to assess interventions as discussed in the modeling section of this chapter.

Figure 5.5 presents the map of financial access, defined as the percentage of children with public or private financial access, pointing to both urban and rural communities with a large percentage of children with no financial access to preventive dental care. Such a map can be used to identify areas in most need for providing care to children whose parents cannot afford dental care for their children. These population can also be targeted through school-based programs supported by the state departments of public health.

Figure 5.6 presents the maps with the travel distance to preventive dental care differentiated by those with public insurance and those with other types of financial

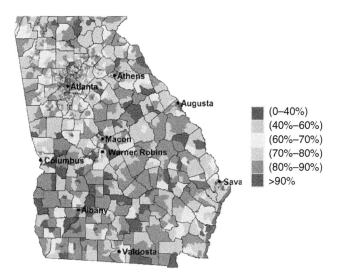

FIGURE 5.5 Geographic distribution of the percentage of children with financial access, including both public insurance and private affordability at the census tract level.

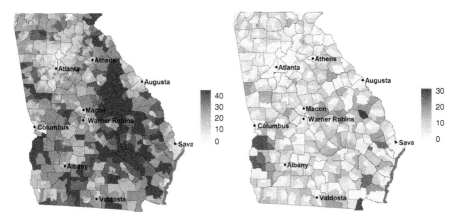

FIGURE 5.6 Geographic distribution of the average travel distance across all children with access to dental care in each census tract for the (a) Medicaid and (b) non-Medicaid population.

access or affordability. Overall, the child population with ability to afford dental care had significantly better access than the child population with public insurance. There were also communities where access to dental care is low for all children.

Figure 5.7 provides a series of maps which can assist in designing interventions. It includes two maps with the location of communities where the difference in the travel distance between private and public insured child populations is significantly larger than 2 or 10 miles. It also provides a map combining the financial and spatial access to identify served, underserved, and unserved communities for pediatric preventive dental care. For comparison, a map of the counties identified as Dental Shortage Area by the Health Resources and Services Administration (HRSA) is included.

Comparing the significance maps (Figure 5.7a,b), even at a difference of 10+ miles, there are many communities in need of intervention. The difference between the designated dental areas based on HRSA's approach versus the designation of unserved communities based on the access model presented here is striking. Importantly, there are many more areas that are unserved, primarily because of the lack of access for those with public insurance. This set of intervention maps demonstrate that rigorous methodology and extensive data are needed to provide meaningful inferences to target interventions.

The maps in Figures 5.5–5.7 can be used to identify "where" there is need for interventions as well as "which" sub-populations and "what" access dimension to target. Such information is very valuable in designing interventions. However, the remaining question is "how" interventions impact the healthcare system in terms of improving access with limited resources?

Access Inference: *How Much* to Intervene?

An important advantage of using the mathematical optimization model for measuring access is its flexibility to integrate and evaluate system changes by varying parameters in the model constraints, also interpreted as system levelers.

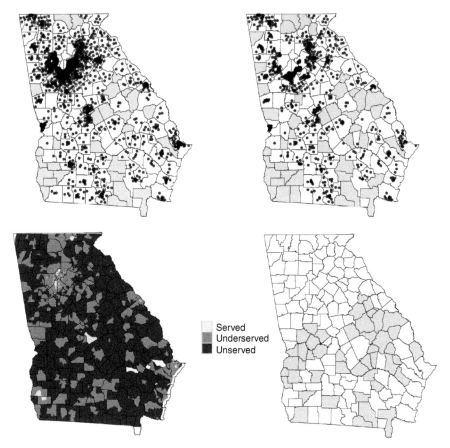

FIGURE 5.7 *Intervention maps.* Significance maps for distance difference of (a) 2+ miles or (b) 10+ miles for non-Medicaid versus Medicaid access. (c) Map of community categorization for interventions. (d) Health Resources and Services Administration designation of dental shortage areas shown in gray.

While there are many policies that could conceivably improve access to dental care, in this section, I will discuss the effect of interventions that increase participation in and/or caseload for the Medicaid program, an important area of improvement in dental care access. To evaluate the impact of increasing physician participation in Medicaid programs, we considered two types of policy implementation:

1. Varying the Medicaid participation rate among the active dental care providers assuming similar caseload of dental care providers already participating in Medicaid.
2. Varying the caseload of Medicaid-participating dentists dedicated to children with public insurance while also varying the Medicaid participation rate.

Different policies and interventions will incentivize providers to accept a higher caseload and/or to participate in Medicaid. I will touch upon such interventions in the last case study of this chapter. In the collaborative research paper (Cao et al. 2017b), we examined the impact of varying provider acceptance rates of public insurance for children from 20 to 80%. I will note that for Georgia, the status quo of the participation rate was higher than 20%; we set a participation rate at a lower rate to also quantify the effect of a decrease in Medicaid participation on access. For the second implementation, we first set the acceptance rate to a given value and then sampled the Medicaid caseload differently for providers in urban (caseload ranged from 35 to 50%) and rural (caseload ranged from 55 to 65%) tracts.

Figure 5.8 presents the variations in three access measures with respect to changes in both the Medicaid participation rate and in the caseload dedicated to preventive dental care for children with public insurance. The figure presents the changes in three different access measures:

- *Percentage of met need*: total met need divided by pediatric need for preventive services. Met need refers to need served within the state access standards. High values indicate high met need.
- *Travel distance*: average distance in miles a child must travel to visit the dentist. The travel distance is provided only for those children with travel distances within the state access standards (10). High values indicate large travel distances.
- *Provider scarcity*: patient caseload served by dentists divided by maximum patient caseload. High values indicate high scarcity of providers.

We considered the impact for the child population living in urban or rural communities; we also differentiated by financial access, with public (Medicaid/CHIP) insurance and private insurance (including out-of-pocket).

Important findings from this analysis are as follows:

- Increasing dental caseload available to publicly insured children could increase their access to preventive dental care.
- Eighty-nine percent of children eligible for public insurance in Georgia would have met preventive dental needs if providers currently taking Medicaid/CHIP increased their caseload to this group to at least 75%.
- Alternatively, increasing the percentage of providers accepting public insurance from 28 to 80% would increase the percentage of children with no unmet preventive dental care need to 97.2%.
- Increasing the Medicaid participation rate from its current state level of 28–50% could decrease the travel distance for a dental visit from 40 to 25 miles and from 12 to 10 miles for publicly insured children living in rural and urban census tracts, respectively.

Such findings are important since they provide the level of intervention enactment that is needed to improve access. They pinpoint what types of interventions or

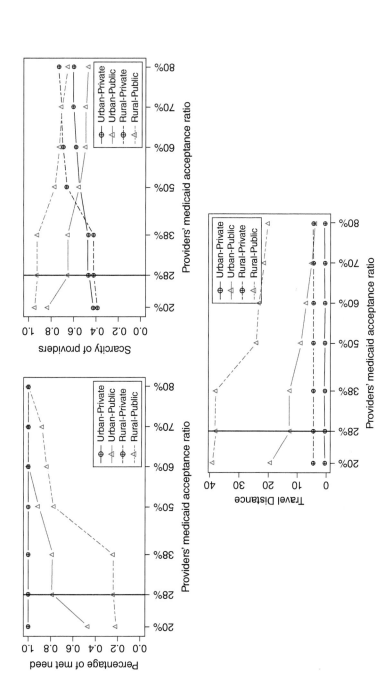

FIGURE 5.8 Changes in access measures with varying Medicaid participation rate assuming also a higher Medicaid caseload differentiated by sub-populations in rural and urban communities and for the child population with public or private insurance. The access measures are: (a) met need, (b) scarcity of providers and (c) distance traveled.

policies are needed. For example, doubling dentist participation in Medicaid would have negligible impact on privately insured children's access, suggesting that there is extra caseload that could become available if the Medicaid program were to provide incentives to participate. Thus incentivizing providers to increase their current caseload of Medicaid-insured children will have a high impact on improving access.

Access Inference: Do the Interventions Have an Impact on Outcomes and Cost?

In this section, I will directly address a critical aspect in deciding on what interventions to pursue: *Are the interventions effective and efficient?* Since preventive dental care is at the core of many interventions targeted to the child population, I will begin by posing a fundamental question: *What is the return on investment of preventive dental care? Is it worth investing in preventive care?* In this section, I will provide examples on the analysis of interventions from this perspective.

Basic pediatric dental preventive services include dental prophylaxis (teeth cleaning), topical fluoride application, and dental sealants. Such services are quite inexpensive and they can be applied in various forms of healthcare settings, including dental care offices, school-based programs, and pediatrician offices. They can also be provided by dentists and dental hygienists when state health policies allow. Thus, there is great flexibility in designing interventions to improve access to preventive dental care for children.

There is strong evidence for the relevance of preventive care in reducing severe health outcomes, with programs promoted through national (Koh and Sebelius 2010; Anderko et al. 2012) and/or state health policies. However, there is not a consensus on whether the cost of prevention leads to savings in downstream healthcare costs (Russell 1993; Task Force on Community Preventive Services 2005; Maciosek et al. 2006; Russell 2007; Cohen et al. 2008; Congressional Budget Office 2009; Rouse and Serban 2014). The Congressional Budget Office (CBO) (Congressional Budget Office 2009) reported that for most preventive services, expanding utilization led to higher medical spending. In a recent book, my co-author and I argued that CBO's evaluation does not hold if prevention is targeted at high-risk populations (Rouse and Serban 2014). I also conjecture that preventive care may be cost-saving for specific types of healthcare services, such as dental care, or for specific sub-populations, such as children.

For insured children, one study found that placing sealants resulted in reduced expenditures and increased the average number of caries-free months per tooth (Quinonez et al. 2005). Other studies suggested that targeting at-risk children, such as the Medicaid-enrolled, may be an effective strategy (Dennison et al. 2000; Leskinen et al. 2008). Studies of preventive care for Medicaid-enrolled children for states such as Alabama, North Carolina, and Iowa have provided evidence for effectiveness of such services, however there are not consistent results on the cost savings (Quinonez et al. 2006; Sen et al. 2013; Chi et al. 2014; Blackburn et al. 2017). These studies neither considered the impact of multiple preventive services jointly nor made comparisons across states with different oral health policies, particularly, across a larger population of children receiving care in different oral healthcare delivery environments. One study focused on the very young (prior to age two years), concluding that preventive care at this early age is neither effective nor cost-saving. However, their sample of children primarily included those with severe dental outcomes; few parents, particularly, those of children with Medicaid insurance, consider dental care prior to age two years unless severe dental problems arise.

In a recent research publication, my collaborators and I have revisited this question by addressing some of the limitations of prior studies (Lee et al. 2018). In this study, we followed about 1 million Medicaid-enrolled children (three to six years old) for several years, from 2005 to 2011. We used patient-identifiable Medicaid Analytic Extract (MAX) claims data of Alabama, Georgia, Mississippi, North Carolina, South Carolina, and Texas. We clustered each state's study population into four groups based on utilization of topical fluoride and dental sealants before caries-related treatment by using machine learning algorithms. We evaluated utilization rates and expenditures across the four groups, and quantified the cost reduction due to preventive care for different levels of penetration. The study was from the perspective of the Medicaid programs. The cost reduction was thus estimated as the difference between the Medicaid expenditure per child in the group receiving preventive before restorative care (if any) versus the cost of those children who didn't. Other important consideration in our study were as follows:

- The study population only included those children who are relatively healthy or with some minor to moderate chronic conditions to avoid bias due to complex health conditions (Herndon et al. 2015).

- We considered the economic evaluation for two dental care services recommended for children in the study population: topical fluoride application (FL) and dental sealants (SE), which can be easily delivered in school-based programs by dentists and/or dental hygienists.

- Other dental care events included in the utilization sequence of each individual child were: evaluation (EV), restorative care events include office visit (OV), severe outcome office visit (SevOV), outpatient (Out), hospitalization (HO). We also extracted monthly enrollment records and added enrollment (EN) and unenrollment (UN) events. We introduced two artificial events, LC (left censoring) and RC (right censoring), for the entry and exit point, respectively. For each child in the study population, we used dental care events and their chronologically ordered time stamps to define the child's longitudinal utilization sequence during the enrollment years. Examples of utilization sequences are shown in Figure 5.9.

- In order to quantify the impact of preventive care, we classified the utilization sequences based on whether the child received repeated FL and/or SE before their first caries treatment event.

- The use of claims data prevented us from observing caries in children who did not receive caries-related treatments, which may have been due to access barriers (Government Accountability Office 2010). To address this limitation, we also estimated the proportion of children that experienced caries among

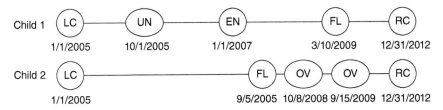

FIGURE 5.9   Examples of utilization sequences of dental care for individual children.

the Medicaid population from the NHANES (Centers for Disease Control and Prevention 2016).

- The Medicaid expenditure per child was measured as the expenditure per member per year (PMPY), computed as the total amount paid by Medicaid due to the event type for the population divided by the total enrollment years of the population.

- All dollar amounts were converted to 2015 US dollars by using the medical cost inflation (Bureau of Labor Statistics 2013).

The proposed model for utilization patterns accounted for the order of events and the time between events. A simple but useful model for summarizing time-ordered events with varying time intervals between events is the Markov renewal process (MRP) (Foufoula-Georgiou and Lettenmaier 1987). For each pair of event types (e.g. EV and SE), a transition probability is estimated along with an inter-event time distribution. For example, the transition probability from EV to SE is the probability of a patient having sealants applied after an oral examination with the inter-event time between EV and SE being a random variable, assumed to have a parametric distribution, for example, exponential. Although the Markov assumption (upon entry to an event, future events, and future inter-event times depend only on the current event) is restrictive, the MRP model has advantages over more advanced statistical models; for example, the model output can be visualized using simple network graphs (e.g. Figure 5.10).

The proposed MRP modeling was integrated within a machine learning algorithm (Hilton et al. 2017) that captures heterogeneity of children's utilization behaviors, inspired from existing research on modeling longitudinal, categorical data (Schach and Schach 1972; Smyth 1997; Ramoni et al. 2002; Pamminger and Frühwirth-Schnatter 2010). The unsupervised classification algorithm grouped children with similar longitudinal utilization patterns, for example, children who regularly receive FL and children who see dentists only for restorative care.

The results on the projected caries reduction and cost-savings are shown in Table 5.1. The results were only for the population of children three to six years old who are relatively healthy or with some minor to moderate chronic conditions; the number of children who are candidates for intervention is in the first column. We also assumed varying levels of penetrations of interventions targeting delivery of preventive dental care; the penetration levels vary from 10 to 30%, meaning

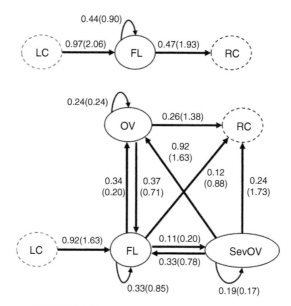

FIGURE 5.10   MRP model output illustrations.

the percentage of children receiving the intervention. The cost savings across the six states were substantive, ranging from $1.1 million per year in Mississippi to $12.9 million per year in Texas at the 10% penetration level, assuming a seven-year time horizon for the impact of the intervention. The level of cost reduction differed among the states due to differences in child population size, utilization rates, and state reimbursement fees for dental procedures.

Access Inference: *How* to Intervene? *Which* Intervention Is Most Effective and/or Efficient?

In the previous case study, I presented an economic evaluation of preventive dental care for young children. While this study showed substantive cost reduction due to preventive dental care, a key question is whether interventions for improving the utilization of preventive dental care also present economic benefits. As I discussed earlier in this chapter, consideration of interventions with some form of economic benefits, not necessarily in expenditure, is part of the decision making. Ideally, expenditure will be reduced along with improvements in outcomes for all in need of care, going back to the trade-off between the 3 Es: efficiency, effectiveness, and equity.

   In the last part of this section, I will present an economic evaluation of three common interventions targeting improvement in access to dental care: (i) loan repayment program; (ii) Medicaid reimbursement; and (iii) school-based programs. This research is based on one of my collaborative research articles (Johnson et al. 2017).

TABLE 5.1 Projected Caries Reduction and Medicaid Cost Savings Associated with Changes in Utilization of Dental Preventive Services

State	N*	Baseline caries† (per year)	Baseline Medicaid cost (per year)	Caries reduction/cost savings (per year)					
				If the percentage starts utilizing fluoride repeatedly			If the percentage starts utilizing fluoride and dental sealants		
				10%	20%	30%	10%	20%	30%
Alabama	140 086	71.9 k	$21.1 M	3.6 k/$0.8 M	7.1 k/$1.6 M	10.7 k/$2.4 M	6.3 k/$1.2 M	12.6 k/$2.5 M	18.9 k/$3.7 M
Georgia	301 469	110.8 k	$51.3 M	5.0 k/$2.2 M	10.0 k/$4.5 M	15.0 k/$6.7 M	10.3 k/$3.5 M	20.6 k/$7.0 M	30.9 k/$10.5 M
Mississippi	70 879	27.9 k	$15.0 M	1.2 k/$0.5 M	2.3 k/$1.1 M	3.5 k/$1.6 M	2.6 k/$1.1 M	5.1 k/$2.2 M	7.7 k/$3.3 M
North Carolina	297 397	131.6 k	$65.1 M	5.4 k/$2.5 M	10.9 k/$4.9 M	16.3 k/$7.4 M	11.1 k/$4.0 M	22.1 k/$8.1 M	33.2 k/$12.1 M
South Carolina	142 113	75.2 k	$30.1 M	3.5 k/$1.2 M	6.9 k/$2.4 M	10.4 k/$3.6 M	7.2 k/$2.2 M	14.4 k/$4.4 M	21.7 k/$6.7 M
Texas	882 878	447.0 k	$237.5 M	11.1 k/$4.6 M	22.3 k/$9.3 M	33.4 k/$13.9 M	34.7 k/$12.9 M	69.4 k/$25.8 M	104.1 k/$38.7 M

*Children enrolled in Medicaid in 2011, three to six years old in 2011, and in clinical risk groups 1–5a.
†The total number of caries-related treatments per year.

The three interventions selected for the economic evaluation are most popular in the delivery of dental care. Loan repayment is commonly used to encourage providers to choose areas of practice with higher need, such as rural areas (Geletko et al. 2014; Nicholson et al. 2015). The increase in the acceptance of public insurance could affect the availability of providers for children with public insurance, referred to as Medicaid herein (Griffin et al. 2007; Borchgrevink et al. 2008; Centers for Medicare & Medicaid Services 2011). Many factors affect a dentist's willingness to participate in the Medicaid program, including paperwork associated with filing claims, low service payment fees, and substantial "no-shows" among the Medicaid-eligible population (Kelly et al. 2005). Last, relaxing independent practice for dental hygienists from direct or indirect supervision (where a dentist needs to be present for the service delivery) to general supervision (when the dentists need not be present) has been undertaken in many states. Currently, three states do not allow general supervision, and five states allow general supervision only for some services and under specific settings (American Dental Hygienists' Association n.d.-a).

In this research, we considered three outcomes derived from the potential implantation of the three interventions: (i) met need, defined as the number of additional children receiving care through an intervention, who are otherwise unserved; (ii) intervention cost, estimated as the total cost of intervention implementation incurred by the state; and (iii) cost-saving from providing preventive care for children eligible for Medicaid/CHIP compared with treatment costs under no prevention. The study also focused only on the child population eligible for Medicaid in Georgia. The study used the access measures for preventive dental care and the Medicaid expenditure for dental care services for the child population from prior studies (Cao et al. 2017b; Lee et al. 2018). The study also was informed by multiple data sets from multiple sources including the ADA (Health Policy Institute 2015), the Agency for Healthcare Research and Quality (2016), and the Kaiser Family Foundation (n.d.), among others.

To evaluate the dentist loan repayment program we considered data specific to the state of Georgia. Loan repayment programs can vary in the annual loan repayment amount and the percentage of the dentist's caseload involving Medicaid children. We considered annual loan repayments in the range $0–60 000 annually, in increments of $10 000. The impact of a loan repayment program was scaled by the number of participating providers. The Georgia Dental Association (GDA) estimated that using loan repayments would encourage 8–12 dentists to practice in rural areas and accept publicly insured children (Georgia Dental Association 2016).

Dental loan repayment programs range from total loan forgiveness after a specified period to a fixed amount per year in exchange for a short-term commitment to practice in shortage areas. The intervention cost was computed as the amount contributed annually by the program. Potential cost savings were based on the additional number of publicly insured children served, based on the intervention setting and the publicly insured population in the service area. The cost saving equaled the number of eligible publicly insured children served multiplied by the potential savings per year per child for providing preventive services.

In order to evaluate the outcomes of interest for the intervention of increasing the Medicaid reimbursement rates for dental care services, we used multivariate linear regression models where the response variable was the state-level Medicaid acceptance rate or utilization of preventive care services (past year dental visit) and the explanatory variable of interest was the fee-for-service reimbursement rate. The objective of this modeling procedure was to assess whether higher reimbursement rates result in improved utilization of preventive care or higher Medicaid acceptance rates. We controlled for confounding from: (i) the structure of the Medicaid program in each state, including whether dental care was included in a state's managed care organizations (MCOs), number of MCOs, and whether the state participated in Medicaid expansion; (ii) the dentist per 100 000 population ratio; (iii) the median family income; (iv) race/ethnicity; and (v) Medicaid enrollment.

We determined the impact of raising Medicaid reimbursement rates by 10 percentage points (53–63% in Georgia). We estimated met need by the increase in utilization by taking the change in utilization multiplied by the number of publicly insured children. The intervention cost was the percentage increase in fees across the publicly insured children already utilizing preventive care plus the total increase in costs of the additional met need. We estimated cost savings by summing the potential savings across the met need satisfied through the provision of additional preventive services.

For the third intervention, we primarily focused on the implementation of school sealant programs under direct and general supervision of dental hygienist. We targeted schools with at least 60% of children participating in the free and reduced meal program since they are most in need of such programs due to limited access to dental care.

Under "direct supervision," we assumed that the dentist undertook all screenings and ensured that sealants were placed correctly, while the dental hygienists applied the sealants. Under "general supervision," the hygienists performed screenings and sealant placement.

We estimated cost savings from the number of children sealed and the averted treatment costs per child from prior research (Lee et al. 2018). Cost savings to the state were based on students who qualified for free or reduced lunch (family income less than 185% of the Federal Poverty Level), which is below the requirement for Medicaid (Centers for Medicare & Medicaid Services 2014). The impact of the school sealant programs was determined for all schools as well as targeting a specific percentage of schools. Details on the implementation of the sealant programs, and the associated costs and assumptions are provided in the collaborative research paper (Johnson et al. 2017).

Table 5.2 summarizes the three outcomes of interest for all three interventions where the third intervention is consider under both direct and general supervision. The take-home points from these results are:

- All three interventions improved met need for preventive dental care.
- Raising the reimbursement rate alone would marginally affect utilization of Medicaid services but would not substantially increase acceptance of Medicaid by providers.
- Both loan repayment programs and amending supervision requirements are potentially cost-saving interventions. Loan repayment programs provide complete care to targeted areas, while amending supervision requirements of dental hygienists could provide preventive care across the state.

TABLE 5.2 Comparison of the Interventions for Improving Access to Preventive Dental Care

Intervention	Met need	Intervention cost ($)	Cost savings ($)
Loan repayment	12 915	400 000	175 909
Reimbursement rate	7 366	38.3 M	200 660
Direct supervision sealant program	27 197	1 274 743	1 087 675
General supervision sealant program	27 197	566 129	1 087 675

Our results on increasing the Medicaid reimbursement rates are not consistent with another recent study, which compared three states (Connecticut, Maryland, and Texas) that have increased the reimbursement rates between 2005 and 2012, to a control group of 14 states that have not had significant changes in oral health policy for the Medicaid program during the same time period (Nasseh and Vujicic 2015). The study found that Connecticut and Texas have experienced a statistically significant increase in utilization of preventive dental care for Medicaid-enrolled children compared with the control group of states.

The findings from this study have several important implications for oral healthcare policy. Implementing loan repayment programs, raising Medicaid reimbursement rates, and relaxing dental hygienist supervision all improve access for Medicaid-insured children. Moreover, both loan repayment programs and relaxing supervision requirements were potentially cost-saving.

CONCLUSIONS

Healthcare interventions are at the core of transforming the healthcare system, potentially with both intended and unintended consequences. This chapter has provided an overview of healthcare interventions, particularly targeting improvements in healthcare access, where the overarching objective is understanding the scope of interventions and their ability to intercede in the delivery of healthcare, which is paramount in informed decision making.

As presented in this chapter, healthcare interventions take various forms, with different requirements needed in their implementation. Most importantly, the implementation of healthcare interventions requires knowledge about the system, extensive data along with rigorous methodologies. The concepts, principles, models, methods, and tools needed to implement healthcare interventions, while complex and challenging, make the transformation of healthcare delivery an achievable goal.

ACKNOWLEDGMENTS

The author is thankful to Jean O'Connor for providing suggestions for improving the presentation of this chapter. This chapter draws substantially upon the recent research presented in three journal articles. In this regard, the author gratefully acknowledges the contributions of Shanshan Cao, Paul Griffin, Susan Griffin, Ben Johnson, Ilbin Lee, Sean Monahan, and Scott Tomar, who have been given their permission to illustrate the concepts and methodologies presented in this chapter using the studies from our collaborative work.

REFERENCES

Agency for Healthcare Research and Quality (2016). Medical Panel Expenditure Survey. https://meps.ahrq.gov/mepsweb (accessed February 2019).

Allison, R.A. and Manski, R.J. (2007). The supply of dentists and access to care in rural Kansas. *Journal of Rural Health* **23**(3): 198–206.

American Dental Hygienists' Association (n.d.-a). Direct Access.http://www.adha.org/direct-access (accessed February 2019).

American Dental Hygienists' Association (n.d.-b). "Reimbursement. http://www.adha.org/reimbursement (accessed November 2018).

American Pharmacists Association (2015). Pharmacist-administered immunizations: What does your state allow?. https://www.pharmacist.com/article/pharmacist-administered-immunizations-what-does-your-state-allow.

American Pharmacists Association (2016). Lawmakers vote to let New Jersey pharmacists prescribe contraception. https://www.pharmacist.com/article/lawmakers-vote-let-new-jersey-pharmacists-prescribe-contraception (accessed Novemebr 2018).

Amir, A., Seyedi, S., and Syam, S.S. (2017). A survey of healthcare facility location. *Computers & Operations Research* **79**: 223–263.

Anderko, L., Roffenbender, J.S., Goetzel, R.Z. et al. (2012). Promoting prevention through the affordable care act: workplace wellness. *Preventing Chronic Disease* **9**: 1–5.

Anderson, A. (2014). *The Impact of the Affordable Care Act on the Health Care Workforce.* The Heritage Foundation.

Anselin, L. (1988). *Spatial Econometrics: Methods and Models.* Dordrecht: Kluwer.

Arifkhanova, A. (2017). The impact of nurse practitioner scope-of-practice regulations in primary care. PhD thesis. RAND Graduate School, Santa Monica, CA.

Baker, C.D., Kamke, H., O'Hara, M.W. et al. (2009). Web-based training for implementing evidence-based management of postpartum depression. *The Journal of the American Board of Family Medicine* **22**(5): 588–589.

Balcik, B., Iravani, S.M.R., and Smilowitz, K. (2010). A review of equity in nonprofit and public sector: a vehicle routing perspective. In: *Wiley Encyclopedia of Operations Research and Management Science.* Wiley.

Barrios, J.M.R., Alcántara, F.P., Crespo, C. et al. (2012). The use of cost per life year gained as a measurement of cost-effectiveness in Spain: a systematic review of recent publications. *The European Journal of Health Economics* **13**(6): 723–740.

Bashshur, R.L. and Shannon, G.W. (2009). *History of Telemedicine: Evolution, Context, and Transformation.* New Rochelle, NY: Mary Ann Liebert, Inc.

Beazoglou, T., Bailit, H., Myne, V., and Roth, K. (2010). Supply and Demand for Dental Services: Wisconsin 2010–2020. Report to the Wisconsin Dental Association.

Benjamini, Y. and Hochberg, Y. (1995). Controlling the false discovery rate: a practical and powerful approach to multiple testing. *Journal of the Royal Statistical Society, Series B* **57** (1): 289–300.

Bennett, A. R. (2010). Home health care logistics planning. PhD thesis. Georgia Institute of Technology, Atlanta.

Bergmo, T.S. (2015). How to measure costs and benefits of eHealth interventions: an overview of methods and frameworks. *Journal of Medical Internet Research* **17**(11): e254.

Berman, S., Dolins, J., Tang, S.-f., and Yudkowsky, B. (2002). Factors that influence the willingness of private primary care pediatricians to accept more Medicaid patients. *Pediatrics* **110**(2 Pt 1): 239–248.

Blackburn, J., Morrisey, M.A., and Sen, B. (2017). Outcomes associated with early preventive dental care among Medicaid-enrolled children in Alabama. *JAMA Pediatrics* **1**(4): 335–341.

Blount, F.A. and Miller, B.F. (2009). Addressing the workforce crisis in integrated primary care. *Journal of Clinical Psychology in Medical Settings* **16**(1): 113–119.

Bodenheimer, T. (2008). Coordinating care-a perilous journey through the health care system. *New England Journal of Medicine* **358**(10): 1064.

Borchgrevink, A., Snyder, A., and Gehshan, S. (2008). The effects of medicaid reimbursement rates on access to dental care. *NASHP*: 1–41.

Box, G.E.P., Jenkins, G.M., and Reinsel, G.C. (1994). *Time Series Analysis: Forecasting and Control*. Englewood Cliffs, NJ: Prentice Hall.

Brailsford, S. and DeSilva, D. (2015). How many dentists does Sri Lanka need? Modelling to inform policy decisions. *Journal of the Operational Research Society* **66**(9): 1566–1577.

Briggs, R.D., Racine, A., and Chinitz, S. (2007). Preventive pediatric mental health care: a CO-LOCATION model. *Infant Mental Health Journal* **28**(5): 481–495.

Brindis, C.D. (2016). The "state of the state" of school-based health centers achieving health and educational outcomes. *American Journal of Preventive Medicine* **51**(1): 139–140.

Brockwell, P.J. and Davis, R.A. (1991). *Introduction to Time Series and Forecasting*. New York: Springer-Verlag.

Bureau of Labor Statistics (2013). Consumer Price Index. http://www.bls.gov/cpi (accessed June 2016).

Cao, S., Gentili, M., Griffin, P. et al. (2017a). Identifying shortage areas for preventive dental care for children using high geographic granularity estimates of need and supply. *Public Health Reports*: 132–132.

Cao, S., Gentili, M., Griffin, P.M. et al. (2017b). Disparities in preventive dental care among children in Georgia. *Preventing Chronic Disease* **14**: 170176.

Centers for Disease Control and Prevention (2009a). Part IV: Benefit-Cost Analysis Outcomes Quantified in Dollars: The Fourth of a Five-Part Series. https://www.cdc.gov/dhdsp/programs/spha/economic_evaluation/docs/podcast_iv.pdf (accessed February 2019).

Centers for Disease Control and Prevention (2009b). Part V: Cost-Effectiveness Analysis. Outcomes in Natural Units: The Fifth of a Five-Part Series. https://www.cdc.gov/dhdsp/programs/spha/economic_evaluation/docs/podcast_v.pdf (accessed February 2019).

Centers for Disease Control and Prevention (2016). National Health and Nutrition Examination Survey. http://www.cdc.gov/nchs/nhanes.htm (accessed October 2016).

Centers for Medicare & Medicaid Services (2011). Improving access to and utilization of oral health services for children in Medicaid and CHIP programs. https://www.medicaid.gov/medicaid/quality-of-care/downloads/cms-oral-health-strategy.pdf (accessed June 2019).

Centers for Medicare & Medicaid Services (2014). State Medicaid, CHIP and BHP Income Eligibility Standards. https://www.medicaid.gov/medicaid/program-information/medicaid-and-chip-eligibility-levels/index.html (accessed June 2019).

Centers for Medicare & Medicaid Services (2016). Quality of Care for Children in Medicaid and CHIP. https://www.medicaid.gov/medicaid/quality-of-care/downloads/performance-measurement/2018-child-chart-pack.pdf (accessed September 2018).

Chi, D.L., van der Goes, D.N., and Ney, J.P. (2014). Cost-effectiveness of pit-and-fissure sealants on primary molars in Medicaid-enrolled children. *American Journal of Public Health* **104**(3): 555–561.

Cissé, M., Yalcindag, S., Kergosien, Y. et al. (2017). OR problems related to home health care: a review of relevant routing and scheduling problems. *Operations Research for Health Care* **13–14**: 1–22.

Cohen, J., Neumann, P.J., and Weinstein, M.C. (2008). Does preventive care save money? Health economics and the presidential candidates. *New England Journal of Medicine* **358** (7): 661–663.

Colwill, J.M., Cultice, J.M., and Kruse, R.L. (2008). Will generalist physician supply meet demands of an increasing and aging population? *Health Affairs* **27**(3): w232–w241.

Community Preventive Services Task Force (2016). School-based health centers to promote health equity. *American Journal of Preventive Medicine* **51**(1): 27–128.

Congressional Budget Office (2009). Letter to Congress on Preventative Medical Care and Wellness Services. Washington, DC.

Cressie, N.A.C. (1993). *Statistics for Spatial Data*. New York, NY: Wiley.

Czako, K. and V. Poreisz (2013). Theory and empirics of horizontal and spatial integration of local communal services. European Regional Science Association.

Daskin, M.S. (1995). *Network and Discrete Location: Models, Algorithms, and Applications.* Wiley-Interscience.

Daskin, M.S. and Dean, L.K. (2004). Location of healthcare facilities. In: *Handbook of OR/MS in Health Care: A Handbook of Methods and Applications* (eds. F. Sainfort, M. Brandeau and W. Pierskalla), 43–76. Kluwer Academic Publishers.

De la Torre-Díez, I., López-Coronado, M., Vaca, C. et al. (2015). Cost-utility and cost-effectiveness studies of telemedicine, electronic, and mobile health systems in the literature: a systematic review. *Telemedicine Journal and e-Health* **21**(2): 81–85.

Decker, S.L. (2011). Medicaid payment levels to dentists and access to dental care among children and adolescents. *Journal of the American Medical Association* **306**(2): 187–193.

Dennison, J.B., Straffon, L.H., and Smith, R.C. (2000). Effectiveness of sealant treatment over five years in an insured population. *The Journal of the American Dental Association* **131** (5): 597–605.

Diaz, R., Behr, J.G., and Tulpule, M. (2015). A system dynamics model for simulating ambulatory health care demands. *Simulation in Healthcare: The Journal of the Society for Simulation in Healthcare* **7**(4): 243–250.

Emilianoa, W., Telhada, J., and do Sameiro Carvalho, M. (2017). Home health care logistics planning: a review and framework. *Procedia Manufacturing* **13**: 948–955.

Estrin, D. and Sim, I. (2010). Open mHealth architecture: an engine for health care innovation. *Science* **330**: 759–760.

Federal Communications Commission (2010). Connecting America: The National Broadband Plan.

Feinberg, E. and Shwartz, A. (2002). *Handbook of Markov Decision Processes*. Springer US.

Fisher, M.A. and Mascarenhas, A.K. (2007). Does Medicaid improve utilization of medical and dental services and health outcomes for Medicaid-eligible children in the United States? *Community Dentistry and Oral Epidemiology* **35**(4): 263–271.

Flores, G. and Tomany-Korman, S.C. (2008). Racial and ethnic disparities in medical and dental health, aceess to care, and use of services in US children. *Pediatrics* **121**(2): e286–e298.

Foufoula-Georgiou, E. and Lettenmaier, D. (1987). A Markov renewal model for rainfall occurrences. *Water Resources Research* **23**(5): 875–884.

Garcia, E., Serban, N., Swann, J., and Fitzpatrick, A. (2015). The effect of geographic access on severe health outcomes for pediatric asthma. *Journal of Allergy and Clinical Immunology* **136**(3): 610–618.

Geletko, K., Brooks, R.G., Hunt, A., and Beitsch, L.M. (2014). State scholarship and loan forgiveness programs in the United States: forgotten driver of access to health care in underserved areas. *Health* **6**: 1994–2003.

Gentili, M., Isett, K., Serban, N., and Swann, J. (2015). Small-area estimation of spatial access to pediatric primary care and its implications for policy. *Journal of Urban Health* **92**(5): 864–909.

Georgia Dental Association (2016). Georgia's Action for Dental Health. http://www.gadental .org/docs/librariesprovider16/default-document-library/dental-health-action-plan-final-10142015.pdf?sfvrsn=6 (accessed September 2018).

Georgia Health Policy Center (2012). A study of Georgia's dental workforce 2012. Presented to the Georgia Dental Association.

Goad, B.A. (2015). The role of community pharmacy-based vaccination in the USA: current practice and future directions. *Integrated Pharmacy Research and Practice* **4**: 67–77.

Goodell, S., Cohen, J.T., and Neumann, P.J. (2009). *Cost Savings and Cost-Effectiveness of Clinical Preventive Care*. Robert Wood Johnson Foundation.

Government Accountability Office (2010). Oral Health: Efforts Under Way to Improve Children's Access to Dental Services, but Sustained Attention Needed to Address Ongoing Concerns. Washington, DC.

Greenberg, B.J.S., Kumar, J.V., and Stevenson, H. (2008). Dental case management – increasing access to oral health care for families and children with low incomes. *The Journal of the American Dental Association* **139**(8): 1114–1121.

Griffin, S., Jones, K.A., Lockwood, S. et al. (2007). Impact of increasing Medicaid dental reimbursement and implementing school sealant programs on sealant prevalence. *Journal of Public Health Management and Practice* **13**(2): 202–206.

Griffin, P.M., Scherrer, C.R., and Swann, J.L. (2008). Optimization of community health center locations and service offerings with statistical need estimation. *IIE Transactions* **40**(9): 880–892.

Griffin, S., Naavaal, S., Scherrer, C. et al. (2016a). School-based dental sealant programs prevent cavities and are cost-effective. *Health Affairs* **35**(12): 2233–2240.

Griffin, S.O., Wei, L., Gooch, B.F. et al. (2016b). Vital signs: dental sealant use and untreated tooth decay among US School-aged children. *MMWR Morbidity and Mortality Weekly Report* **65**: 1141–1145.

Guagliardo, M.F. (2004). Spatial accessibility of primary care: concepts, methods and challenges. *International Journal of Health Geographics* **3**(3): 1–13.

Gutiérrez, E.V. and Vidal, C.J. (2013). Home healthcare logistics management problems: a critical review of models and methods. *Revista Facultad de Ingeniería Universidad de Antioquia* **68**: 160–175.

Hartigan, J.A. (1975). *Clustering Algorithms*. New York, NY: Wiley.

Hastie, T., Tibshirani, R., and Friedman, J. (2009). *The Elements of Statistical Learning: Data Mining, Inference, and Prediction*. New York, NY: Springer-Verlag.

Health Policy Institute (2015). The Oral Health Care System: A State by State Analysis. American Dental Association.

Health Policy Institute (2017). Webinar: Measuring What Matters – A New Way of Measuring Geographic Access to Dental Care Services. http://www.ada.org/en/science-research/health-policy-institute/publications/webinars/measuring-access-to-dental-care-in-every-state. (accessed June 2017).

Herndon, J.B., Tomar, S.L., Catalanotto, F.A. et al. (2015). The effect of Medicaid primary care provider reimbursement on access to early childhood caries preventive services. *Health Services Research* **50**(1): 136–160.

Hilton, R., Zheng, Y.R., Fitzpatrick, A. et al. (2017). Patient-level longitudinal utilization for pediatric asthma healthcare: drawing inferences from millions of claims. *Medical Decision Making* **38**(1): 107–119.

Hilton, R., Zheng, Y., and Serban, N. (2018). Modeling heterogeneity in healthcare utilization using massive medical claims data. *Journal of the American Statistical Association* **113** (521): 111–121.

Hofer, A.N., Abraham, J.M., and Moscovice, I. (2011). Expansion of coverage under the patient protection and affordable care act and primary care utilization. *The Milbank Quarterly* **89**(1): 69–89.

Holm, S. (1979). A simple sequentially rejective multiple test procedure. *Scandinavian Journal of Statistics* **6**(2): 65–70.

Homik, J. and Suarez-Almazor, M. (2004). An economic approach to health care. *Best Practice & Research Clinical Rheumatology* **18**(2): 203–218.

Horner, M. and Mascarenhas, A. (2007). Analyzing location-based accessibility to dental services: an Ohio case study. *Journal of Public Health Dentistry* **67**(2): 113–118.

HRSA (2013). Projecting the Supply and Demand for Primary Care Practitioners Through 2020. Health Resources and Services Administration Bureau of Health Professions, National Center for Health Workforce Analysis.

Hughes, D.C., Duderstadt, K.G., Soobader, M.-P. et al. (2005). Disparities in children's use of oral health services. *Public Health Reports* **120**(4): 455–461.

Husereau, D., Drummond, M., Petrou, S. et al. (2013). Consolidated health economic evaluation reporting standards (CHEERS) statement. *BMJ* **346**: f1049.

Jefferson, T., Demicheli, V., and Vale, L. (2002). Quality of systematic reviews of economic evaluations in health care. *JAMA* **287**(21): 2809–2812.

Johnson, B., Serban, N., Griffin, P.M., and Tomar, S.L. (2017). The cost-effectiveness of three interventions for providing preventive services to low-income children. *Community Dentistry and Oral Epidemiology* **45**(6): 522–528.

Johnson, B., Ngueyep, R., Schechter, M. et al. (2018). A study of the impact of geographic access on health outcomes for cystic fibrosis. *Pediatric Pulmonology* **53**(3): 284–292.

Johnson, B., Serban, N., Griffin, P. et al. (2019). Projecting the economic impact of silver diamine fluoride on caries treatment expenditures and outcomes in young U.S. children? *Journal of Public Health Dentistry* https://doi.org/10.1111/jphd.12312.

Joint Commission on Accreditation of Healthcare Organizations (2016). Standards FAQ Details. https://www.jointcommission.org/mobile/standards_information/jcfaqdetails .aspx?StandardsFAQId=1857&StandardsFAQChapterId=74&ProgramId=5&=74& IsFeatured=False&IsNew=False&Keyword= (accessed January 2019).

Kaiser Family Foundation (2012). "Medicaid Benefits: Nurse Practitioner Services. https:// www.kff.org/medicaid/state-indicator/nurse-practitioner-services (accessed September 2018).

Kaiser Family Foundation (2017). "Medicare Advantage. https://www.kff.org/medicare/fact-sheet/medicare-advantage (accessed October 2018).

Kaiser Family Foundation (n.d.). Medicaid and CHIP. https://www.kff.org/state-category/ medicaid-chip (accessed September 2018).

Kelly, S., Binkley, C.J., Neace, W.P., and Gale, B.S. (2005). Barriers to care-seeking for children's oral health among low-income caregivers. *American Journal of Public Health* **95** (8): 1345–1351.

Khazeni, N., Hutton, D.W., Garber, A.M. et al. (2009). Effectiveness and cost effectiveness of vaccination against pandemic influenza (H1N1) 2009. *Annals of Internal Medicine* **151**: 1909–1916.

Kirkizlar, E., Serban, N., Sisson, J.A. et al. (2013). Evaluation of telemedicine for screening of diabetic retinopathy in the veterans health administration. *Ophthalmology* **120**(12): 2604–2610.

Knopf, J.A., Finnie, R.K., Peng, Y. et al. (2016). School-based health centers to advance health equity a community guide systematic review. *American Journal of Preventive Medicine* **51** (1): 114–126.

Koh, H.K. and Sebelius, K.G. (2010). Promoting prevention through the affordable care act. *New England Journal of Medicine* **363**(14): 1296–1299.

Koike, S., Matsumoto, M., Ide, H. et al. (2016). The effect of concentrating obstetrics services in fewer hospitals on patient access: a simulation. *International Journal of Health Geographics* **15**(4) https://doi.org/10.1186/s12942-016-0035-y.

Kwong, J.C., Ge, H., Rosella, L.C. et al. (2010). School-based influenza vaccine delivery, vaccination rates, and healthcare use in the context of a universal influenza immunization program: an ecological study. *Vaccine* **28**(15): 2722–2729.

Landers, S. (2010). Why health care is going home. *New England Journal of Medicine* **363** (18): 1690–1691.

Larson, R.C. and Nigmatulina, K.R. (2010). *Engineering Responses to Pandemics*. IOS Press.

Lee, I., Monahan, S., Serban, N. et al. (2018). Estimating the cost savings of preventive dental services delivered to medicaid-enrolled children in six Southeastern states. *Health Services Research* **53**(5): 3592–3616.

Leskinen, K., Salo, S., Suni, J., and Larmas, M. (2008). Comparison of dental health in sealed and non-sealed first permanent molars: 7 years follow-up in practice-based dentistry. *Journal of Dentistry* **36**(1): 27–32.

Liao, C.-C., Ganz, M.L., Jiang, H. et al. (2008). The impact of the public insurance expansions on children's use of preventive care. *Maternal and Child Health Journal* **14**(1): 58–66.

Maciosek, M.V., Coffield, A.B., Edwards, N.M. et al. (2006). Priorities among effective clinical preventive services: results of a systematic review and analysis. *American Journal of Preventive Medicine* **31**(1): 52–61.

Mallender, J., Tierney, R., Gontzes, D. et al.(2018). Cost-effectiveness and Return on Investment (ROI) of interventions associated with the Best Start in Life. Public Health England.

Mandell, M.B. (1991). Modelling effectiveness-equity trade-offs in public service delivery systems. *Management Science* **37**(4): 467–482.

McDonald, K.M., Sundaram, V., Bravata, D.M. et al. (2007). *Closing the Quality Gap: A Critical Analysis of Quality Improvement Strategies*. Agency for Healthcare Research and Quality.

MedicineNet (n.d.) Medical definition of intervention. https://www.medicinenet.com/script/main/art.asp?articlekey=34214 (accessed June 2019).

Mehrotra, A. (2014). Expanding the Use of Telehealth. http://docs.house.gov/meetings/if/if14/20140501/102173/hhrg-113-if14-wstate-mehrotraa-20140501.pdf (accessed September 2018).

Mishan, E.J. (1982). *Cost-Benefit Analysis*. London, UK: George Allen & Unwin.

Mitzner, T.L., Beer, J.M., McBride, S.E. et al. (2009). Older Adults' needs for home health care and the potential for human factors interventions. *Proceedings of the Human Factors and Ergonomics Society Annual Meeting* **53**(1): 718–722.

Moran, A., Serban, N., Danielson, M. et al. (2019). Adherence to recommended care guidelines in the treatment of preschool-age Medicaid-enrolled children with a diagnosis of ADHD. *Psychiatric Services* **70**(1): 26–34.

Munson, B. and Vujicic, M. (2018). Supply of Full-Time Equivalent Dentists in the U.S. is Expected to Increase Steadily. Health Policy Institute, American Dental Association Research Brief.

Murawski, L. and Church, R.L. (2009). Improving accessibility to rural health services: the maximal covering network improvement problem. *Socio-Economic Planning Sciences* **43**: 102–110.

Nasseh, K. and Vujicic, M. (2015). The impact of Medicaid reform on children's dental care utilization in Connecticut, Maryland, and Texas. *Health Services Research* **50**(4): 1236–1249.

Nasseh, K., Eisenberg, Y., and Vujicic, M. (2017). Geographic access to dental care varies in Missouri and Wisconsin. *Journal of Public Health Dentistry* **77**(3): 197–206.

National Alliance of State Pharmacy Associations (2018). Pharmacists Authorized to Prescribe Birth Control in More States. https://naspa.us/2017/05/pharmacists-authorized-prescribe-birth-control-states (accessed November 2018).

National Association of State Boards of Education (n.d.). State School Health Policy Database: Counseling and Mental Health Services. http://www.nasbe.org/healthy_schools/hs/bytopics.php?topicid=4120&catExpand=acdnbtm_catD (accessed February 2019).

Naughton, D.K. (2014). Expanding oral care opportunities: direct access care provided by dental hygienists in the United States. *Journal of Evidence Based Dental Practice* **14**: 171–182. e171.

Newacheck, P.W., Hughes, D., Hung, Y.Y. et al. (2000). The unmet health needs of America's children. *Pediatrics* **105**(4): 989–997.

Nicholson, S., Vujicic, M., Wanchek, T. et al. (2015). The effect of education debt on dentists' career decisions. *The Journal of the American Dental Association* **146**(11): 800–807.

Nobles, M., Serban, N., and Swann, J. (2014). Measurement and inference on pediatric healthcare accessibility. *Annals of Applied Statistics* **8**(4): 1922–1946.

Owen, S.H. and Daskin, M.S. (1998). Strategic facility location: a review. *European Journal of Operational Research* **111**(3): 423–447.

Pamminger, C. and Frühwirth-Schnatter, S. (2010). Model-based clustering of categorical time series. *Bayesian Analysis* **5**(2): 345–368.

Pathman, D.E., Konrad, T.R., King, T.S. et al. (2004). Outcomes of states' scholarship, loan repayment, and related programs for physicians. *Medical Care* **42**(6): 560–568.

Penchansky, R. and Thomas, J.W. (1981). The concept of access: definition and relationship to consumer satisfaction. *Medical Care* **19**(2): 127–140.

Pendharkar, S.R., Bischak, D.P., Rogers, P. et al. (2015). Using patient flow simulation to improve access at a multidisciplinary sleep centre. *Journal of Sleep Research* **24**(3): 320–327.

Peng, Z. (1997). The jobs-housing balance and urban commuting. *Urban Studies* **34**: 1215–1235.

Petterson, S.M., Liaw, W.R., Phillips, R.L. Jr. et al. (2012). Projecting US primary care physician workforce needs: 2010–2025. *The Annals of Family Medicine* **10**(6): 503–509.

Pham, H.H., Schrag, D., O'Malley, A.S. et al. (2007). Care patterns in medicare and their implications for pay for performance. *New England Journal of Medicine* **356**(11): 1130–1139.

Philips, K. and Holtgrave, D. (1997). Using cost-effectiveness/cost-benefit analysis to allocate health resources: a level playing field for prevention. *American Journal of Preventive Medicine* **13**(1): 18–25.

Pierskalla, W. (2009). Examples of operational systems engineering applications relevant to traumatic brain injury care. In: *Systems Engineering to Improve Traumatic Brain Injury Care in the Military Health System* (eds. J. Buono, D. Butler, F. Erdtmann and P. Reid), 49–69. Washington, DC: The National Academies Press.

Pierskalla, W. and Brailer, D. (1994). Applications of operations research in healthcare delivery. In: *Handbooks in Operations Research and Management Science* (ed. S.M. Pollock), 469–505. Elsevier Science.

Praxia Information Intelligence and Gartner Inc. (2011). *Telehealth Benefits and Adoption: Connecting People and Providers across Canada*. Stamford, CT: Gartner, Inc.

Qiang, C. Z., Yamamichi, M., Hausman, V., and Miller, R. (2011). Mobile Applications for the Health Sector. World Bank.

Quinonez, R.B., Downs, S.M., Shugars, D. et al. (2005). Assessing cost-effectiveness of sealant placement in children. *Journal of Public Health Dentistry* **65**(2): 82–89.

Quinonez, R.B., Stearns, S.C., Talekar, B.S. et al. (2006). Simulating cost-effectiveness of fluoride varnish during well-child visits for Medicaid-enrolled children. *Archives of Pediatrics and Adolescent Medicine* **160**(2): 164–170.

Rahman, S. and Smith, D. (2000). Use of location-allocation models in health service development planning in developing nations. *European Journal of Operational Research* **123**(3): 437–452.

Ramoni, M., Sebastiani, P., and Cohen, P. (2002). Bayesian clustering by dynamics. *Machine Learning* **47**(1): 91–121.

Ramsay, J.O. and Silverman, B.W. (2010). *Functional Data Analysis*. New York, NY: Springer.

Ran, T., Chattopadhyay, S., and Hahn, R.A., and the Community Preventive Services Task Force (2016). Economic evaluation of school-based health centers: a community guide systematic review. *American Journal of Preventive Medicine* **51**(1): 129–138.

Rodriguez, M.I., Anderson, L., and Edelman, A.B. (2016). Pharmacists begin prescribing hormonal contraception in Oregon: implementation of house bill 2879. *Obstetrics and Gynecology* **128**(1): 168–170.

Romagnoli, K.M., Handler, S.M., and Hochheiser, H. (2013). Home care: more than just a visiting nurse. *BMJ Quality & Safety* **22**(12): 972–974.

Rouse, W. and Serban, N. (2014). *Understanding and Managing the Complexity of Healthcare*. MIT Press.

Rouse, W.B. and Serban, N. (2015). *Understanding and Managing the Complexity of Healthcare*. Cambridge, MA: MIT Press.

Rudner, N. and Kung, Y.M. (2017). An assessment of physician supervision of nurse practitioners. *Journal of Nursing Regulation* **7**(4): 22–29.

Rumball-Smith, J., Wodchis, W.P., Koné, A. et al. (2014). Under the same roof: co-location of practitioners within primary care is associated with specialized chronic care management. *BMC Family Practice* **15**(1): 1–8.

Russell, L.B. (1993). The role of prevention in health reform. *New England Journal of Medicine* **329**(5): 352–354.

Russell, L.B. (2007). *Prevention's Potential for Slowing the Growth of Medical Spending*. Washington, DC: National Coalition on Health Care.

Schach, E. and Schach, S. (1972). A continuous time stochastic model for the utilization of health services. *Socio-Economic Planning Sciences* **6**(3): 263–272.

Seale, N.S. and Casamassimo, P.S. (2003). Access to dental care for children in the United States – a survey of general practitioners. *Journal of the American Dental Association* **134** (2): 1630–1640.

Sempowski, I.P. (2004). Effectiveness of financial incentives in exchange for rural and underserviced area return-of-service commitments: systematic review of the literature. *Canadian Journal of Rural Medicine* **9**(2): 82.

Sen, B., Blackburn, J., Morrisey, M.A. et al. (2013). Effectiveness of preventive dental visits in reducing nonpreventive dental visits and expenditures. *Pediatrics* **131**(6): 1107–1113.

Serban, N. and Tomar, S. (2018). ADA health policy Institute's methodology overestimates spatial access to dental care for publicly insured children. *Journal of Public Health Dentistry* **78**(4): 291–295.

Serban, N., Bush, C., and Tomar, S.L. (2019). Medicaid caseload for pediatric dental care. *Journal of the American Dental Association* **150**(4): 294–304.

Smyth, P. (1997). Clustering sequences with hidden Markov models. In: *Advances in Neural Information Processing Systems*, 648–654. MIT Press.

Soares, N.S., Johnson, A.O., and Patidar, N. (2013). Geomapping telehealth access to developmental-behavioral pediatrics. *Telemedicine Journal and e-Health* **19**(8): 585–590.

Sullivan, G., Kanouse, D., Young, A.S. et al. (2006). Co-location of health care for adults with serious mental illness and HIV infection. *Community Mental Health Journal* **42**(4): 345–361.

Suter, E., Oelke, N.D., Adair, C.E., and Armitage, G.D. (2009). Ten key principles for successful health systems integration. *Healthcare Quarterly* **13**: 16–23.

Svensson, M. and Hultkrantz, L. (2017). A comparison of cost-benefit and cost-effectiveness analysis in practice: divergent policy practices in Sweden. *Nordic Journal of Health Economics* (2): 41–53.

Task Force on Community Preventive Services (2005). *The Guide to Community Preventive Services: What Works to Promote Health?* Oxford University Press.

The National Association for Home Care & Hospice (2010). Basic Statistics About Home Care.

Topol, E. (2010). *The Creative Destruction of Medicine: How the Digital Revolution Will Create Better Health Care*. New York, NY: Basic Books.

Tracy, M., Cerdá, M., and Keyes, K.M. (2018). Agent-based modeling in public health: current applications and future directions. *Annual Review of Public Health* **39**: 77–94.

Tukey, J. (1949). Comparing individual means in the analysis of variance. *Biometrics* **5**(2): 99–114.

US Department of Health and Human Services (2000). Oral Health in America: A Report of the Surgeon General. National Institute of Dental and Craniofacial Research, National Institutes of Health.

US Department of Health and Human Services (2014). 2014 Annual Report on the Quality of Care for Children in Medicaid and CHIP. Department of Health and Human Services, Washington, DC.

Uzsoy, R. (2005). Supply-chain management and health care delivery: pursuing a system-level understanding. In: *Building a Better Delivery System: A New Engineering/Health Care Partnership* (eds. W.D. Compton, P.P. Reid, J.H. Grossman and G. Fanjiang), 143–147. Washington, DC: The National Academies Press.

Verter, V. and Lappiere, S.D. (2002). Location of preventive health care facilities. *Annals of Operations Research* **110**: 123–132.

Waller, L. and Gotway, C.A. (2004). *Applied Spatial Statistics for Public Health Data*. Hoboken, NJ: Wiley-Interscience.

Wasserman, L. (2004). *All of Statistics: A Concise Course in Statistical Inference*. New York, NY: Springer.

Wassertein, R. and Lazar, N. (2016). The ASA's statement on p-values: context, process, and purpose. *The American Statistician* **70**(2): 129–133.

Weinstein, M., Siegel, J.E., Gold, M.R. et al. (1996). Recommendations of the panel on cost-effectiveness in health and medicine. *JAMA* **276**: 1253–1258.

Wichmann, A.B., Adang, E.M.M., Stalmeier, P.F.M. et al. (2017). The use of quality-adjusted life years in cost-effectiveness analyses in palliative care: mapping the debate through an integrative review. *Palliative Medicine* **31**(4): 306–322.

Widener, M.J., Metcalf, S.S., and Bar-Yam, Y. (2018). Agent-based modeling of policies to improve urban food access for low-income populations. *Applied Geography* **40**: 1–20.

Wishner, J.B. and Marks, J. (2017). *Ensuring Compliance with Network Adequacy Standards: Lessons from Four States*. Robert Wood Johnson Foundation.

World Health Organization (2009). TELEMEDICINE: Opportunities and Developments in Member States: Report on the Second Global Survey on eHealth. https://www.who.int/goe/publications/goe_telemedicine_2010.pdf (accessed June 2019).

World Health Organization (2015). The growing need for home health care for the elderly: Home health care for the elderly as an integral part of primary health care services http://applications.emro.who.int/dsaf/EMROPUB_2015_EN_1901.pdf?ua=1 (accessed June 2019).

World Health Organization (n.d.). Health policy. http://www.who.int/topics/health_policy/en (accessed November 2018).

Zarnke, K.B., Levine, M.A.H., and O'Brien, B.J. (1997). Cost-benefit analyses in the health-care literature: don't judge a study by its label. *Journal of Clinical Epidemiology* **50**(7): 813–822.

Zilberberg, M.D. and Shorr, A.F. (2010). Understanding cost-effectiveness. *Clinical Microbiology and Infection* **16**: 1707–1712.

6

DATA ANALYTICS

Healthcare delivery can be thought of as a continual series of information-processing procedures, from the initial collection of data (the patient's history, physical exam, and diagnostic tests), a hypothesis (diagnosis) is formed and then validated by further data collection (Reid et al. 2005). Disease-specific registries, interactive voice response, computer touch screens, hand-held computer devices, mobile phones, and web-based applications have enhanced our caseload to collect health outcomes information in an efficient and effective manner (Statistics Canada and Canadian Institute for Health Information 2008). Public health also sets numerous "experiments," testing and implementing policies and interventions, with both intended and unintended consequences, creating data collection environments for population health and health policy making. Thus, in healthcare systems, data, and knowledge are acquired in many forms at every step within the healthcare delivery process. Current information technologies greatly facilitate this data acquisition process. Billions of pieces of data are generated by the healthcare system every day. Every individual interacting with the healthcare system, every provider contributing to healthcare delivery, and every intervention tested and implemented generates invaluable data that can contribute to understanding *what works, for who, and where.*

The large amount of data collected within the healthcare system can be used to advance personalized medicine, target interventions, evaluate guidelines and practices, and identify fraud, among many others. It can provide opportunities to set up "policy labs" where policies and interventions can be tested without their direct deployment to the public; to a great extent, the methodologies presented in this book have wide applicability in such policy-making labs, where retrospective and prospective data analysis can be used to evaluate "what-if" scenarios of policies and interventions.

While there are enormous opportunities, generating massive amounts of healthcare data does come with a price to be paid. Because much of the healthcare data provide individual-detailed information, ensuring privacy and confidentiality of the health information of each individual is paramount. This significantly deters access to such

Healthcare System Access: Measurement, Inference, and Intervention, Nicoleta Serban.
© 2020 John Wiley & Sons, Inc. Published 2020 by John Wiley & Sons, Inc.

data, regardless of the benefits to the overall population. But not only data safeguards restrict access to health(care) data. The right of information, "who to use it," "how to use it," and "who owns it" is highly prevalent in health-related data access.

The fragmentation of the healthcare system implicitly results in fragmentation of data as well as information-poor and low quality data (Tien and Goldschmidt-Clermont 2009). Therefore, despite the abundance of data in the field of public health and healthcare, it is often very difficult to obtain relevant, meaningful, and quality health(care) data. Moreover, integrating fragmented data, observed at different scale and resolution levels, and with different quality levels, requires a broad knowledge about the healthcare system, health analytics, and data science.

Along with the increase in the abundance of data, the caseload to analyze the data grows faster than our ability to understand it. Data analysis techniques also change with the availability of massive data sets. Traditional statistical methods were developed to handle data shortage. Modern data analysis based on big data poses new challenges, including the need for computational innovation, cross-disciplinary methodologies, statistical inference for big data, and high-dimensional data visualization, among others (National Research Council 2013). Such challenges are no less relevant to decision making in healthcare delivery and public health if data-driven.

These challenges are particularly relevant to investigations on health(care) outcomes and healthcare access, due to the complexity of the data needed to inform policies and interventions, spanning all four levels of the healthcare system, people, processes, organizations, and ecosystem. The overarching objective of this book is to contribute to the integration of domain-specific knowledge, data and methodologies in these fields of research.

Specifically, the goal of this chapter is to lay out the grounds for understanding healthcare data along with a description of common data (re)sources that could be useful in a wide range of methodological implementations of policies and interventions for improving healthcare access and health outcomes. The chapter will expand on the modern paradigm of data science, integrating all data processes from data acquisition and processing to data translation, to data modeling and finally decision making as illustrated in Figure 6.1. The overarching message is that data science is at the core of informed decisions, interventions, and ultimately at the core of system's transformations.

HEALTHCARE DATA SOURCES

In the case studies presented in the previous chapters, I have demonstrated how each specific healthcare access problem tackled requires data collected from multiple sources. Examples of data sets in these studies include the Medicaid Analytic Extract (MAX) data files acquired from the Centers for Medicare & Medicaid Services (CMS); the National Plan and Provider Enumeration System (NPPES); the United States Census Bureau data; the Behavioral Risk Factor Surveillance System (BRFSS); the H1N1 vaccine shipment data obtained from the Centers for Disease

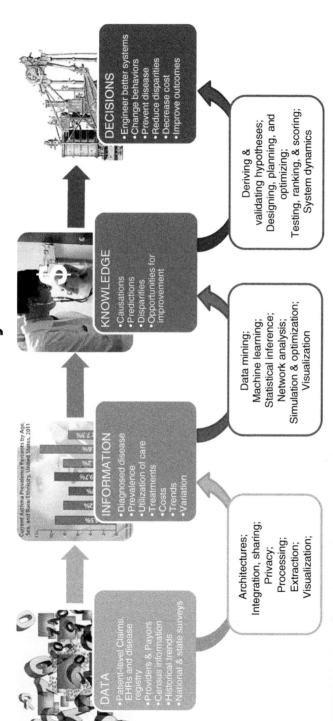

FIGURE 6.1 Data science framework encompassing all data processes from data acquisition and processing to data translation, to data modeling and finally decision making, where at each step several data tools and methodologies need to be integrated and implemented. EHRs, electronic health records.

Control and Prevention; the cystic fibrosis (CF) Registry data acquired from the Cystic Fibrosis Foundation (CFF); the Online Analytical Statistical Information System (OASIS) database; the Healthcare Cost and Utilization Project (HCUP) state database by the Agency for Healthcare Research and Quality; the Health Policy Institute (HPI) of the American Dental Association (ADA) reports and data sets; the InsureKidsNow.gov database; the National Health and Nutrition Examination Survey (NHANES) by the National Center for Health Statistics (NCHS); the Kaiser Family Foundation reports and data; among many other databases, reports, and publications specifying information on various aspects about providers' characteristics and caseload, patients' preferences, and guidelines or legislation.

Moreover, many of the models introduced in these case studies rely on specifications of a series of structural parameters representing model assumptions and approximations. They are often drawn from a wide range of published documents or simply input using expert knowledge. This is common practice because of the lack of relevant data needed to produce estimates about patients' behaviors and preferences, providers' constraints, and network structures. Therefore, data inputs for models measuring and making inference on healthcare access and health outcomes come from many sources, with different levels of accuracy and aggregation. Identifying the appropriate sources of data inputs and understanding their limitations are overarching aspects of data analytics for public health and for decision making as I will expand on in this chapter.

Overview of Healthcare Data Sources

The scope of data sources used in healthcare access and health outcome studies includes many types of data set, some larger and some smaller in size, some are derived from observational studies while others from randomized trials, and some may be surveys of a sample of the study population while others may cover the entire study population. Below I overview three types of data set I have used extensively in my research related to healthcare access and health(care) outcomes.

Protected health information (PHI) patient-detailed data consist of individual-level records about the health status, healthcare delivery, or healthcare expenditure collected by a healthcare provider or organization. Most common PHI data are *electronic health records (EHRs)*, collected by large or small providers, e.g. Kaiser Permanente, Veterans Health Administration (VHA), Community Health Centers as well as small physician offices; *administrative claims data*, the larger provider collecting such data being the CMS covering the Medicaid-insured and Medicare-insured populations; and *clinical registry data*, commonly focusing on patients who share a common reason for needing healthcare or with a specific condition, e.g. CFF Registry, Colon Cancer Family registry and many others.

PHI data are subject to many regulations to protect individuals' identity, which can be derived from the data. Such regulations can specify safeguards on physical storage, access, share, transmit, and distribution along with specifications related to data reporting and publication. Individual-level data can be made available in three format types, non-identifiable data set files, limited data set (LDS) files or identifiable data set files. Non-identifiable data set files contain non-identifiable person-specific information and are commonly made available within the public domain. LDS files have been stripped of data elements that might permit identification of beneficiaries following the specifications of the Health Insurance Portability and Accountability Act (HIPAA) Privacy Rule. Identifiable data files are different from LDS files in that they contain actual beneficiary-specific and provider-specific information, thus requiring stricter safeguards than LDS format. The level of safeguards to protect personal health information depends on the data format. Moreover, availability of LDS or identifiable data is limited since few information technology (IT) systems can accommodate the safeguards required to protect PHI data.

EHRs are the major source of data used to derive clinical outcomes. EHRs are digital records of patient health information generated by encounters in any care delivery setting. They include demographics, progress notes, diagnoses, medications, vital signs, medical history, immunizations, laboratory data, and radiology reports. They are the backbone of information-driven health practices.

EHRs are widespread around the world. In Canada, Health Infoway, Inc., has been working in collaboration with Canada's 14 provinces and territories to establish the framework and standards for an interoperable, nationwide EHR system based on interconnected regional systems. The United Kingdom's National Health Service (NHS) has implemented a nationwide EHR system under the umbrella of the NHS Care Record Service. In the United States, in 2004 President George W. Bush established a national goal of universal adoption of EHRs and health information exchanges by 2014. This initiative was followed with a financial commitment in 2009 under federal legislation, the Health Information Technology for Economic and Clinical Health (HITECH) Act (US Department of Health and Human Services 2009). With the advancement of HITECH, currently most healthcare providers have moved away from the paper-based medical record to electronically recorded information at the point of care.

EHRs are the main sources of data for clinical and wellbeing outcomes. They can provide rich information about an individual's health with respect to a specific condition and/or healthcare setting. Most common EHRs are one-time snapshots of an individual's health, recorded by providers contracted by a health insurance program to deliver care without coordination of the overall healthcare of the individual receiving care across multiple providers and care settings. In this case, because the EHRs only reflect one's health for a specific condition at one point in time, they are limited in deriving meaningful data on health outcomes. However, EHRs can also be longitudinal, comprehensive patient-level medical records, acquired, and maintained by large managed care organizations. One large comprehensive EHR system is the Veterans Information Systems and Technology Architecture (VistA) system, a centralized resource of medical records for all veteran-related care and services. Because the VHA provides care for the veteran population on a continuum of care, coordinating multiple care services and providers, the VistA EHRs can be used to draw inferences on the overall health of the veterans, being relevant to the study of health outcomes in relation to healthcare access.

Administrative claims data consist of billed medical claims for delivery of care for patients insured by a health insurance program. Generally, each encounter with the healthcare system generates multiple claims, each claim being submitted for reimbursement for delivery of a specific service. Each claim record can specify information about the diagnosis (e.g. specified by ICD-9 or ICD-10 codes), procedure performed (e.g. based on the National Procedure Codes), provider taxonomy (e.g. National Provider Index, NPI), the cost submitted for reimbursement and how much of the cost was actually reimbursed, date of service, place of service (e.g. hospital, physician office), type of service (e.g. emergency department), type of claim (e.g. fee-for-service [FFS], encounter) and other information about the patient, provider, and payment. Thus a claim record is a complex piece of information, which can be translated into actual information based on the specifications of each data element in the record provided in a data dictionary and coded by established national codes.

While translating claims records into actual data that can be used in healthcare studies and decision making is challenging, one of the advantages of administrative claims data is standardization; claims records are structured similarly, using common terminology and information models regardless of the organization recording them. Because of this standardization, claims data can be used broadly, in large studies connecting records from private and public insurance programs. One such system is provided by the IBM MarketScan Research Data.

One of the largest providers of administrative claims data is CMS, the largest health insurance provider, covering about 120 million people in the United States in 2018 through three publicly funded programs: Medicaid, Medicare, and the Children's Health Insurance Program (CHIP). There are many forms through which CMS could provide data assistance and resources but among the most sought after data files are the Medicaid and Medicare claims files consisting of individual-level data on eligibility, demographics characteristics, healthcare utilization, and payments. The data files are available for all states and the District of Columbia beginning with calendar year 1999. These data are developed to support research and policy analysis initiatives for Medicaid and Medicare programs, for example, analyzing provider payments, conducting quality or access to care studies, and conducting statistical analysis for public reporting. Many case studies in this book have been informed in part by the MAX claims data acquired from CMS (Centers for Medicare & Medicaid Services n.d.-a).

There are also many limitations in using the EHRs and administrative claims data in health(care) studies. Not all services received are billed and/or not all clinical information is recorded, patients change insurance payers, and a high percentage of United States patients do not have stable insurance coverage and thus incur no utilization record (claim or medical record) when they receive care. Provider information can be incomplete, particularly in claims data, as presented in one of the case studies in this chapter. The claims or medical records only capture information about patients who have been diagnosed and received care, but not those who may be treated but not diagnosed. Therefore, estimates on the healthcare utilization, prevalence, or treatment may be biased for certain subgroups that have difficulty in maintaining healthcare insurance coverage, lack of access, or are susceptible to particularly disparate utilization (DeVoe et al. 2011). Moreover specifically, claims data are collected for administrative purposes thus they do not provide clinical information. Similarly, EHR data are collected for delivery of quality care and thus primarily focus on clinical outcomes, and less so on healthcare outcomes, for example, healthcare expenditure.

There also notable more limitations for the CMS claims data, particularly the MAX files. For example, the number of deaths may be underreported since if a person has a claim but no eligibility information, the data element for death is filled with a zero. Also, previous research has found that MAX data capture approximately 73% of foster care cases (Raghavan et al. 2017). Another possible limitation concerns the fact that the administrative claims in the MAX other therapy (OT) file include limited number of diagnosis codes per claim. Thus if an individual was receiving treatment for multiple co-morbid conditions, it is possible that a condition of interest may not have been included in the codes on the outpatient claim. Furthermore, Medicaid MAX files can have data quality issues, especially for states with large populations on managed care (Byrd and Dodd 2012; Byrd and Dodd 2015). DeVoe et al. (2011) found that relying solely on Medicaid claims data is likely to underestimate substantially the quality of care.

Clinical data registry can be of two types, national registries covering most of the population with a specific condition, or registries including data on a sample population commonly collected using an observational study (National Institutes of Health n.d.). A list of clinical data registry is maintained by the NIH (https://www .nih.gov/health-information/nih-clinical-research-trials-you/list-registries). Below I will illustrate the range of data formats available in registries for two different conditions; these two examples demonstrate the variety of clinical registry data from a national registry including the majority of patients with a rare condition versus a local registry including only a small number of patients with a chronic condition.

The CFF has established a national *CF Registry*, including medical records of CF patients who agree to participate in the CF Registry. Cystic fibrosis is a rare disease that requires sub-specialty care that is available at a small number (~121) of accredited care centers nationally (Knapp et al. 2016). The CFF estimated that the registry currently captures data on 81–84% of all persons with CF in the United States (Knapp et al. 2016). The medical records are acquired from the CFF-accredited care centers and they track patient outcomes and trends in health over many years, starting with 1986 to date. The CF Registry data can be directly acquired from the CFF by submitting a research protocol to the foundation. The data include clinical outcomes such as age at death, the forced expiratory volume in one second as a percentage of predicted volume (%FEV1), body mass index (BMI) for age >2, weight and height for infants (<2 years of age), number of pulmonary exacerbations, recovery of %FEV1 after treatment for pulmonary exacerbations, HgA1c for patients with CF-related diabetes, development of co-morbidities (e.g. diabetes and liver disease); access outcomes such as the location of the care center; and patient characteristics such as zip code of their residence, age, health insurance status, genetic mutation. The data are available in a LDS format and are observed longitudinally.

The *Wisconsin Diabetes Registry Study* was funded by the National Institute of Diabetes, Digestive, and Kidney Diseases (part of the NIH) starting in 1987 to understand the complications and co-morbidities associated with diabetes. The sample set consists of 733 men and women from a 28-county region in south-central Wisconsin. The long-term goal of the registry was to prevent or delay the progression of the complications that arise over time from diabetes. Since type 1 and type 2 diabetes have similar complications, this data set has also been used for analyses of type 2 diabetes mellitus, usually developed in later life due to a relative inability to produce sufficient insulin for the person's body mass (BMI). The main complications studied by the Wisconsin Diabetes Registry Study include nerve disease (neuropathy), kidney disease (nephropathy), eye disease (retinopathy), and cardiovascular disease.

Survey data collected by public and private organizations are public health data sets collected from phone or in-person interviews, sometimes cross references with physical examinations, and they can be acquired for specific years, or as cross-sectional or longitudinal surveys. Three of the most popular national health surveys are BRFSS, National Health Interview Survey (NHIS) by the NCHS, and NHANES by the NCHS. *BRFSS* is a telephone survey collected at the state level, providing information about health risk behaviors, clinical preventive practices, and health care access and use (Centers for Disease Control and Prevention 2010). *NHIS* is a face-to-face survey, monitoring the United States population health by collecting information on a wide range of health topics (National Center for Health Statistics n.d.-b). *NHANES* combines interviews and physical examinations, focusing on different population groups or health conditions or settings (National Center for Health Statistics n.d.-a).

Other national surveys include the National Ambulatory Medical Care Survey (NAMCS); The National Survey of Children's Health (NSCH) Surveys; and the Medical Expenditure Panel Survey (MEPS) (Centers for Disease Control and Prevention n.d.-a), among many others. The surveys developed by NSCH provide information for physical and mental health status, access to quality healthcare, as well as information on the child's family, neighborhood, and social context (National Survey of Children's Health n.d.). The *MEPS* collects data from individuals, employers, and medical providers, and it provides information about healthcare use and costs, as well as health insurance use and costs. The *NAMCS* collects data on utilization and provision of care primarily provided in physician offices and emergency departments.

Generally, most surveys are randomized studies, covering a small sample of the population and covering a small proportion of the United States communities. For example, NHANES has limited geographic coverage with little more than 1% of 3141 United States counties sampled. In the formats available to the public, the surveys do not provide location information about the individuals surveyed to keep their identity protected. Thus data from such surveys have limited applicability in healthcare access studies.

Secondary health and healthcare data are available from public and private organizations, national, or state level. Federal or governmental providers and organizations collecting such data include CMS, Centers for Disease Control and Prevention (CDC), Agency for Healthcare Research and Quality (AHRQ), Health

Resources and Services Administration (HRSA), NIH, NCHS, National Cancer Institute (NCI), among many others. Secondary public health data are commonly collected by state and local departments of public health. Data may be also collected by non-profit associations, for example, the American Medical Association (AMA), American Hospital Association (AHA), Medical Group Management Association (MGMA), Kids Data, and UCLA Center for Health Policy Research. Public health data may also be collected by foundations, for example, the Robert Wood Johnson Foundation, the Commonwealth Fund, the Annie E. Casey Foundation, the Kaiser Family Foundation, and the Pew Foundation.

Many states and local districts collect their own data and house data registries, disease surveillance systems, and healthcare utilization measures by sub-populations and geographic regions. These data systems are commonly managed by state departments of public health. Examples are the OASIS of Georgia state (https://oasis.state .ga.us); the Indicator-Based Information System of New Mexico state (https://ibis .health.state.nm.us); the county and sub-county data and reports of the Department of Health in New York State (https://www.health.ny.gov/statistics); the Data and Health Reports such as the Comprehensive Hospital Abstract Reporting System (CHARS) of Washington state (https://www.doh.wa.gov/dataandstatisticalreports).

With the initiation of HITECH, health information exchanges have been developed across the country, allowing interoperability among data systems, however with limited applicability to state and local district data because states have implemented different data operability systems and formats. This in turn may result in limited ability to compare health outcomes and access measures derived from such data sources across states

Figure 6.2 displays a summary of the data sources and how they can be used for measuring and making inference on healthcare access. As highlighted in this figure, the data sources can inform multiple aspects of healthcare access, health disparities and outcomes, with the overarching objective to inform healthcare interventions. I will expand on the use of these multiple data sources in the remaining sections of this chapter. Specifically, I will present how all such data sources can be used to evaluate the provider-level supply of healthcare, to estimate the need or demand of specific healthcare services at a geographically granular level, to specify constrains in the delivery of care and patients' or providers' preferences, to identify health outcomes to be targeted with improvement in healthcare access, and to design and evaluate interventions to achieve such improvements.

Access Measurement: Supply Network

One very useful source of data for detailed information on the supply of healthcare services is the NPPES (Centers for Medicare & Medicaid Services n.d.-b), which includes provider-level information on their unique NPI used for reimbursement, their business practice addresses, the taxonomy of their type of services provided, and whether a sole or group provider, specified by the Entity field, among other data elements. The NPI coding system was created because the HIPAA (in 1996) required a unique health care provider identifier to facilitate electronic transmission of claims and other health care information. Hence, the NPI code is used in every billing claim.

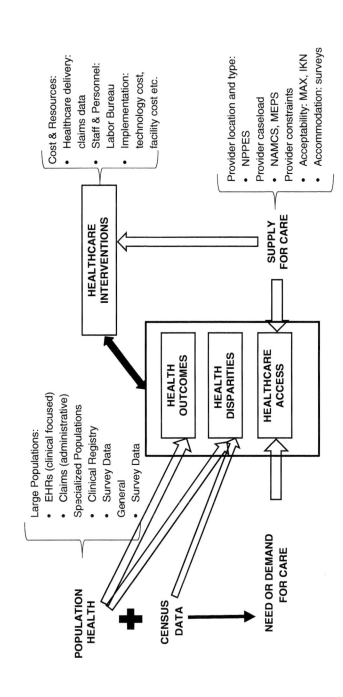

FIGURE 6.2 Data sources for measurement of and inference on healthcare access, healthcare disparities and health outcomes, informing the design and evaluations of healthcare interventions. IKN, InsureKidsNow.org.

Important provider-level data elements available in the NPPES and used in measuring supply of healthcare are described in Table 6.1.

Depending on the type of healthcare services of interest, the taxonomy of healthcare providers can be selected from the list of Health Care Provider Taxonomy Code Set maintained by the CMS and the National Uniform Claim Committee (NUCC). Moreover, the addresses need to be geocoded to latitude and longitude information. In my research, I commonly use the Texas A&M Geocoding Services (http://geoservices .tamu.edu/Services/Geocode/) and the census.gov for geocoding, and the ArcGIS Network Analyst to compute the street-network distances.

Other sources of data on provider census are available (Health Resources and Services Administration 2013aa); however, they particularly target specific types of care and/or are aggregated within specific geographic units, for example, county; many of them also are not made publicly available and/or for free use. For example, the state boards of physicians and of dentists generally keep a census of the healthcare providers; however, such data are not readily available and/or are not easy to link to medical administrative data, which include information on the NPI providers delivering the healthcare services. Another example is the AMA Masterfile. The Masterfile contains demographic, educational, and current professional activity on more than 1 million medical and osteopathic physicians, including AMA members and non-members. Hence, records in this data base correspond to Entity 1 type of records in the NPPES database. However, the AMA files are not publicly available. They also do not include exact location information about the providers; only the practice zip code is available. In most healthcare access studies, exact provider practice information is essential.

In my research, I used the NPPES data because they are observed at the provider level, with very detailed information about the providers, and are comprehensive across all types of care. However, there are some challenges in using the NPPES data to specify the network of healthcare providers. Generally, as a provider changes its location and/or other fields in the data, if the provider submits this information to the NPPES, then it is updated immediately. However, providers do not make revisions to their NPI data immediately as they come up, thus there may be inconsistencies in the reporting. There is no direct link or information that can reveal any association between the record of a provider (an Entity 1 type of record) and the record of the group or hospital where the provider works (an Entity 2 type of record). The Healthcare Provider Taxonomy Group attribute can reveal whether the entity has multiple locations, however, in the case of multiple locations, there is no information about where the additional practice locations are. The only available information is related to the primary business practice location, which is indicated in the practice address. Because of this, in my collaborative research, we used the Business Practice address as the primary location of a provider. Last, these data provide detailed information on healthcare providers reimbursed for their services; however, they do not include information about the mid-level licensed providers working under the supervision of physicians or dentists, which are not directly reimbursed for their services.

Information on the location and taxonomy of the healthcare providers is necessary but not sufficient to fully specify supply of healthcare. Providers have different

TABLE 6.1 List of Attributes for each Record of the NPPES Database that are of Relevance in Healthcare Access Case Studies

Attribute	Description	Related entity	Additional comments
NPI	The unique 10-digit identifier		
Entity type code	Code describing the type of health care provider that is being assigned an NPI. Codes are 1 = (person): individual human being who furnishes health care; 2 = (non-person): entity other than an individual human being that furnishes health care (for example, hospital, SNF, hospital subunit, pharmacy, or Health Maintenance Organization [HMO])		
Provider organization name (legal business name)	The name of the organization provider, this is the legal business name	Only entity 2	
Provider last name (legal name)	The last name of the provider this is the legal name	Only entity 1	
Provider first name	The first name of the provider, if the provider is an individual	Only entity 1	
Provider middle name	The middle name of the provider, if the provider is an individual	Only entity 1	
Provider other organization name	The name by which the organization provider is or has been known	Only entity 2	
Provider other organization name type code	Code identifying the type of other name. Codes applicable for this field are: 3 = doing business as (d/b/ a) name; 4 = former legal business name; 5 = other	Only entity 2	Required if "Provider other organization name" contains data. Codes 1–2 apply to individuals; codes 3–4 apply to organizations; code 5 applies to both
Provider other last name	Last name associated with another name the provider has used, if applicable	Only entity 1	

(continued overleaf)

TABLE 6.1 *(Continued)*

Attribute	Description	Related entity	Additional comments
Provider other first name	First name associated with another name the provider has used, if applicable	Only entity 1	
Provider other last name type code	Code identifying the type of other name. Codes applicable for this field are: 1 = former name; 2 = professional name; 5 = other	Only entity 1	Required if "Provider other last name" contains data. Codes 1–2 apply to individuals; codes 3–4 apply to organizations; code 5 applies to both
Provider first line business mailing address	The first line mailing address of the provider being identified. This data element may contain the same information as "Provider first line business practice location address"		
Provider second line business mailing address	The second line mailing address of the provider being identified. This data element may contain the same information as "Provider second line business practice location address"		
Provider business mailing address city name	The city name in the mailing address of the provider being identified. This data element may contain the same information as "Provider business practice location address city name"		
Provider business mailing address state name	The State or Province name in the mailing address of the provider being identified. This data element may contain the same information as "Provider business practice location address state name."		Required if the address has no state code but contains a state or province name
Provider business mailing address postal code	The postal ZIP or zone code in the mailing address of the provider being identified. Note: ZIP code plus 4-digit extension, if available. This data element may contain the same information as "Provider business practice location address postal code"		

TABLE 6.1 *(Continued)*

Attribute	Description	Related entity	Additional comments
Provider first line business practice location address	The first line location address of the provider being identified. For providers with more than one physical location, this is the primary location. This address cannot include a Post Office box		
Provider second line business practice location address	The second line location address of the provider being identified. For providers with more than one physical location, this is the primary location. This address cannot include a Post Office box		
Provider business practice location address city name	The city name in the location address of the provider being identified		
Provider business practice location address state name	The state abbreviation in the location of the provider being identified		
Provider business practice location address postal code	The postal ZIP or zone code in the location address of the provider being identified. Note: ZIP code plus 4-digit extension, if available		
Last update date	The date that a record was last updated or changed		
NPI deactivation reason code	The reason that the provider's NPI was deactivated in the NPS. Codes are: 1 = death of entity type "1" provider; 2 = entity type "2" provider disbandment; 3 = fraud. 4 = other (for example, retirement)		
NPI deactivation date	The date that the provider's NPI was deactivated in the NPS		
NPI reactivation date	The date that the provider's NPI was reactivated in the NPS		

(continued overleaf)

TABLE 6.1 (*Continued*)

Attribute	Description	Related entity	Additional comments
Provider gender code	The code designating the provider's gender if the provider is a person	Only entity 1	
Healthcare provider taxonomy code	Code designating the provider type, classification, and specialization. Codes are from the Healthcare Provider Taxonomy code list. The NPS will associate these data with the license data for providers with entity type code = 1.		
Is sole proprietor	A sole proprietor/sole proprietorship is eligible for a single NPI. A sole proprietor/sole proprietorship cannot have subparts and cannot designate subparts. In terms of NPI assignment, a sole proprietor/sole proprietorship is an entity type I (individual). A sole proprietor can have employees		A sole proprietorship is a type of business entity that is owned and run by one individual and in which there is no legal distinction between the owner and the business. It is a "sole" proprietorship in contrast with partnerships. A sole proprietor may use a trade name or business name other than his or her legal name
Healthcare provider taxonomy group	Multi-specialty group (193200000X) or single specialty group (193400000X) or multi single specialty group (193400000X) • Single specialty groups have members with one taxonomy • Multi-specialty groups have members with more than one taxonomy • Multi single specialty groups have more than one location and the members have one taxonomy		

caseloads, measured in number of patients or visits, allocated for specific services (e.g. preventive vs specialized), sub-populations (e.g. children vs adults), provider type (e.g. general vs pediatric), by location (e.g. rural vs urban practice location), by state, or other provider characteristics. Such specifications or caseload constraints require using additional data sources, including HRSA Bureau of Health Professions, National Center for Health Workforce Analysis (Health Resources and Services Administration 2013bb); Organization for Economic Co-operation and Development (OECD)'s Health Care Resources (Organization for Economic and Co-operative Development n.d.); the NAMCS (National Center for Health Statistics 2015); and administrative claims or other data sources (Altschuler et al. 2012).

Medical claims data such as those available from the CMS can also be used to specify provider-level information on the realized caseload for specific sub-populations and services. But realized caseload as observed from claims data or EHRs is not potential caseload; to address the difference between realized and potential caseload, an excess number of patients or visits may be added to the realized caseload because not all patients in need of care may access the healthcare system, particularly for sub-populations with limited access. Some access measurement approaches assume a pre-specified caseload for all providers, for example, the HRSA assumes a provider per 1000 population ratio as one criterion to define medically underserved areas (MUAs). Generally, obtaining provider-level caseload estimates is one of the challenging aspects in estimating access; because of this, few studies incorporate such information in the access estimates while it can impact the accuracy of the access estimates greatly, with implication in deriving policies and interventions (Serban and Tomar 2018; Serban et al. 2019).

Access Measurement: Need/Demand Network

As I mentioned earlier in this book, health economics differentiate between need and demand for healthcare. I will expand on these concepts in this section with reference to data analytics approaches to evaluate them in healthcare access studies.

Demand measures the quantity of health services the population is willing to consume and purchase given cost and access constraints, preferences, or other related behaviors. A sub-population's demand for medical services depends on cultural, religious, educational, and social status as well as on perceived physical or mental distress (Jeffers et al. 1971). For example, demand can be estimated from EHRs or claims data based on the realized utilization of the healthcare system for a study population. It can be quantified based on the number of services or the number of visits for a specific type of care for the patients in a sub-population defined by various characteristics and/or a given geographic region. Alternatively, utilization rates per patient per year (PPPY) or per patient per month (PPPM) can be obtained from existing studies, which can be used as multipliers on the study population stratified by various characteristics.

Need consists of health(care) services that a healthcare professional finds necessary to deliver following specific health indicators or recommended care guidelines. Need for a particular service is determined by healthcare professionals based on demographics, clinical risk factors, health status, and genetic background, among others. Need commonly consists of two data inputs: the size of the population in need for care: and the recommended care level by patient characteristics. Thus the difference in estimation of demand versus need is in the multiplier to the population in need for care; for demand, it is derived from realized utilization of healthcare while for need, it is based on recommended practice guidelines. For example, the number of preventive care visits for Medicaid-insured children aged three to six years is between 0.69 and 1.01 per Medicaid child per year as provided by a study on the utilization of dental care for six southeast states (Lee et al. 2018) versus two or more visits per year as recommended for Medicaid-insured children due to their higher risk for caries (American Academy of Pediatric Dentistry 2013). Recommended practices are generally established by medical and dental national associations, which can be easily accessible from reports published and disseminated widely by the associations. For example, asthma guidelines are published by the National Heart Blood and Lung Institute (National Heart Blood and Lung Institute 2007); preventive dental care guidelines are published by the American Academy of Pediatric Dentistry (American Academy of Pediatric Dentistry 2013); and pediatric primary care guidelines are published by the American Academy of Pediatrics (American Academy of Pediatrics 2014).

Need for healthcare can also be "felt need," when an individual assesses his/her health status and finds a lower or higher need for healthcare than recommended by a medical professional. This is different from demand in that felt need may not be pursued or consumed due to access or cost constraints, for example. Generally, most public health studies, particularly those related to healthcare access, focus on demand or need but not on felt need. This is because demand and need are quantifiable or measurable. Moreover, "demand" is most frequently used by medical economists, while "need" is most frequently used by health professionals, commissions, and agencies (Jeffers et al. 1971).

Regardless of whether demand or need is considered against existing supply in measuring healthcare access, detailed information about the study population is required. Such detailed information can be derived from census data such as the American Community Survey (ACS), administrative claims data, and EHRs. Prevalence of a condition for a study population can be obtained from surveillance studies such as those conducted by CDC or state-level secondary data as described in the previous section. However, such data are not commonly available at low geographic granularity, such as census tracts. For example, projections about the risk or prevalence of a condition at low geographic granularity can be derived using survey data such as NHANES and micro-simulation models (Davila Payan et al. 2014; Cao et al. 2017a,b).

It is important to distinguish between demand and need in health services research because the gap between them depends greatly by population characteristics, with one of the most substantive contributor being health education. Medical professional standards of what constitutes "good health" and the extent and limitations of the preventive, therapeutic, and rehabilitative capabilities of healthcare are not widely known and understood. In general, most people do not recognize symptoms of ill health until they manifest as pain, or other obvious abnormalities (Jeffers et al. 1971). The difference between the two can be both positive and negative. When individuals demand health services they do not need, it can cause waste of resources. On the other hand, if individuals do not demand health services, which they medically require, it will lead to worsening of their health, and if that disease is communicable, then of others too.

When measuring healthcare access, public health researchers commonly prefer to use the need instead of demand to contrast it to the supply of healthcare. This is because need is not subjective to patient's characteristics such as socioeconomic, education, or geographic location. Need is based on what professional healthcare providers find necessary to deliver to meet patients' needs for care and not what they can access or afford. However, need evaluated based on recommended care guidelines can also be an overestimate of "true" need, where "true" refers to needed care at the level that one can prevent severe outcomes and ill health. For example, in one of my collaborative research papers, we found that children diagnosed with persistent asthma generally do not have emergency room visits and hospitalizations if they regularly take asthma controller medication, and do not necessarily need to visit a physician for their asthma diagnosis at the level recommended by practice guidelines (Hilton et al. 2017). Thus consideration of both demand and need of healthcare may provide a more appropriate level of needed care when evaluated against existing supply in a system with limited resources and already escalating costs.

Access Measurement: Constraints and Preferences

As I presented earlier in this book, healthcare access is a multidimensional construct within a complex system. Depending on the access dimension of interest, various constraints and preferences impact the extent of healthcare access greatly.

Because affordability of healthcare has been at the forefront of the national and local health policy agenda, many data sources provide information on the uninsured population as well as on Medicaid, Medicare, and the exchange insurance programs. Common data sources providing summary facts, reports, and granular geographic data or estimates on healthcare insurance are available from the United States Census Bureau, CMS and Kaiser Family Foundation, among others. Extensive data for the uninsured population are available at the national level for various population characteristics (United States Census Bureau 2017), as small area estimates for the United States counties (United States Census Bureau 2016) or derived based on community survey data. Extensive data for the population with public insurance are available at the state level from the Kaiser Family Foundation and at the county or census tract level from community survey data.

For specific healthcare services, for example dental care for children, estimates on affordability of care are challenging to derive because affordability takes various forms, including public and private insurance as well as out-of-pocket expenditure. Preventive dental care is primarily covered by out-of-pocket expenditure for a large proportion of the population without public insurance, thus estimation of the child population percentages with parents with ability to afford preventive dental care for their children requires information on parents' income as well as data on utilization of dental care by income to estimate the income levels at which parents afford dental care for their children (Cao et al. 2017a,b).

Health insurance, or lack of it, becomes a necessary constraint when measuring access for other dimensions. Lack of affordability could deem healthcare services inaccessible regardless of the extent of the access with respect to other dimensions. Access to different health insurance programs is also strongly related to the acceptability dimension. Healthcare providers commonly accept only a handful of health insurance programs, with a smaller percentage of providers accepting public insurance. Seeking care at a provider not accepting a specific health insurance program involves higher out-of-pocket expenses, in some cases, making healthcare not affordable.

Thus data on health insurance, more specifically, on affordability of healthcare and acceptability of insurance programs specify important constraints in the measurement of access dimensions, such as accessibility and availability. Acceptability of public insurance along with its implications in public health is one of the primary emphases in health services research. Data on acceptability of public insurance vary depending on the healthcare service of interest. For example, the database available from InsureKidsNow.gov reports all the dentists who accept public insurance. Such databases are not readily available for other services.

The MAX claims data can also be a data source for identifying which healthcare providers accept public insurance; if this data set is used, then it needs to be linked to the NPPES data for location and taxonomy information, thus requiring accurate NPI records for the providers recorded in the MAX data, who provide healthcare services to the Medicaid-insured population. However, not all states have complete and accurate data on NPIs of the Medicaid providers in the MAX files; the accuracy of the data also depends on the type of healthcare service. For example, mental and behavioral health services for public insurance may be delivered under carve-out managed care, a Medicaid financing model where some portion of the healthcare benefits are separately managed and/or financed by another organization or retained by the state Medicaid agency on a FFS basis (Mandros 2014). When the behavioral health benefits are carved out of the overall public healthcare system, the claims for such services may be underreported, thus the information on the behavioral health providers accepting Medicaid may also be underreported.

Many other constraints on the network of providers are specified in regulations and guidelines on access for the Medicaid managed care, established both at the national and local/state level (Centers for Medicare & Medicaid Services 2016b, 2017a). Such regulations and guidelines are used in contracting insurance providers in Medicaid managed care. In addition to the number of network providers who are not accepting new Medicaid patients mentioned above, examples of access constraints provided in the final law established in 2016 by CMS include state standards for timely access to care and services, taking into account the urgency of the need for services; and the means of transportation ordinarily used by Medicaid enrollees.

Access standards generally establish some level of accountability for managed care organizations in providing timely healthcare access. Such standards assume some maximum level of one's willingness to travel a specific distance or to wait a specific time for receiving healthcare services, depending on whether residing in a rural or urban community, and depending on whether seeking primary, specialized, or urgent care. Access standards vary by state and they can specify travel distance, travel time, appointment wait time and/or maximum number of patients a provider may have, differentiated by service type. The Department of Health and Human Services compiled all access standards by state in 2013 (DHHS 2014); however the standard may have changed for some states in response to the final law established in 2016 (Centers for Medicare & Medicaid Services 2016b).

State Medicaid agencies are required by the CMS to enact access standards for managed care organizations (Ndumele et al. 2017) and are starting to be rated in managed care contracts on or after July 2018; thus states will need to report how well the contracted managed care providers perform with respect to many regulations on availability of services. More data will be available on these aspects as the rating will start to take shape.

The means of transportation can be limiting in terms of accessibility of services for sub-populations with public insurance; if an individual does not have access to a car or has disabilities that restrict use of a car, then public or Medicaid transportation are the only options if the services are not accessible within walking distance. Data on poverty along with data on ownership of cars available in the ACS can be used to estimate access to private transportation means for the population eligible for Medicaid; these data can be combined with access standards to determine the extent of accessibility for specific services.

Medicaid transportation has been one of the main means of transportation for specialized services requiring long travel distances for the Medicaid population. Qualifying for Medicaid or non-emergency medical transportation does come with some restrictions, varying by state (Centers for Medicare & Medicaid Services 2016a). Such restrictions can be documented directly from the state regulatory reporting systems. Constraints due to these restrictions can also limit accessibility to some healthcare services.

Other examples of system constraints discussed in previous chapters include policies on independent practice and scope of practice for licensed professionals such as nurse practitioners, physician assistants, or dental hygienists, among many others. Regulations in practice acts vary by state and they can change from one year to another since practice acts are the current focus of health policy making in many states. Information on current policies are available from the supporting associations, such the American Association of Nurse Practitioners, the American Dental Hygienists' Association, and the American Pharmacists Association, among others. When incorporating information on the practice of licensed medical providers in access estimates, these associations can provide the most up-to-date practice acts and specifications.

Examples of patient preferences impacting the extent of healthcare access include trade-off between travel distance and wait time; the choice of physicians versus licensed medical professionals in provision of primary care; the choice of a provider because of language or ethnical preference; the availability of a provider after hours; among many others.

The trade-off between travel distance and wait time can be subjective, depending on one's willingness to travel, the severity of the condition, the type of healthcare services sought, and the provider's ability to manage multiple services. In measuring access using the optimization modeling approach presented in previous chapters, the trade-off between travel distance and wait time is specified through a penalty that is the same across all providers and communities; it can be set using sensitivity analysis. The optimization approach allows for varying the trade-off by community specifications or provider characteristics; however, this would result in significantly higher computational efforts that can be overcome only by using distributed optimization (Palomar and Mung 2006; Nedic and Ozdaglar 2009; Boyd et al. 2011).

Many access constraints and preferences point to the interdependence between multiple access dimensions. For example, the choice of a provider allowing visits after hours or during the weekend is a form of the accommodation dimension. The choice of a provider because of language or ethnical preferences as well as participation of providers in different health insurance programs belong to the acceptability dimension. The trade-off between travel and wait time reflects the trade-off between availability and accessibility dimensions. Policies on independence practice impact both affordability and availability dimensions. Thus, as highlighted throughout this book, access is a multidimensional construct, going beyond its (mis)interpretation as a financial barrier in the existing political discourse on national healthcare policy. All access dimensions are fundamental in providing quality healthcare for all.

Inference on Disparities

Measuring disparities with respect to healthcare access involves data analytics in both approaches discussed in Chapter 3. A first approach is to group a study population in such a way the groups reflect sub-populations for which systematic health disparities are believed to be significant and unfair. For this approach, access measurements are derived for each sub-population, based on detailed data on supply, need/demand and access constraints or preferences. As discussed in the previous section, acquiring detailed access measurement data for each sub-population can be challenging; this is particularly a challenge for sub-populations vulnerable to health disparities since they may be under-represented in many data sources.

A second approach in assessing systematic health disparities discussed in Chapter 3 is using regression models to evaluate how access measurements vary with multiple potential contributors to disparities in health. This approach involves measurement of access for the entire sup-population but varying by geography, then modeling the relationship of the access measure to multiple factors, such as education level, median income, race/ethnicity, among others. Data on such factors can be acquired primarily from census data, for example, the ACS, complemented by other public data sources, for example, CDC, AHRQ, NIH, NCHS, among many other sources.

An important data analytics consideration in the latter approach is that not all factors may be observed on the same geographic granularity as the access measures; for example, if observed at higher geographic resolution (e.g. census tract), then the predicting factors need to be aggregated into the lower geographic resolution (e.g. county) with consideration of the challenges of combining incompatible spatial data, particularly the modifiable areal unit problem (Gotway and Young 2002).

Thus, while for the former approach, the main challenge is the availability of detailed data for access measurement for multiple sub-populations, for the second approach, the main challenge is the need for advanced modeling to estimate the relationship between access measures and multiple demographic and socioeconomic factors.

Health(care) Outcome Data

Health(care) outcome data cover many outcome types, many conditions, sub-populations and multiple aspects about health and healthcare as presented in Chapter 4. Data sources and analytics are specific to each of these outcome considerations.

Clinical outcomes, referring to clinical measures of organs' functionality, commonly tailored to a specific condition as introduced in Chapter 4, are commonly derived from EHRs and from clinical data registries. For most part, these data sources provide clinical information for a small subset of a population of interest, e.g. patients treated by the Rural Health Center, and/or within one care setting, e.g. home-based psychological services. Such data sources have limited applicability in healthcare access studies. There are however large managed care organizations, for example, Kaiser Permanente, VHA, and Children's Healthcare providers in many large cities (e.g. Atlanta, Cincinnati, Los Angeles), which have compiled EHRs for large samples of sub-populations (e.g. children, veterans) and across many healthcare settings. There are also national clinical data registries, for example, the Cystic Fibrosis Registry, covering the majority of the population with a specific condition. These data sources have relevance in studies of the relationship between access and outcomes because they are comprehensive in the information provided, particularly when the healthcare organizations join to create a larger network of health information exchange. One challenge however is accessing such data sources due to the safeguard requirements for PHI and due to the proprietary aspects associated with such patient-detailed information.

Wellbeing outcomes refer to health status measures, e.g. BMI, risk of a condition; individual-reported measures, e.g. level of pain; and population health measures, e.g. mortality, prevalence of a condition. Because these outcomes are mostly based on individual-reported information about one's health and wellbeing, they are primarily derived from survey data, or derived as measures based on clinical outcomes thus informed by EHRs or clinical registry data. In the overview of data sources provided earlier in this chapter, many survey data sources collected by public and private organizations were presented, which are commonly used in health services research, particularly in studies of health outcomes. EHRs can also be used in deriving wellbeing outcome measures, particularly if the measures are derivatives of clinical outcomes to portray health status, for example, clinical health risk. However, due to the challenge of accessing EHRs from large managed care organization, (public) survey data are the most common data sources in deriving wellbeing outcomes.

Healthcare outcomes refer to utilization of healthcare services, such as emergency department visits, physician office visits, and medication adherence. There are many disperse sources of data that can be used to derive healthcare outcomes. However, few data sources are available at a granular geographic level. Examples of such data sets commonly available at the county level in the United States are as follows:

- The HCUP, available from the AHRQ, is the largest longitudinal hospital care data in the United States. It is a set of annual databases with encounter-level data including both clinical and non-clinical information for each patient record. Different databases contain annual records by state, outcome type, and age category. The HCUP data are made available directly from AHRQ HCUP for most states. However, for some states, the data could only be acquired directly from the states under (restrictive) data acquisition conditions.

- MEPS, available from the AHRQ, is a national survey collecting data from individuals, employers, and medical providers (Centers for Disease Control and Prevention n.d.-a). It provides information about healthcare use, health insurance use, and costs. MEPS data are available for public use, with different data files available each year. The MEPS website makes available publications, reports, charts, and data tables.

- The largest health information system of administrative claims files has been supported and maintained by CMS, consisting of person-level data on eligibility, service utilization, and payments. The data come in three formats that also define the level of access: non-identifiable data set files, LDS files, and identifiable data set files. Non-identifiable data set files contain non-identifiable person-specific information and are within the public domain; examples include, among others, the Prescription Drug Plan Formulary and Pharmacy Network File containing formulary and pharmacy network data for Medicare Prescription Drug Plans and Medicare Advantage Prescription Drug; and the Hospital Service Area File containing number of discharges, length of stay, and total charges summarized by provider number and zip code of the Medicare beneficiary. LDS files are available for the Medicare Current Beneficiary Survey (MCBS), the Health Outcomes Survey (HOS), and for the Standard Analytical Files among other files that contain various levels of data on the Medicare beneficiaries. The HOS LDSs consist of the national sample for a two-year cohort and specify Medicare health plan identifiers, as well as several additional variables describing plan characteristics. The MCBS is a survey of a representative national sample of the Medicare population where the objective is to evaluate expenditures, sources of payment, and all types of health insurance coverage for Medicare beneficiaries and to assess processes longitudinally for identifying changes in the Medicare healthcare system. Identifiable data files are different from LDS files in that they contain actual beneficiary-specific and physician-specific information. They are available for the MAX data, a set of person-level data files on Medicaid eligibility, service utilization, and payments. MAX files are not available in LDS format. Because identifiable files contain beneficiary-specific information, which could be used to identify the individuals in the data, they are subject to very stringent access rules.

- The Dartmouth Institute has derived multiple healthcare outcomes for the Medicare population using the Medicare claims data acquired from CMS under the program called the Dartmouth Atlas Data. Within this program, healthcare outcomes for the Medicare-insured population are available in aggregate at the state level as well as at varying geographic granularity. This data science program is an important shift in the approach to data sharing, particularly, in the context when many healthcare data sources are challenging to acquire, with the data translation process requiring additional extensive computing resources.

- Many states also maintain their own data systems, which provide county-level data on hospital discharges, emergency department encounters, and other healthcare outcomes; these local data sources can complement the HCUP database for states where the HCUP data are not directly available from AHRQ. An example is the OASIS data for Georgia (Georgia Department of Public health n.d.) – for this state, HCUP data can only be acquired from the Georgia Hospital Association under a series of data acquisition constraints.

System outcomes refer to overall outcomes at the system or society level, measuring, for example, performance of the system, disparities in wellbeing or healthcare outcomes; or risk of chronic conditions by race, income; but also referring to organizational and provider outcomes such as emergency department volume. All data sources described above provide valuable information in developing and analyzing system outcomes because such outcomes are derivatives of other outcome types and/or they involve data derived at the organization or ecosystem levels. For example, population risk of chronic conditions for sub-populations requires first establishing a risk measure of chronic disease derived from clinical registry data or EHRs, then informed with data on disease progression and management. Performance of healthcare delivery can be measured in terms of cost, benefits, effectiveness, and impact on improving access and other outcomes. To measure performance, data on specifications of a healthcare setting, for example, telemedicine, are accompanied with data on healthcare utilization and expenditure and on the disease progression and management if the healthcare setting targets a specific condition. Thus, system outcomes are used to synthesize data on clinical, wellbeing and healthcare outcomes, data on diseases and conditions, and data on specifications of the healthcare system.

Designing and Evaluating Interventions

In Chapter 5, I expanded on a wide range of potential healthcare interventions, including health policies, network interventions, community-based healthcare and e-healthcare. Generally, designing and evaluating interventions starts with assessing the status quo, requiring measurement of healthcare access, quantification of health disparities, and assessment of the relationship between health outcomes and healthcare access. Thus, all data ingredients discussed so far are needed for informed and targeted interventions.

Addressing healthcare access through interventions is a more complex endeavor, going beyond the assessment of the existing gaps in access. Depending on the type of interventions, various sources of information may be considered.

Health Policies Because legislation is at the basis of most health policies, knowledge about the existing local and national laws, guidelines, and recommendations is key to decision making. The potential impact of health policies is also in the details; for example, there is a wide variation in the specifications of independent practice policies for dental hygienists across the states in the United States, ranging from being able to have their own practice in Colorado to requiring supervision from a dentist in many settings including schools in North Carolina.

Translating policy specifications requires knowledge about the healthcare settings in which they apply along with data on outcomes derived with and without the specifications. To illustrate, specifications of supervision of a dental hygienist when providing preventive dental care to children in school can impact the intervention cost of school sealant programs as demonstrated in the case study in Chapter 5, with further details in one of my collaborative research papers (Johnson et al. 2017). One approach to translating policy specifications is to identify similar settings where similar policy specifications have been implemented; data on real-practice policy impact can be used to understand "what works and for who" using simulation in a "policy lab" setting. However, such information and data are not readily available.

Network Interventions Network interventions include opening new facilities or expanding the caseload at some of the existing facilities given an expandable budget. For the healthcare system, facilities can be clinics, provider groups, individual practices, public health department centers, or school centers but also telemedicine sites. Important data analytics efforts in network interventions are toward selection of locations, implementation, and evaluation with other services. While implementation is a major effort in network interventions, I will primarily focus on the other two efforts because they are directly related to healthcare access.

Selection of sites for implementation and/or integration of healthcare services falls under the more general approach of facility location. In facility location, a first step is assessment of the status quo of healthcare delivery, specifically, the gaps in healthcare access. Thus data on the existing network of providers as well as on the need/demand for healthcare as discussed in the previous section are of great relevance. Furthermore, the methodologies discussed in Chapter 5 can be used to identify sub-populations and/or healthcare services to be targeted for intervention. A second step in selection of optimal location-allocation of resources is identifying best opportunities (e.g. site location, additional services to be provided at a specific location) to improve access based on the information about resources for each potential opportunity and the benefits of an intervention.

Quantifying the benefits and resources or costs of an intervention is at the core of an economic analysis. As discussed in Chapter 5, there are three specific types of costs: *direct* costs, *indirect* costs, and *intangible*. Data on the three cost types come from different sources. The direct costs can be obtained from similar programs that have already been implemented, if any, or estimated by considering the main ingredients for the delivery, such as cost of healthcare utilization and for the implementation, e.g. cost for staffing a program, technology, rents, and transportation, among others.

Cost of healthcare delivery can be derived from claims data in the form of healthcare expenditure for the delivered services. One challenge with using these data is that the actual cost for healthcare delivery is neither the amount charged nor the payment reimbursed as commonly recorded in claims data since it depends on the insurance program (e.g. Medicaid generally has low reimbursement rates) and the type and place of service (e.g. emergency vs primary care). They also do not account for the cost to the patient. Making adjustments to obtain cost of care rather than expenditure for care requires additional data analytics considerations, commonly not considered in many health economic evaluations.

Generally, data on direct implementation cost is publicly available from many sources, based on surveys on labor or staffing needs (e.g. United States Labor Bureau, NAMCS, MEPS), and costs of technology acquired from the technology providers. To acquire such information, one must first distinguish among different important implementations, the cost of a new facility or the cost of expansion of an existing practice, then search for data on each programmatic component; there is not one source of data specifying such information unless other researchers have performed similar research.

Data on indirect and tangible costs are much harder to obtain, particularly, since they reflect subjective views on personal losses and suffering. One of the most common indirect costs counted in economic evaluations is loss of productivity, with several existing approaches to quantifying it (Gandjour 2014). Intangible costs are however not commonly included in the overall cost evaluation since they quantify personal experiences.

Benefits of the outcomes of interest can be quantifiable as savings to the system due to an intervention using administrative claims data. For example, if a specific service is used for prevention, for example, dental preventive care for young children, a comparison of healthcare expenditure for the cohorts with and without the service provision can provide an estimate of the cost savings due to the utilization of such services as shown in a case study in Chapter 5. However this approach requires access to individual-level claims data, commonly not available due to the challenges of acquiring PHI. Alternatively, costs of care with and without intervention can be estimated from data provided by the existing literature.

In cost-effectiveness evaluation studies, the focus is not on a cost reduction due to an intervention but the effectiveness of an intervention to improve quality of life. In such studies, the quality-adjusted life years (QALYs) are often used as the outcome measure of effectiveness. The QALY takes into account two factors: the quality (of life; "Q") and the quantity (life years gained; "LY") due to healthcare interventions. In the QALY, the length of time spent in a certain health state is weighed by a utility score given to that health state. For instance, one year of perfect health is worth one QALY, a year of less than perfect health could be worth less than one QALY, and death is considered to be equivalent to zero QALYs (Phillips and Thompson 2009). It is not uncommon to approximate the QALYs based on patient-reported survey data, for example, using the EuroQol-5D (EQ-5D), the Short-Form Health Survey-6D (SF-6D), extracted from the 36-item Short-Form Health Survey (SF-36), and the 12-item Short-Form Health Survey (SF-12) (EuroQol Group EuroQol 1990; Brazier and Roberts 2004). The quality weights derived from such surveys are multiplied with the duration of each health state experienced by the patients under a given health state. For example, four years in a 0.5 quality state is two QALYs.

Community-Based Healthcare: In-home and In-school Healthcare Community-based healthcare, specifically, in-home and in-school healthcare, have recently had extensive support from both national and local decision makers. The growing support comes from a better understanding of the impact of such healthcare approaches on the trade-off between the 3 E's, efficiency, effectiveness, and equity (Britto et al. 2001; Kwong et al. 2010; Landers 2010; Brindis 2016; Knopf et al. 2016; Ran et al. 2016). Because this area of healthcare intervention has been investigated locally and because large organizations only recently have begun to build on medical records reflecting the use of in-home and in-school approaches to healthcare delivery, access to comprehensive data for such programs is currently limited.

CMS has launched many surveys on the patients' experience with home healthcare programs for the Medicare-insured population, the most comprehensive one being the Home Health CAHPS, covering topics such as communication about care, pain, and prescription medication use, the care received from the home health agency, staying informed about scheduling, and global ratings. CMS also makes available the Home Health Compare data sets, comparing the quality of care provided by Medicare-certified home health agencies throughout the nation, a list of all agencies providing home health for the Medicare population, and many other data sets related to home health for elderly population (Centers for Medicare & Medicaid Services 2019).

There are no similar surveys for other populations because home healthcare has had most expansion for the older adult population. For children, surveys primarily cover in-school healthcare. The School Health Profiles is a system of surveys assessing school health policies and practices (Centers for Disease Control and Prevention n.d.-b). The surveys are conducted biennially by education and health agencies among middle and high school principals and lead health education teachers. The School-Based Health Alliance (SBHA) has performed a national census covering more than 80% of school healthcare (2013). SBHA can make available data based on this census subject to some data sharing policies; for example, the list of school-based health center (SBHCs) is not made available. This restricts access to data needed for healthcare access studies since location of SBHCs is necessary in such studies.

Other sources of data related to in-home and in-school healthcare are EHRs and administrative claims. For example, in the MAX claims, two data fields, type of service and place of service, can be used to identify claims submitted for in-home and in-school delivery of care. However, the healthcare providers only recently have begun to accurately specify the care provided within such programs in the MAX files because of recent changes in the specification of procedure codes or in reimbursement fees. In contrast, EHRs are generally more accurate in the specification of care provided at home or in school, however they are generally available from smaller providers and/or over shorter periods of time, thus with limited applicability in the analysis of effectiveness of such programs.

HEALTHCARE DATA ANALYTICS

Overall Challenges

In previous sections of this chapter, the complexity in data sources needed for various aspects related to healthcare access has been underlined, such as measurement, disparities, and interventions, particularly in the context when health(care) data are scattered and fragmented, available from various sources, including governmental or nongovernmental health organizations, commercial or noncommercial sources, and nationwide or statewide sources. Data also come in different structures and forms while lacking integration with outside sources and being distributed among a wide range of different providers and stakeholders including physicians, nurses, payers, patient advocates, and policy makers. These challenges can be addressed using advanced data science for data interoperability, integration, translation and processing within a complex IT system.

An important aspect to the complexity of the IT system is that access to many data sources discussed in this chapter requires prior safeguards to physically store, access, share, transmit, and distribute data along with specifications related to data reporting and publication. For example, claims and patient-detailed data often are needed in the identifiable or limited format, called PHI, requiring Health Insurance Portability and Accountability Act (HIPAA) protection.

To acquire PHI data, several steps need to be followed, such as submitting a study protocol for approval to the institution in charge with the data provision and to the institutional review board (IRB). The study protocol may include but not be limited to a proposal describing the research that will be carried out with the requested data; a data management plan laying out the terms under which data will be safeguarded; and a data use agreement between the organization providing the data and that acquiring the data, among others. Depending on the extent of the research, whether the data are identifiable or limited, and the risks for a potential breach of the data safeguards, the completion of the data acquisition process and fully implementing the data safeguards specified in the data management plan could be very involved. This challenge can be addressed by developing an adaptive IT system. The IT system needs to be adaptive to changes in the data structures, size, and access restrictions.

In the case studies presented in the previous chapters, I presented how each specific healthcare problem requires data collected from multiple sources, some of small size while others derived from massive data sets, and recorded with different levels of accuracy, at various temporal levels (event-level, monthly, or yearly), and at various aggregation spatial levels (individual, census tract, zip code, county, state, or national). Data analytics thus involves advanced modeling to process data acquired at multiple scales, to translate data into meaningful information, to combine incompatible spatial data (Gotway and Young 2002), to visualize complex data, and to develop computational and inferential approaches to deal with massive data sets (National Research Council 2013).

Many of the models introduced in these studies rely on specifications of a series of structural parameters representing model assumptions and approximations. They are often drawn from a wide range of published documents or simply input using expert knowledge. This is common practice because of the lack of relevant data necessary in assessing patients' behavior, flow of processes, or interconnectivity between organizations. Therefore, despite the abundance of data in the field of public health and healthcare, it is often very difficult to obtain relevant and quality health data. Reliance on such model assumptions and approximations is only noted as a limitation in most health services research and public health studies although it can have great implications in decision making.

Quantifying how sensitive the decisions are to assumptions and approximations is paramount because they can inform whether a decision is to be made or whether further data should be acquired for reducing the uncertainty in decision making. Advanced simulation modeling approaches can be used; however they require rigorous considerations of the computational effort. In my recent research, I have considered how theoretical results can be used to improve the computation of a large number of optimization models such as those used in measuring access when the models vary in input parameters and input data (Lee et al. 2018). While the development of such advanced computational methodology is generally difficult to motivate in public health studies due to limited resources and advanced modeling knowledge, it is important to acknowledge it as an overarching objective in future development of decision tools for decision makers.

Such data science, IT and modeling advancements are generally challenging to employ because they require multidisciplinary knowledge and skills, and computational resources along with an understanding of public health and healthcare delivery. However, it is my hope that this book will raise awareness on these challenges as well as provide knowledge which researchers can use to promote their research toward making reliable and accurate decisions. Making a decision is more meaningful when there is broad knowledge and an overall appreciation of the challenges behind the machinery of the decision making tool and the overall efforts required.

Data Science: Acquisition, Processing, and Translation

Data alone have limited use unless access to data in all its forms is in real time or at least within a meaningful time frame. Access to data commonly available from different non-homogeneous sources is the first step in the analysis to be undertaken to translate them into information for input to modeling efforts. But access takes multiple forms: availability of data (i.e. data may not be electronically stored but stored on paper in filing cabinets, or access may be limited due to privacy and patient confidentiality constraints), affordability of data (i.e. some organizations rely on expensive processes to derive, store, and extract data resulting in large costs for end users), and accessibility of data (i.e. knowing where data are available and from what source, or lack of interoperability between data sources). All three forms of data access – availability, affordability, and accessibility – require orchestrated efforts in the *data acquisition* process.

Acquisition of appropriate data is a necessary step in healthcare access studies; it requires not only broad knowledge about the data landscape as extensively presented in this chapter but also an understanding on important characteristics of the data, for example, if derived from randomized or observational studies, whether representing a sample or the entire study population, whether requiring PHI data safeguards, and whether available at the individual level or in aggregate. Thus the data acquisition process involves rigorous considerations, with implications in the later steps in data analytics, including data translation, data modeling, and informed decision making.

The translational process, data translated into knowledge, involves the processing, analysis and integration of data from many sources of information. Simmons and Davis (1993) distinguish between *actual knowledge* and *representation of knowledge*. Actual knowledge describes the attributes of a concept (e.g. the diabetes diagnosis) where its representation consists of the symbols and language used to encode the knowledge in the information system (e.g. the ICD-9 code of a diagnosis). It is common for healthcare data sets to be accompanied by hundreds of pages of data dictionary, describing complex data representations. Along with the data dictionary, the data sets are also commonly linked with lists of codes (e.g. National Drug Codes [NDCs], ICD-10 Diagnosis Codes, Provider Taxonomy Codes, Zip Codes) to map representations of the information available in healthcare data sets into actual knowledge about a healthcare event, a clinical decision, or a self-reported health status, among others. This translational process is paramount in deriving meaningful data that can be used in data modeling and informed decision making.

Data Analytics: Modeling and Inference

Data analytics in healthcare is an enormous opportunity but it is not without a price to be paid. Tien and Goldschmidt-Clermont (2009) call it the "data rich, information poor conundrum." As more data are observed and recorded, the number of possible questions to be addressed, and the combinations of information bits increase exponentially. The priorities now shift from simply getting and managing data to making it understandable.

Making data understandable involves data translation and data modeling, both being closely interrelated. Data translation needs to be tailored to the data modeling and the decision making. While the scope of modeling methods for addressing healthcare challenges is broad, here I will only share considerations and challenges in data modeling for improving healthcare, as experienced in my research programs to date.

Data Science Efforts   Data modeling in "old times" (20 or so years ago!) was generally disconnected from data science efforts. There were clear boundaries between skills and areas of research; training was generally a deep dive into one area without a broad understanding of the bridge between disciplines. With the advent of the World

Wide Web, ready access to knowledge, open access to many data sources, and increasing opportunities for collaboration, research in healthcare has seen a leap in collaborative research. Synthesizing and cross-pollinating data acquisition, data translation, data modeling and decision making is now a common approach to research in data analytics. Thus, data modeling cannot be removed from the overall end point of a research program, instead it needs to be integrated with all other components. John Tuckey, one of the most established statisticians to date, said "Embrace your data, not your models."

Massive Data   Along with the increase in the abundance of data, the caseload to analyze the data grows faster than our ability to understand it. Data analysis techniques also change with availability of massive data sets (National Research Council 2013). Traditional statistical methods were developed to handle data shortage. Confidence intervals, p-values, and the notion of statistical significance were adopted to answer specific questions about large populations based on small samples. These concerns are becoming less relevant, and modern data analysis is instead designed to find answers to questions we never thought to ask (Kairos Future 2011).

Methodological Rigor   A popular quote among statisticians by George Box is "All models are wrong, but some are useful." There are several important considerations in making a model "useful." First, it needs to have statistical power to identify statistically significant heterogeneous effects, meaning that a large enough sample size is needed to satisfy a minimum level of statistical power. Most importantly in large and complex data sets, the model needs to capture the data dependencies rigorously. The common assumption of independence in many quantitative analyses is a rough simplification of reality. Healthcare data can vary in time, geography, and between groups of people, and are observed at multi levels of scales and aggregations. Health outcomes, costs, and access have different spatial patterns depending on whether one state is compared with another, or whether one neighborhood is compared with another; they evolve in time with various trends, and they display disparities across population groups. Moreover, the associations between variables are highly nonlinear, and co-variations are highly dynamic. One of the limitations of not rigorously accounting for relationships, dependence, and dynamics in the data is that statistical inference leads to misleading results.

Methodological rigor goes beyond goodness of fit and statistical power of modeling approaches however. It is also important in identifying system constraints and patient preferences in measuring access; distinguishing between confounding and explanatory factors in modeling relationships with outcome measures; establishing the type of economic evaluation appropriate for the study at hand; understanding the limitations of the data, modeling approaches and their implications in the interpretation of the findings; and quantifying the variations in the estimates of measures and relationships due to data uncertainty, among many others.

Computing Resources and Efforts   The considerations discussed above, such as data science efforts, dealing with massive data and methodological rigor, require extensive computational efforts. An important aspect acknowledged in the discourse about "big data" is the need for computational capabilities and resources that are required in the process of transforming information into knowledge. This is particularly important in the word of healthcare, where the patient information is protected by HIPAA and other regulatory policies. Many existing platforms for data storage, indexing, and processing (e.g. Hadoop) may not apply in a data environment requiring high levels of data safeguards.

In such an environment, process decisions need to be made for physical and computing resources, database backbone and knowledge sharing process to facilitate smooth access to information while containing the PHI safeguards. Moreover, developing tools and procedures on process mining are needed to translate and analyze data, with the goal of managing and making discoveries from the data aggregations. Thus, the IT system needs to accommodate not only storage and wrangling of massive, heterogeneous data sets, but also to accommodate queries, data translation, and data analytics using rigorous modeling. However, without the investment in IT and computing systems required by large-scale data science and analytics programs, knowledge about the healthcare system is limited, without the ability to draw inferences on healthcare interventions locally and nationally.

Deriving Knowledge While data translation and modeling are essential to informed decision making, without appropriate tools, interpretation, and dissemination, they are simply data analytics exercises. Interpretation of the knowledge derived from data translation and modeling is challenging because it requires various forms of data representation, including visual and interactive displays, summaries, tabulations, aggregations, but ultimately interventions and policies. Deriving knowledge from data analytics, particularly, in decision making for healthcare access, requires a broad knowledge about the public health system and how policies and interventions are implemented and enacted. Integrating data science, data analytics and public health is however challenging. Which intervention to target and how to target? Can change be driven by data-supported findings? What are the barriers to change? Are decision makers willing to change course given the availability of data-driven results? How to interpret and present to decision makers? Such questions go beyond academic initiatives of developing research programs and pursuing publication of the research results. They concern translation and dissemination of research to make the case for change in healthcare as illustrated in the case studies in Chapter 5.

Dissemination: Data Portals

Large data require well-endowed IT systems that offer the needed security, space, access, and readiness in working with the data. Because of the sophisticated infrastructure involved in the process of data acquisition, storage, use, and access in large studies, only few institutions can leverage their resources to research such data, giving them a competitive advantage in research and/or education while creating a space of "exclusivity" in healthcare research. One way to overcome this "exclusivity" in healthcare research is to create a community of data sharing, where data initiatives and systems, such as CDC, AHRQ, NIH, the state data reporting systems, the Dartmouth Atlas Data, the Kaiser Family Foundation, among many other, disseminate data broadly. "Data is the new resource, and unlike money or oil sharing doesn't deplete it" (Kairos Future 2011).

Sharing the data is a necessary step toward overcoming this "exclusivity" in healthcare research, however it is not sufficient. Because of the data fragmentation across so many sources and initiatives, it is difficult to identify appropriate sources of data to inform models, interventions, and decisions. One approach to addressing the data fragmentation is to develop open data portals, which can synthesize data from multiple sources, particularly those not accessible to the public at large. Several ingredients are desirable when developing data portals:

- The interface of the portal needs to be user friendly, with fast data query and retrieval, and an easy-to-navigate data menu, possibly accompanied with a README file providing navigation directions along with a list of all data elements available and how they can be accessed.

- The right amount of data needs to be made available through the portal while being comprehensive in covering many data elements within a specific public health initiative, including data from multiple sources, measures derived from existing methodologies, and different types of outcomes.

- The data portal needs to be self-informative, with acknowledgement of the data sources and explicit description of the data, possibly including a data dictionary which can provide information about how various data elements were derived along with references to supporting research and/or sources providing details on the approaches used to derive the data.

- Data sharing can be complemented by visual analytics to help the user perform exploration of the data within the portal without the need of an external visual tool, particularly when the portal is intended for users without data analytics skills.

Implementation of data portals with these ingredients is challenging because they require knowledge and skills in many areas, including web application development, visual analytics, data analytics, and public health. They also require yearly updates and maintenance since most outcome measures change from one year to the next. Last, they need to have a "home" where they can be disseminated and accessed over the course of many years.

In the case studies introduced in this chapter, I will illustrate two data portals derived from my collaborative research, developed to support such data sharing initiatives.

CASE STUDIES: DATA ANALYTICS AND DISSEMINATION

Supply for Mental and Behavioral Healthcare Services

Low-income children tend to experience mental health conditions at higher rates than the general population. Most of these children qualify for public insurance including Medicaid or their State CHIP, being the largest insurer of children (American Academy of Pediatrics 2017) and the single largest payer of mental health services (Centers for Medicare & Medicaid Services 2017b). Studies have documented that many Medicaid-insured children with mental health and behavioral disorders do not receive any psychotherapy (Harris et al. 2012; Cummings et al. 2017). Several studies have found that lack of healthcare access is one of the major barriers to psychotherapy services for this population, due, in part, to low provider participation in the Medicaid program (Bisgaier and Rhodes 2011; Stein ct al. 2013).

In a collaborative research project with a PhD candidate, Pravara Harati, and Dr. Janet Cummings, we estimated the supply of mental health providers for the Medicaid enrollees and the number of psychotherapy visits provided using the 2012 MAX claims files and the 2013 NPPES database. In this section, I will emphasis the approach and the challenges in linking these two data sets to identify the healthcare supply, an illustration of a data translation approach. Results and findings of this research are presented elsewhere (Harati et al., submitted).

When working with the NPPES data, a first step is to identify the taxonomy of providers for a specific healthcare service, for example, mental and behavioral healthcare in this study. Behavioral and mental healthcare providers as provided by HRSA include: Advanced Practice Psychiatric Nurses, Licensed Professional Counselors, Marriage and Family Therapists, Psychiatrists, Psychologists, and Social Workers. These are professionals likely to provide psychotherapy to children. The NPPES taxonomies for these providers are shown in Table 6.2.

Using these taxonomies, the NPPES database is queried to extract all providers with primary taxonomy as provided in the list. Once these providers are identified along with information on their taxonomy, information about their practice address and entity as described earlier in this chapter is also captured. Overall, we identified 344 856 individual providers, small practices, or mental health centers within the 2013 NPPES database nationwide.

However, the NPPES database does not provide information on which providers participate in Medicaid. For this, we need to link this database with the MAX claims data. We thus derive this information from the 2012 MAX data, available for all states in the United States. More specifically, we used information from the MAX Personal Summary file, which contains demographic data for all Medicaid beneficiaries, and the MAX OT file, which contains all claims for services received by Medicaid beneficiaries outside of inpatient hospitals, long-term care facilities, and pharmacies. Each MAX OT claim includes a patient identification number, ICD-9 diagnosis codes, Current Procedural Terminology (CPT) codes, and codes to identify the billing provider who submitted the claim for payment and the service provider who treated the patient.

TABLE 6.2 List of Taxonomies that Identify Mental and Behavioral Healthcare Providers in the NPPES Database

Category	Taxonomy	Name
Advance Practice Psychiatric Nurses	163WP0808X	Psychiatric/Mental Health
	163WP0807X	Psychiatric/Mental Health, Child & Adolescent
Licensed Professional Counselors	101YP2500X	Professional Counselor
	101YM0800X	Mental Health Counselor
Marriage and Family Therapists	106H00000X	Marriage & Family Therapist
Psychiatrists	2084P0800X	Psychiatry
	2084P0804X	Child & Adolescent Psychiatry
Psychologists	103T00000X	Psychologist
	103TC0700X	Clinical Psychologist
	103TC1900X	Counseling Psychologist
	103TC2200X	Clinical Child & Adolescent Psychologist
Social Workers	1041C0700X	Clinical Social Worker
Additional taxonomies found to provide behavior therapy in Medicaid data	251S00000X	Community/Behavioral Health Agency
	261QM0801X	Mental Health Clinic/Center (including Community Mental Health Center)
	261QM0855X	Adolescent and Children Mental Health Clinic/Center
	251300000X	Local Education Agency

To capture providers who delivered psychotherapy, it is more appropriate to use the CPT code rather than the patient's diagnosis. The diagnosis is not an indication of a psychotherapeutic visit; it could also involve an assessment only or prescription of medication. The CPT codes were primarily identified in prior research (Visser et al. 2016) and sub-sampled to focus on psychotherapy only.

The MAX OT file contains two separate identifiers for the billing provider (the NPI number as well as a unique Medicaid ID number) and one identifier for the service provider (a unique Medicaid ID number). Thus, the only NPI information for the Medicaid providers in the MAX files is in the billing provider. However, the Medicaid beneficiary receives services from the provider listed in the "service provider" field, which can differ from the "billing provider." For example, individual providers may work in one location, but bill under a parent organization NPI. To address this challenge, we developed an algorithm to match an NPI to the service provider field using information from the billing provider fields. This algorithm is described below and summarized in Figure 6.3.

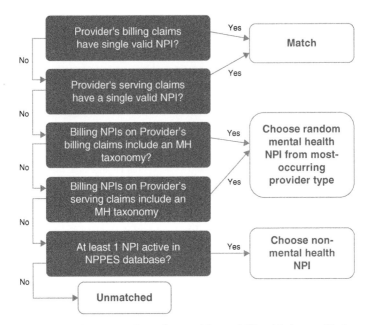

FIGURE 6.3 Procedure to match service providers to NPIs with the specified taxonomy.

For a given service provider (State, SID), we found a matching NPI. Because the Billing NPI in the MAX OT file should correspond to billing providers, we prioritized claims where the service provider of interest acted as a billing provider. If there are multiple potential matches, we additionally prioritized NPI specializing in mental health. This process is detailed in the steps below:

Step 1. Select all claims in the MAX OT file where State Abbreviation Code is the same as the State and Billing Provider Identification Number. If at least one claim was selected, all selected claims have the same Billing NPI, and that Billing NPI is found in the NPPES database, match the service provider to that NPI. If not, continue to step 2.

Step 2. Select all claims in the MAX OT file where State Abbreviation Code is the same as the State and Servicing Provider Identification Number. If all selected claims have the same Billing NPI and that Billing NPI is found in the NPPES database, match the service provider to that NPI. If not, continue to step 3.

Step 3. Again consider the claims selected in step 1. Using the NPPES database, identify the primary taxonomies of all Billing NPI among the selected claims. Consider only the Billing NPI with primary taxonomies. If none exists, continue to step 5. Otherwise, continue to step 4.

Step 4. Categorize each of the mental health Billing NPI into one of four mutually exclusive groups using their primary taxonomy and entity code found in the NPPES database. These groups are centers and Entity 2 providers,

Entity 1 nurses, Entity 1 psychiatrists, and Entity 1 therapists. From the group containing the Billing NPI (or the union of all the groups with the highest number of Billing NPI if there is a tie), randomly select one of the Billing NPI. Match the service provider to this NPI.

Step 5. Repeat steps 3–4 using the claims selected in step 2. If a match still did not occur, continue to step 6.

Step 6. Using the claims selected in both steps 1 and 2, check if any of the Billing NPI are listed in the NPPES database. If so, match the service provider to a randomly selected Billing NPI. If not, declare the service provider unmatched.

If a service provider was matched in steps 1 or 2, we say they are matched to a single NPI. If they were matched in steps 3–6, we say they have multiple potential matches. The state-level results from this algorithm are provided in Table 6.3. According to this analysis, only 27 states and Washington, DC had a matching of at least 75% of the service providers.

States with lower matching than 75% either had a large number of service providers each with multiple potential NPI (e.g. Indiana, Nebraska, and Wyoming) or had a large number of billing NPI not listed in the NPPES database and therefore service providers could not be matched to any NPI (e.g. Iowa, New Hampshire, and Utah). I will highlight here that the low rates of matching for some states are also due to the fact that mental and behavioral health services for public insurance may be delivered under carved-out managed care, a Medicaid financing model where some portion of the healthcare benefits are separately managed and/or financed by another organization or retained by the state Medicaid agency on a FFS basis (Mandros 2014). When the behavioral health benefits are carved out of the overall public healthcare system, the claims for such services may be underreported, thus the information on the behavioral health providers may also be underreported. However, there are also states that have underreported NPI information for providers billing for Medicaid services overall services.

Informing Medicaid participation of mental and behavioral health providers using the MAX claims data and the NPPES databases comes with many challenges and limitations. One challenge is the derivation of the NPIs and the associated taxonomies of providers identified in the MAX data as provided by the matching algorithm above. The matching algorithm makes some assumptions related to the billing versus practice addresses of providers, which may not hold in all cases. There are also some limitations in matching entity 1 (individual) and entity 2 (organization) providers. Specifically, some providers who work for an organization may still bill as individuals, thus being double counted. Finally, we must emphasize that we are only examining the caseload of psychotherapeutic/psychosocial services. Some providers bill solely through their organization NPI. The matching algorithm would link these providers only to the organization NPI, preventing from correctly identifying what type of practitioner (e.g. psychiatrist, psychologist, or primary care physician) is actually providing the service. These challenges and limitations must be well understood, particularly, with respect to their implications in obtaining access estimates for mental and behavioral health.

TABLE 6.3 Matching Results between the NPPES Database and the MAX Files by State

	All ages						Children					
	Service	% Single match		% Random match			Service	% Single match		% Random match		
State	providers	Overall	MH	Overall	MH	% Unmatched	providers	Overall	MH	Overall	MH	% Unmatched
AL	801	95.6	53.4	3.9	2.4	0.5	511	96.1	46.2	3.5	2.0	0.4
AK	297	60.3	27.6	28.3	21.2	11.4	184	53.8	23.9	32.6	25.5	13.6
AZ	1208	93.0	69.6	3.2	2.1	3.8	670	96.3	75.4	2.4	1.8	1.3
AR	2768	16.0	6.3	50.7	48.2	33.3	2404	13.4	3.8	52.1	49.9	34.5
CA	4002	50.1	39.4	24.9	11.2	25.0	2288	63.3	51.0	16.2	7.7	20.5
CT	2088	95.1	72.7	3.8	3.1	1.1	1531	95.9	77.9	3.7	3.3	0.4
DE	813	58.4	44.6	40.7	29.5	0.9	492	56.9	46.5	42.7	37.0	0.4
DC	219	90.0	41.6	6.8	3.7	3.2	112	87.5	40.2	6.3	4.5	6.3
FL	4811	89.9	58.9	1.6	1.2	8.5	3323	91.2	60.0	1.5	1.1	7.3
GA	3266	97.3	71.2	0.2	0.1	2.4	2771	97.3	70.1	0.2	0.1	2.5
HI	141	94.3	45.4	3.5	0.0	2.1	45	93.3	20.0	6.7	0.0	0.0
IL	3560	83.1	36.9	5.4	1.6	11.5	2353	89.3	28.3	6.2	2.0	4.5
IN	1479	8.0	4.3	77.9	48.7	14.1	1138	6.3	2.5	77.2	49.4	16.5
IA	2435	30.5	10.8	3.2	0.4	66.3	1700	20.8	2.4	3.4	0.2	75.8
KY	883	88.8	43.6	1.5	0.6	9.7	452	80.5	36.3	2.0	0.9	17.5
LA	904	69.4	51.7	30.3	22.7	0.3	670	67.8	52.4	31.8	24.9	0.4
ME	233	76.4	34.3	23.2	22.3	0.4	94	43.6	35.1	56.4	55.3	0.0
MD	2214	78.1	67.5	20.0	12.8	1.9	1409	83.3	72.5	15.6	12.1	1.1
MA	13 634	78.9	58.4	8.5	5.3	12.7	5660	75.8	54.5	10.6	6.2	13.6
MI	5894	30.6	17.6	15.1	8.6	54.3	4063	29.4	17.8	14.1	7.9	56.6
MN	2721	86.5	35.6	8.3	6.6	5.2	1028	81.7	46.1	14.5	12.5	3.8
MS	595	98.8	60.7	0.3	0.2	0.8	346	98.6	67.1	0.6	0.3	0.9
MO	4898	32.8	22.8	11.0	7.6	56.2	3995	34.2	23.7	11.0	7.6	54.9
MT	1250	97.9	58.1	0.4	0.2	1.7	1023	98.0	55.3	0.4	0.3	1.6

NE	3035	12.0	9.7	66.3	54.2	21.6	2059	13.0	11.2	67.6	59.1	19.4
NV	3649	99.5	29.9	0.0	0.0	0.5	3203	99.7	30.0	0.0	0.0	0.3
NH	1188	1.3	1.0	27.6	9.8	71.0	887	0.9	0.5	30.0	9.7	69.1
NJ	1051	76.8	58.8	21.6	13.5	1.6	503	66.0	53.1	30.8	21.3	3.2
NM	5648	94.8	63.6	4.6	3.3	0.6	3103	93.9	63.4	5.8	4.4	0.3
NY	15 548	74.4	52.0	19.2	14.3	6.4	6718	75.3	51.3	19.9	15.8	4.8
NC	5825	98.4	79.0	1.3	1.0	0.3	4341	98.4	80.5	1.2	1.0	0.4
ND	648	11.7	7.9	61.9	48.8	26.4	514	10.9	6.6	58.9	46.3	30.2
OH	4298	97.8	48.6	1.8	1.3	0.4	2515	98.0	44.4	1.6	1.2	0.4
OK	7769	99.5	71.1	0.2	0.1	0.3	6630	99.5	72.6	0.2	0.1	0.3
OR	1617	84.6	66.5	8.2	3.5	7.2	820	90.7	73.7	5.9	3.4	3.4
PA	1134	90.4	33.3	6.4	1.0	3.2	887	94.1	34.7	4.7	1.1	1.1
SC	1304	29.3	9.4	48.8	23.7	21.9	928	29.1	9.3	48.9	25.4	22.0
SD	402	71.1	57.0	28.1	23.6	0.7	311	66.9	53.1	32.2	27.3	1.0
TN	1987	88.4	66.0	11.2	2.2	0.4	1189	93.5	75.7	6.1	2.7	0.3
TX	6751	95.5	76.1	2.1	1.2	2.5	5350	95.4	76.7	2.0	1.2	2.6
UT	1782	30.1	20.0	3.7	3.0	66.2	1093	29.3	19.1	3.8	3.0	67.0
VT	1459	40.8	34.7	57.4	48.9	1.8	825	35.8	31.2	61.7	56.6	2.5
VA	3384	98.6	81.2	0.0	0.0	1.4	2538	99.1	82.2	0.0	0.0	0.9
WA	1305	98.3	67.1	1.6	1.2	0.1	922	98.9	66.3	1.0	0.7	0.1
WV	428	98.1	72.2	1.6	1.2	0.2	277	98.2	72.9	1.4	1.1	0.4
WI	4306	97.5	74.5	2.3	1.7	0.2	2893	98.0	78.4	1.9	1.5	0.1
WY	1003	32.5	20.0	66.9	48.0	0.6	719	26.6	19.5	72.7	53.1	0.7

Total service provider and the percent of service providers seeing patients of any age ("All ages") or seeing at least one child ("Children") for psychotherapy that were matched to a single NPI of any primary taxonomy ("Overall") and mental health primary taxonomy ("MH"), randomly matched to an NPI, or left unmatched.

The objective of this case study is to highlight an approach for linking information between two data sets commonly employed in evaluating healthcare supply but also to point to potential limitations. While many healthcare data sets are available, they may require extensive efforts toward data translation of the representations of knowledge into useful, actual data. They also may not be consistently reliable across states and sub-populations. All these aspects are important considerations in healthcare access studies.

Georgia Web Data Portal

Research in community health has emerged as economic and social equity advocates recognized that where people live influences their opportunities for economic development, access to quality health care, and political participation (Jackson and Kochtitzky 2002; Frumkin et al. 2004; Flournoy and Treuhaft 2005; Morland et al. 2006; Lee and Rubin 2007; Auchincloss et al. 2008; Blackwell and Treuhaft 2008). Community health is a broad concept, referring not only to health outcomes and healthcare opportunities of the people living within a geographic area but also to their wellbeing and economic opportunities. When designing interventions for improving community health, transformations need to be reflected in a multidimensional construct, including dimensions of access to healthcare and other fundamental services; wellness factors; socioeconomic environment factors; and social determinants of health, among others. Data and methodologies for such a multidimensional construct require access to multiple sources of data, IT for analyzing the data, and advanced knowledge for deriving meaningful measures.

For many communities, undertaking a data science initiative at the scale needed for building such a multidimensional construct can be prohibitive because of lack of access to data resources, lack of knowledge on appropriate measures, and/or lack of technical assistance. Moreover, it is not only important to measure the health of one specific community but to benchmark with other communities that can be similar or dissimilar with respect to the rurality level, demographics, policies, and socioeconomic environment. Benchmarking allows identification of both positive-deviance and negative-deviance communities (Rust et al. 2012).

To disseminate meaningful and integrated data to communities broadly, my research team in collaboration with the Healthcare Georgia Foundation has developed a comprehensive measurement approach for disseminating baseline measures of community health and for identifying measures that are most relevant to specific interventions or policies. We have implemented a web-based visual interactive application for accessing such baseline measures in Georgia; the web data portal is available at https://www.healthanalytics.gatech.edu/georgia-map-visualizations. Within this web data platform, interactive maps are freely available and online queries can be easily visualized to help decision makers better understand both the needs of their community and how to intervene.

Health interactive maps are a well-recognized and suitable tool in dissemination (Shneiderman et al. 2013). Their importance lies in the possibility of connecting the geographic characteristics of a community with health indicators of health services and/or outcomes, among others. Since it is crucial for policy makers and researchers to have the availability of analysis tools useful both for providing health information at different geographic levels and for understanding the available options for addressing disparities, the web platform can be a useful tool. It is a tool to integrate data from different sources, visualize measures, compare and evaluate needs of the population, and visualize the effects of possible interventions.

The end point of the web-based data portal is for communities in Georgia to have access to health(care) measures to inform interventions and policies that can improve the community health. Particularly, the measures can be selected from a drop down menu, differentiated into Healthcare Measures and Health Determinants. The layout of the web data portal is provided in Figure 6.4, which displays one particular example. In this example, the selection of the healthcare measure is the utilization of psychological services for Medicaid-insured children, measured as the percent of children receiving such services; and the health determinant is the percent of the population receiving food stamps and SNAP (Supplemental Nutrition Assistance Program). The selection of the two measures is shown in the drop down menu on the left, displaying many possible options, where the measures could be provided at the county or census tract level, and for pediatric or adult population. The two maps can be downloaded as maps or as raw data.

The *healthcare measures* available through the web portal include:

1. Health outcomes primarily derived from the Georgia County Health Rankings, a Robert Wood Johnson Foundation program.
2. Healthcare access measures for affordability by sub-populations, and for accessibility and availability for multiple healthcare services, including primary, specialized, and emergency care derived from the MAX claims data.
3. Medicaid disease prevalence for multiple conditions for the Medicaid-insured pediatric and adult population derived from the MAX claims data.
4. Medicaid healthcare utilization measured as percent utilization (percentage of population using a specific type of care) and per member per year (number of care visits per Medicaid member per year) for multiple types of services.

The *health determinants* available through the web portal include:

1. Demographic factors including age, disability, race, veteran population.
2. Local economy factors including county charges, expenditure and investment, county revenue and taxes, as well as farm acres, expenses, income, and production.
3. Education factors including education attainment and enrollment as well as K-12 education availability.
4. Housing factors including market value, building permits, mobile homes, and housing costs.
5. Socioeconomic factors including crime rates, percent on food stamp and SNAP, labor force participation, percent of people under poverty level, and unemployment rate.
6. Workforce factors including healthcare provider count or by population, and other professions by industry.

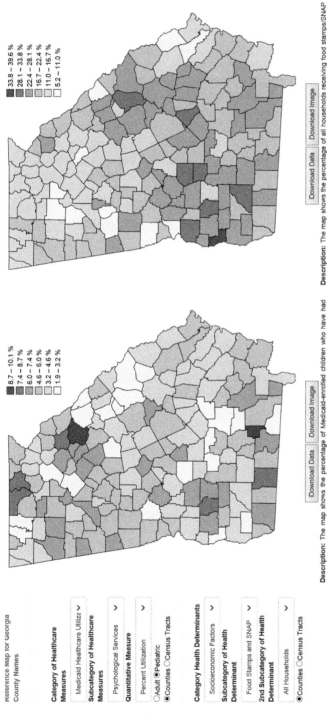

Reference Map for Georgia
County Names

■ 8.7 – 10.1 %
▦ 7.4 – 8.7 %
▨ 6.0 – 7.4 %
▧ 4.6 – 6.0 %
▫ 3.2 – 4.6 %
□ 1.9 – 3.2 %

Category of Healthcare Measures

Medicaid Healthcare Utiliz ⌄

Subcategory of Healthcare Measures

Psychological Services ⌄

Quantitative Measure

Percent Utilization ⌄

○Adult ◉Pediatric
○Counties ◉Census Tracts

Category Health Determinants

Socioeconomic Factors ⌄

Subcategory of Health Determinant

Food Stamps and SNAP ⌄

2nd Subcategory of Health Determinant

All Households ⌄

◉Counties ○Census Tracts

■ 33.8 – 39.6 %
▦ 28.1 – 33.8 %
▨ 22.4 – 28.1 %
▧ 16.7 – 22.4 %
▫ 11.0 – 16.7 %
□ 5.2 – 11.0 %

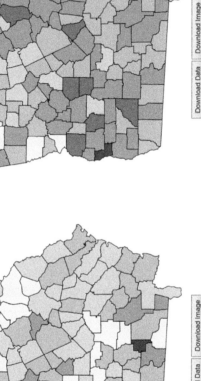

Download Data   Download Image

Description: The map shows the percentage of Medicaid-enrolled children who have had psychological services at least once during the year by county. The darker the color, the higher the utilization percentage of psychological services.

Source: 2012 Medicaid Analytic eXtract claims data available from the Centers for Medicare

Download Data   Download Image

Description: The map shows the percentage of all households receiving food stamps/SNAP assistance at the county level.

Source: 2011-2015 US Census Bureau American Community Survey (ACS) 5-Year Estimates for 2015

FIGURE 6.4   Georgia web data portal: the drop down menu is shown on the left; the two maps are illustrations of the selection of a measure within each of the two categories, healthcare measures and health determinants. Below each map, there is the option to download raw data or the map of the measure as well as the description of the measure and the source of the data.

Additional features of the data portal include the ability to scroll through the maps to look up the measure of interest for specific counties or census tracts, with comparison with the range for the entire state provided in the key. Figure 6.5 illustrates an example of how such features can be used to draw inferences on various access measures. The figure shows the maps of the percent adult population with Medicaid or Medicare insurance as well as the uninsured population. Comparing with the key that shows the range of values for each map, the selected county has the maximum percent of population on Medicaid as compared with the entire state but is somewhere in the middle for the other two categories.

Medicaid Prevalence Data Portal

As I mentioned earlier in this chapter, large data require well-endowed IT systems that offer the needed security, space, access, and readiness in working with the data. The MAX claims data available nationwide is a massive database, consisting of individual claims records for each Medicaid-insured adult and child at each interaction with the healthcare system. Altogether, the MAX database built at Georgia Tech including multiple years of MAX claims files has more than 1 trillion such records, accessed under a very restrictive data protection environment. Navigating such a large database under a constrained IT system is more like finding a needle in a haystack. Dealing with a massive database of claims records, acquiring the data and building the IT infrastructure, and developing the knowledge to derive meaningful information from such data can take years and significant institutional investment.

Because of these challenges, few research teams have the ability to have access to important information about the Medicaid population. To support the community of data sharing, my research team has begun a program of Medicaid data dissemination. One illustration is the Prevalence Mapping Portal (available at https://www .healthanalytics.gatech.edu/data/prevalence-mapping-portal).

For this web data portal, we compiled unique (in-treatment) prevalence data on multiple chronic conditions common in children. We focused on children age 0–17. The prevalence data are derived from patient-identifiable medical claims from the 2012 MAX files acquired from the CMS.

The prevalence data are census tract estimates of the percentage of Medicaid-enrolled children diagnosed with a chronic condition. We derived the prevalence estimates using the 3M Clinical Risk Grouping software (Neff et al. 2002). Episode Diagnostic Categories (EDCs) are derived for each child enrolled in Medicaid using the child's diagnosis codes, procedure codes, and NDCs found in the recorded medical claims in the MAX files. EDCs are used to determine a patient's Primary Chronic Disease, which is the most significant chronic disease actively being treated, and its severity for each organ system.

We considered EDCs for 22 conditions; these conditions were selected due to their high prevalence among children enrolled in the Medicaid program. (Lower prevalence conditions cannot be captured due to the restriction of meeting a minimum cell size of 11 patients required by the data use agreement with CMS.) For each condition or EDC, we obtained the population of Medicaid-enrolled children with the condition along with the number of enrollment months of these children within each zip code

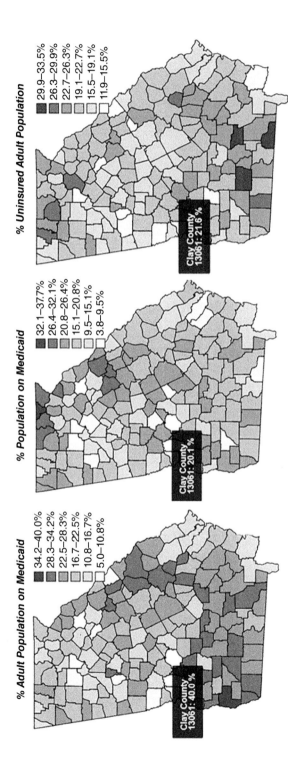

FIGURE 6.5 Illustration of how the Georgia web data portal can be used to understand the level of healthcare access and health outcomes, benchmarking with other counties in the state. The web data portal allows scrolling through the map to find the values of the measure of interest for specific counties. A county reference map is also provided as part of the portal for reference on the location of the counties.

and county. We derived the prevalence of conditions by dividing the total number of member months of patients treated for a given condition by the total number of member months of all children on Medicaid for each county and zip code area. We further estimated the census tract prevalence using the zip code and county estimates along with geographic information of the boundaries of the different geographic divisions (county, zip code, census tracts) and the information on the population count across the geographic divisions. For cells with less than 11 patients, we used the mean estimation at the state level, along with a generated beta distribution noise term.

The prevalence estimates are derived at the census tract level, where census tracts are commonly used as proxies of communities. We have a total of 64 873 census tracts for which we have obtained prevalence estimates for all conditions. The census tracts cover the entire United States excluding Colorado and Idaho due to data unavailability at the point of implementing this research program.

Figure 6.6 illustrates the data portal, with the selection of a specific condition (e.g. asthma) and of a specific state (e.g. Texas). The national map shows the in-treatment prevalence for asthma at the county level while the state-level data display also provides benchmarking with the national level as well as within state. Thus, the prevalence data can be used for local decision making, for example, at the county level, with benchmarks within and between states.

The prevalence data can also be used to make inference on the burden of pediatric chronic conditions using clustering algorithms. In one of my collaborative research papers, we derived the clustering of communities (using census tracts as proxies) nationwide using a model-based clustering algorithm, which accounts for spatial dependence (Zheng and Serban 2018). Using this approach, we derived three clusters profiling the burden of chronic conditions locally. The three clusters are as follows:

- *Cluster 1* consists of communities, predominantly with chronic and moderate mental health diseases, along with some acute and major conditions.
- *Cluster 2* consists of communities, where the prevalence of mental diseases is mostly low, with moderate prevalence in some respiratory and skin related diseases.
- *Cluster 3* consists of communities, where moderate prevalence for all conditions exists, except for some severe chronic mental conditions, diabetes, and dental diseases.

Figure 6.7 presents the distribution of three clusters for Georgia. Most rural Georgia is predominantly in Cluster 3, with a mix of both mental health and respiratory chronic conditions, while suburban and urban areas are predominantly in Cluster 1 or 2, pointing to either heavily weighted mental and behavioral conditions or severe chronic conditions. In the metropolitan Atlanta area, several communities are assigned to Cluster 1 or 2. Similar inferences can be made for all other states.

The web data portals introduced in this chapter are two examples among many others. Many foundations, organizations, and research teams are now placing substantive emphasis on dissemination of data derived from research and surveys. Many of the data sources mentioned in this chapter are data portals, some providing national-level or state-level data, aggregated measures, focusing on specific

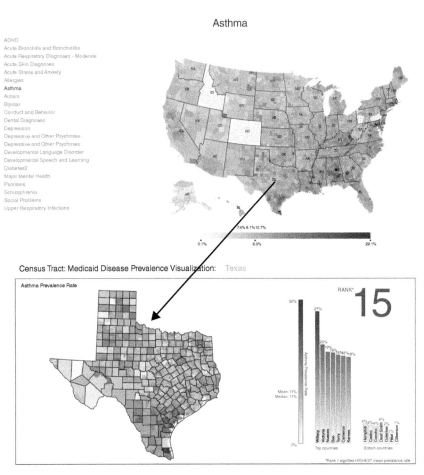

FIGURE 6.6 Illustration of the prevalence web data portal, showing the selection of asthma condition along with the detailed information provided for the selection of the Texas state.

sub-populations or on specific aspects of healthcare. It is important however to highlight the need of centralizing data, to allow public health decision makers to acquire the data in support of targeted interventions and decisions from one single source, without the need to navigate multiple web data portals and websites. It also important to accompany raw data and information with interactive visualization; decision makers do not have ready access to visual analytics tools and thus are without the ability to benchmark and to visualize trends and patterns that can be meaningful in the decision-making process. These are substantive considerations toward wide dissemination of data systems, which can enable informed decision making.

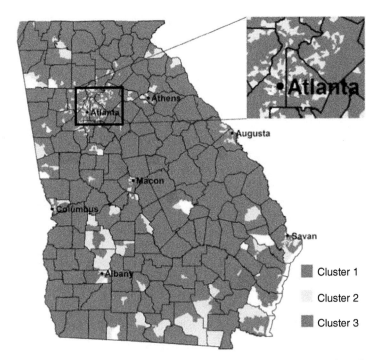

FIGURE 6.7   Illustration of a clustering of communities to infer the burden of pediatric chronic conditions. .Source: Zheng and Serban 2018

CONCLUSIONS

The focus of this chapter is on a summary of data science and analytics used to inform methodologies for measuring and making inference on healthcare access. It provides additional details on what type of data sources are available depending on the context in which they are considered. Specifically, I expanded on the wide range of data sources, with different applicability in healthcare access, healthcare disparities, and health outcomes. The overview on the data sources is not comprehensive but it is meant to guide the reader to relevant resources along with specifications on how such resources might be useful.

In this chapter I also briefly highlighted various challenges in data acquisition, translation, and modeling. In fact, these aspects were covered throughout the entire book, as they are at the core of informed decision making. While many of the challenges discussed here are common to data analytics for managing and transforming complex systems, there are specific challenges that are of particular relevance to healthcare, for example, development of IT systems PHI or data fragmentation across multiple sources, providers, and organizations.

Last, within the case studies provided in this chapter, I illustrated the linking of the two data sets, NPPES and MAX data, to derive information on the Medicaid participation, and the development of data portals for broad dissemination of data not readily accessible to policy makers. These illustrations highlight the challenges in using healthcare data to address healthcare access.

ACKNOWLEDGMENTS

This chapter draws substantially upon the research presented in a recent journal article and from a collaborative effort of data dissemination. In this regard, I gratefully acknowledge the contributions of Pravara Harati for illustration of the data science effort for evaluating supply of mental and behavioral health in the United States. I also knowledge the collaboration and support of the Healthcare Georgia Foundation for the development of the Georgia data portal. The research in the case studies in this chapter was approved by CMS (Data Use Agreement #23621) and by the Institutional Review Board of Georgia Tech (protocol #H11287). All data derived from the MAX files meet a minimum cell size of 11 in terms of the number of patients according to the Data Use Agreement with CMS.

REFERENCES

Altschuler, J., Margolius, D., Bodenheimer, T., and Grumbach, K. (2012). Estimating a reasonable patient panel size for primary care physicians with team-based task delegation. *The Annals of Family Medicine* **10**(5): 396–400.

American Academy of Pediatric Dentistry (2013). Guideline on periodicity of examination, preventive dental services, anticipatory guidance/counseling, and Oral treatment for infants, children, and adolescents. *Pediatric Dentistry* **35**(5): E148.

American Academy of Pediatrics (2014). Maintaining and improving the oral health of young children. *Pediatrics* **134**(6): 1224–1229.

Auchincloss, A., Diez Roux, A.V., Brown, D.G. et al. (2008). Neighborhood resources for physical activity and healthy foods and their association with insulin resistance. *Epidemiology* **19**(1): 146–157.

Bisgaier, J. and Rhodes, K.V. (2011). Auditing access to specialty care for children with public insurance. *The New England Journal of Medicine* **364**: 2324–2333.

Blackwell, A.G. and Treuhaft, S. (2008). *Regional Equity and the Quest for Full Inclusion*. Oakland, CA: PolicyLink.

Boyd, S., Parikh, N., Chu, E. et al. (2011). Distributed optimization and statistical learning via the alternating direction method of multipliers. *Foundations and Trends in Machine Learning* **3**(1): 1–122.

Brazier, J. and Roberts, J. (2004). The estimation of a preference-based measure of health from the SF-12. *Medical Care* **42**(9): 851–859.

Brindis, C.D. (2016). The "state of the state" of school-based health centers achieving health and educational outcomes. *American Journal of Preventive Medicine* **51**(1): 139–140.

Britto, M.T., Klostermann, B.K., Bonny, A.E. et al. (2001). Impact of a school-based intervention on access to healthcare for underserved youth. *Journal of Adolescent Health* **29**(2): 116–124.

Byrd, V. L. H. and A. H. Dodd (2012). Assessing the Usability of Encounter Data for Enrollees in Comprehensive Managed Care across MAX 2007–2009. Mathematica Policy Research.

Byrd, V. L. H. and A. H. Dodd (2015). Assessing the Usability of Encounter Data for Enrollees in Comprehensive Managed Care 2010–2011. Mathematica Policy Research/Centers for Medicare and Medicaid Services.

Cao, S., Gentili, M., Griffin, P. et al. (2017a). Identifying shortage areas for preventive dental care for children using high geographic granularity estimates of need and supply. *Public Health Reports*: 132–132.

Cao, S., Gentili, M., Griffin, P. et al. (2017b). Disparities in preventive dental care among children in Georgia. *Preventing Chronic Disease* **14**: 170176.

Centers for Disease Control and Prevention (2010). Behavioral Risk Factor Surveillance System Survey Data 2010 Child Asthma Data: Prevalence Tables. http://www.cdc.gov/asthma/brfss/2010/child/current/tableC3.htm (accessed September 2018).

Centers for Disease Control and Prevention. n.d.-a Medical Expenditure Panel Survey Data. http://meps.ahrq.gov/mepsweb (accessed February 2019).

Centers for Disease Control and Prevention. n.d.-bSchool Health Profiles. https://www.cdc.gov/healthyyouth/data/profiles/index.htm (accessed March 2019).

Centers for Medicare & Medicaid Services 2016a. Non-Emergency Medical Transportation. https://www.cms.gov/medicare-medicaid-coordination/fraud-prevention/medicaid-integrity-education/downloads/nemt-booklet.pdf (accessed June 2019).

Centers for Medicare & Medicaid Services (2016b). Medicaid and CHIP Managed Care Final Rule https://www.medicaid.gov/medicaid/managed-care/guidance/final-rule/index.html (accessed June 2019)

Centers for Medicare & Medicaid Services (2017a). *Medicaid & CHIP Strengthening Coverage, Improving Health*. Baltimore, MD.

Centers for Medicare & Medicaid Services 2017b. State Guide to CMS Criteria for Medicaid Managed Care Contract Review and Approval. https://www.medicaid.gov/medicaid/managed-care/downloads/mce-checklist-state-user-guide.pdf (accessed September 2018).

Centers for Medicare & Medicaid Services. (2019) Home Health. HealthData.gov (accessed March 2019).

Centers for Medicare & Medicaid Services. (n.d.-a) Medicaid Analytic eXtract (MAX) General Information https://www.cms.gov/research-statistics-data-and-systems/computer-data-and-systems/medicaiddatasourcesgeninfo/maxgeneralinformation.html (accessed September 2018).

Centers for Medicare & Medicaid Services. (n.d.-b) National Plan and Provider Enumeration System. https://nppes.cms.hhs.gov (accessed September 2018).

Cummings, J.R., Ji, X., Allen, L. et al. (2017). Racial and ethnic differences in ADHD treatment quality among Medicaid-enrolled youth. *Pediatrics* **139**(6) https://doi.org/10.1542/peds.2016-2444.

Davila Payan, C., DeGuzman, M., Johnson, K. et al. (2014). Estimating prevalence of obese children in small geographical areas using publicly available data. *Preventing Chronic Disease* **12**: 140229.

DeVoe, J.E., Gold, R., McIntire, P. et al. (2011). Electronic health records vs Medicaid claims: completeness of diabetes preventive care data in community health centers. *Annals of Family Medicine* **9**(4): 351–358.

DHHS (2014). State Standards for Access to Care in Medicaid Managed Care. https://oig.hhs.gov/oei/reports/oei-02-11-00320.pdf (accessed June 2019).

EuroQol Group EuroQol (1990). A new facility for the measurement of health-related quality of life. *Health Policy* **16**(3): 199–208.

Flournoy, R. and Treuhaft, S. (2005). *Healthy Food, Healthy Communities: Improving Access and Opportunities through Food Retailing*. PolicyLink.

Frumkin, H., Frank, L., and Jackson, R. (2004). *Urban Sprawl and Public Health Designing, Planning, and Building for Healthy Communities*. Island Press.

Gandjour, A. (2014). Considering productivity loss in cost-effectiveness analysis: a new approach. *The European Journal of Health Economics* **15**(8): 787–790.

Georgia Department of Public Health (n.d.). Online Analytical Statistical Information System. https://oasis.state.ga.us (accessed February 2019).

Gotway, C.A. and Young, L.J. (2002). Combining incompatible spatial data. *Journal of the American Statistical Association* **97**: 632–648.

Harris, E., Sorbero, M., Kogan, J.N. et al. (2012). Concurrent mental health therapy among medicaid-enrolled youths starting antipsychotic medications. *Psychiatric Services* **63**(4): 351–356.

Health Resources and Services Administration 2013a). Compendium of Federal Data Sources to Support Health Workforce Analysis April 2013. https://bhw.hrsa.gov/sites/default/files/bhw/nchwa/compendiumfederaldatasources.pdf (accessed June 2019).

Health Resources and Services Administration (2013b). Projecting the Supply and Demand for Primary Care Practitioners through 2020. https://bhw.hrsa.gov/health-workforce-analysis/primary-care-2020 (accessed June 2019).

Hilton, R., Zheng, Y.R., Fitzpatrick, A. et al. (2017). Patient-level longitudinal utilization for pediatric asthma healthcare: drawing inferences from millions of claims. *Medical Decision Making* **38**(1): 107–119.

Jackson, R. J. and C. Kochtitzky (2002). Creating a Healthy Environment: The Impact of the Built Environment on Public Health. Sprawl Watch Clearinghouse, Centers for Disease Control and Prevention.

Jeffers, J.R., Bognanno, M.F., and Bartlett, J.C. (1971). On the demand versus need for medical services and the concept of "shortage". *American Journal of Public Health* **61**(1): 46–63.

Johnson, B., Serban, N., Griffin, P.M., and Tomar, S.L. (2017). The cost-effectiveness of three interventions for providing preventive services to low-income children. *Community Dentistry and Oral Epidemiology* **45**(6): 522–528.

Kairos Future (2011). *The Data Explosion and the Future of Health*. Stockholm: Kairos Future.

Knapp, E.A., Fink, A.K., Goss, C.H. et al. (2016). The Cystic Fibrosis Foundation patient registry: design and methods of a National Observational Disease Registry. *Annals of the American Thoracic Society* **13**(7): 1173–1179.

Knopf, J.A., Finnie, R.K., Peng, Y. et al. (2016). School-based health centers to advance health equity a community guide systematic review. *American Journal of Preventive Medicine* **51**(1): 114–126.

Kwong, J.C., Ge, H., Rosella, L.C. et al. (2010). School-based influenza vaccine delivery, vaccination rates, and healthcare use in the context of a universal influenza immunization program: an ecological study. *Vaccine* **28**(15): 2722–2729.

Landers, S.H. (2010). Why health care is going home. *The New England Journal of Medicine* **363**(18): 1690–1691.

Lee, M. and V. Rubin (2007). The Impact of the Built Environment on Community Health: The State of Current Practice and Next Steps for a Growing Movement. https://community-wealth.org/sites/clone.community-wealth.org/files/downloads/report-lee-rubin.pdf (accessed June 2019).

Lee, I., Monahan, S., Serban, N. et al. (2018). Estimating the cost savings of preventive dental services delivered to Medicaid-enrolled children in six southeastern states. *Health Services Research* **53**(5): 3592–3616.

Mandros, A. (2014). Which States Carve Behavioral Health Benefits Out Of Medicaid Managed Care Contracts?. OPEN MINDS Market Intelligence Report.

Morland, K., Diez Roux, A.V., and Wing, S. (2006). Supermarkets, other food stores, and obesity: the atherosclerosis risk in communities study. *American Journal of Preventive Medicine* **30**(4): 333–339.

National Center for Health Statistics (2015). Ambulatory Health Care Data. Centers for Disease Control and Prevention.

National Center for Health Statistics (n.d.-a). National Health and Nutrition Examination Survey. Centers for Disease Control and Prevention.

National Center for Health Statistics (n.d.-b.) National Health Interview Survey. Centers for Disease Control and Prevention.

National Heart Blood and Lung Institute (2007). Expert Panel Report 3: Guidelines for the Diagnosis and Management of Asthma. National Institutes of Health. Technical report.

National Institutes of Health (n.d.). List of Registries. https://www.nih.gov/health-information/nih-clinical-research-trials-you/list-registries (accessed January 2019).

National Research Council (2013). *Frontiers in Massive Data Analysis*. Washington, DC.: National Academies Press.

National Survey of Children's Health n.d.). 2016 and 2016–2017 Combined National Survey of Children's Health Interactive Data Query. The Child & Adolescent Health Measurement Initiative. https://www.childhealthdata.org/browse/survey (accessed January 2019).

Ndumele, C.D., Cohen, M.S., and Cleary, P.D. (2017). Association of state access standards with accessibility to specialists for Medicaid managed care enrollees. *JAMA Internal Medicine* **177**(10): 1445–1451.

Nedic, A. and Ozdaglar, A. (2009). Distributed subgradient methods for multi-agent optimization. *IEEE Transactions on Automatic Control* **54**(1): 48–61.

Neff, J.M., Sharp, V.L., Muldoon, J. et al. (2002). Identifying and classifying children with chronic conditions using administrative data with the clinical risk group classification system. *Ambulatory Pediatrics* **2**: 71–79.

Organization for Economic and Co-operative Development (n.d.). Health care resources: physicians by age and gender. http://stats.oecd.org/index.aspx? DataSetCode=HEALTH_STAT (accessed January 2019).

Palomar, D.P. and Mung, C. (2006). A tutorial on decomposition methods for network utility maximization. *IEEE Journal on Selected Areas in Communications* **24**(8): 1439–1451.

Phillips, C. and Thompson, G. (2009). What is QALY? *Health Economics* **1**: 400–405.

Raghavan, R., Brown, D.S., and Allaire, B.T. (2017). Can Medicaid claims validly ascertain foster care status? *Child Maltreatment* **22**(3): 227–235.

Ran, T., Chattopadhyay, S., Hahn, R.A., and the Community Preventive Services (2016). Economic evaluation of school-based health centers: a community guide systematic review. *American Journal of Preventive Medicine* **51**(1): 129–138.

Reid, P.P., Compton, W.D., Grossman, J.H., and Fanjiang, G. (eds.) (2005). *Building a Better Delivery System: A New Engineering/Health Care Partnership*. Washington, DC: National Academies Press.

Rust, G., Levine, R.S., Fry-Johnson, Y. et al. (2012). Paths to success: optimal and equitable health outcomes for all. *Journal of Health Care for the Poor and Underserved* **23**(2 Suppl): 7–19.

School-Based Health Alliance (2013–2014). National School-Based Health Care Census. https://www.sbh4all.org/school-health-care/national-census-of-school-based-health-centers (accessed March 2019).

Serban, N. and Tomar, S. (2018). ADA health policy Institute's methodology overestimates spatial access to dental care for publicly insured children. *Journal of Public Health Dentistry* **78**(4): 291–295.

Serban, N., Bush, C., and Tomar, S.L. (2019). Medicaid capacity for pediatric oral health care. *Journal of the American Dental Association* **150**(4): 294–304.

Shneiderman, B., Plaisant, C., and Hesse, B.W. (2013). Improving health and healthcare with interactive visualization methods. *IEEE Computer Special Issue on Challenges in Information Visualization* **46**(5): 58–66.

Simmons, R. and Davis, R. (1993). The roles of knowledge and representation in problem solving. In: *Second Generation Expert Systems* (eds. M. David, J.P. Krivine and R. Simmons). New York, NY.: Springer-Verlag.

Statistics Canada and Canadian Institute for Health Information (2008). *A Framework for Health Outcomes Analysis*. Ottawa, ON: Canadian Institute for Health Information.

Stein, B.D., Sorbero, M., Dalton, E. et al. (2013). Predictors of adequate depression treatment among Medicaid-enrolled youth. *Social Psychiatry and Psychiatric Epidemiology* **48**(5): 757–765.

Tien, J.M. and Goldschmidt-Clermont, P.J. (2009). Engineering healthcare as a service system. *Information, Knowledge, Systems Management* **8**: 277–297.

United States Census Bureau (2016). Small Area Health Insurance Estimates. https://www.census.gov/library/publications/2018/demo/p30-03.html (accessed February 2019).

United States Census Bureau (2017). Health Insurance Coverage in the United States. https://www.census.gov/library/publications/2018/demo/p60-264.html (accessed February 2019).

US Department of Health and Human Services (2009). Health Information Technology for Economic and Clinical Health (HITECH) Act. American Recovery and Reinvestment Act of 2009 (ARRA): Public Law 111–5.

Visser, S.N., Danielson, M.L., Wolraich, M.L. et al. (2016). Vital signs: national and state-specific patterns of attention deficit/hyperactivity disorder treatment among insured children aged 2–5 years — United States, 2008–2014. *Morbidity and Mortality Weekly Report (MMWR)* **65**(17): 443–450.

Zheng, Y. and Serban, N. (2018). Clustering the burden of pediatric chronic conditions in the United States using distributed computing. *Annals of Applied Statistics* **12**(2): 915–939.

American Academy of Pediatrics (2017). Medicaid Facts. https://www.aap.org/en-us/Documents/federaladvocacy_medicaidfactsheet_all_states.pdf (accessed June 2019).

Index